Bioactive Compounds from Brown Algae

Bioactive Compounds from Brown Algae

Editor

Roland Ulber

MDPI • Basel • Beijing • Wuhan • Barcelona • Belgrade • Manchester • Tokyo • Cluj • Tianjin

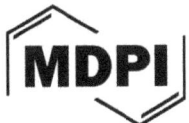

Editor
Roland Ulber
Technische Universität Kaiserslautern
Germany

Editorial Office
MDPI
St. Alban-Anlage 66
4052 Basel, Switzerland

This is a reprint of articles from the Special Issue published online in the open access journal *Marine Drugs* (ISSN 1660-3397) (available at: https://www.mdpi.com/journal/marinedrugs/special_issues/Bioactive_Compounds_Brown_Algae).

For citation purposes, cite each article independently as indicated on the article page online and as indicated below:

LastName, A.A.; LastName, B.B.; LastName, C.C. Article Title. *Journal Name* **Year**, *Volume Number*, Page Range.

ISBN 978-3-0365-2468-9 (Hbk)
ISBN 978-3-0365-2469-6 (PDF)

Cover image courtesy of Roland Ulber and Ahmed Zayed

© 2021 by the authors. Articles in this book are Open Access and distributed under the Creative Commons Attribution (CC BY) license, which allows users to download, copy and build upon published articles, as long as the author and publisher are properly credited, which ensures maximum dissemination and a wider impact of our publications.
The book as a whole is distributed by MDPI under the terms and conditions of the Creative Commons license CC BY-NC-ND.

Contents

About the Editor vii

Preface to "Bioactive Compounds from Brown Algae" ix

Pilar Mercader-Moyano, Oswaldo Morat-Pérez and Carmen Muñoz-González
Diphlorethohydroxycarmalol Attenuates Palmitate-Induced Hepatic Lipogenesis and Inflammation
Reprinted from: *Mar. Drugs* **2020**, *18*, 475, doi:10.3390/md18090475 1

Ahmed Zayed, Mona El-Aasr, Abdel-Rahim S. Ibrahim and Roland Ulber
Fucoidan Characterization: Determination of Purity and Physicochemical and Chemical Properties
Reprinted from: *Mar. Drugs* **2020**, *18*, 571, doi:10.3390/md18110571 17

Philipp Dörschmann, Christina Schmitt, Kaya Saskia Bittkau, Sandesh Neupane, Michael Synowitz, Johann Roider, Susanne Alban, Janka Held-Feindt and Alexa Klettner
Evaluation of a Brown Seaweed Extract from *Dictyosiphon foeniculaceus* as a Potential Therapeutic Agent for the Treatment of Glioblastoma and Uveal Melanoma
Reprinted from: *Mar. Drugs* **2020**, *18*, 625, doi:10.3390/md18120625 49

Liyuan Lin, Shengtao Yang, Zhenbang Xiao, Pengzhi Hong, Shengli Sun, Chunxia Zhou and Zhong-Ji Qian
The Inhibition Effect of the Seaweed Polyphenol, 7-Phloro-Eckol from *Ecklonia cava* on Alcohol-Induced Oxidative Stress in HepG2/CYP2E1 Cells
Reprinted from: *Mar. Drugs* **2021**, *19*, 158, doi:10.3390/md19030158 63

Hui-Hua Hsiao, Tien-Chiu Wu, Yung-Hsiang Tsai, Chia-Hung Kuo, Ren-Han Huang, Yong-Han Hong and Chun-Yung Huang
Effect of Oversulfation on the Composition, Structure, and In Vitro Anti-Lung Cancer Activity of Fucoidans Extracted from *Sargassum aquifolium*
Reprinted from: *Mar. Drugs* **2021**, *19*, 215, doi:10.3390/md19040215 79

Bertoka Fajar Surya Perwira Negara, Jae-Hak Sohn, Jin-Soo Kim and Jae-Suk Choi
Antifungal and Larvicidal Activities of Phlorotannins from Brown Seaweeds
Reprinted from: *Mar. Drugs* **2021**, *19*, 223, doi:10.3390/md19040223 99

Saraswati, Puspo Edi Giriwono, Diah Iskandriati and Nuri Andarwulan
Screening of In-Vitro Anti-Inflammatory and Antioxidant Activity of *Sargassum ilicifolium* Crude Lipid Extracts from Different Coastal Areas in Indonesia
Reprinted from: *Mar. Drugs* **2021**, *19*, 252, doi:10.3390/md19050252 111

Marcelo D. Catarino, Catarina Marçal, Teresa Bonifácio-Lopes, Débora Campos, Nuno Mateus, Artur M. S. Silva, Maria Manuela Pintado and Susana M. Cardoso
Impact of Phlorotannin Extracts from *Fucus vesiculosus* on Human Gut Microbiota
Reprinted from: *Mar. Drugs* **2021**, *19*, 375, doi:10.3390/md19070375 125

Hyunjun Woo, Min-Kyung Kim, Sohyeon Park, Seung-Hee Han, Hyeon-Cheol Shin, Byeong-gon Kim, Seung-Ha Oh, Myung-Whan Suh, Jun-Ho Lee and Moo-Kyun Park
Effect of Phlorofucofuroeckol A and Dieckol Extracted from *Ecklonia cava* on Noise-induced Hearing Loss in a Mouse Model
Reprinted from: *Mar. Drugs* **2021**, *19*, 443, doi:10.3390/md19080443 143

Yanping Li, Yuting Zheng, Ye Zhang, Yuanyuan Yang, Peiyao Wang, Balázs Imre, Ann C. Y. Wong, Yves S. Y. Hsieh and Damao Wang
Brown Algae Carbohydrates: Structures, Pharmaceutical Properties, and Research Challenges
Reprinted from: *Mar. Drugs* **2021**, *19*, 620, doi:10.3390/md19110620 . . . . **155**

About the Editor

Roland Ulber studied chemistry at the University of Hannover. His doctoral thesis (Optimization of Sensor Systems for Biotechnology) was completed at the Institute of Biochemistry of the Westphalian Wilhelms University of Münster and at the Institute of Technical Chemistry of the Leibniz University Hanover. In 2002, he completed his venia legendi in "Technical Chemistry" at the same university. Since 2004, he has been a professor for Bioprocess Engineering at the Technical University of Kaiserslautern. His research focuses on industrial bioprocess engineering. Further information on his fields of research and teaching can be found at https://www.mv.uni-kl.de/biovt/.

Preface to "Bioactive Compounds from Brown Algae"

Brown algae comprise approx. 2040 species grown in various climatic conditions. They represent a reservoir of various bioactive compounds, including fucoidan, alginate, phlorotannins, and fucoxanthins. In the special volume "Bioactive Compounds from Brown Algae", current developments in this exciting field are highlighted by leading scientists. In addition to seven research articles, three review articles summarize current developments, particularly in the field of pharmacological agents. The contributions to the book illustrate, once again, that biological active molecules from marine organisms have a wide range of applications for human health. Of course, great efforts are required to make these substances available in with the necessary purity and quantity. Macroalgae, in particular, present us with major challenges here. However, the examples shown in this special volume encourage us to expect many more active ingredients from marine resources in the future.

Roland Ulber
Editor

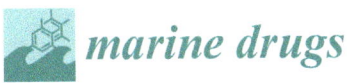

Article

Diphlorethohydroxycarmalol Attenuates Palmitate-Induced Hepatic Lipogenesis and Inflammation

Seon-Heui Cha [1,*], Yongha Hwang [2], Soo-Jin Heo [3,4] and Hee-Sook Jun [2,5,6,*]

[1] Department of Marine Bio and Medical Sciences, Hanseo University, Chungcheongnam-do 31962, Korea
[2] Gachon Medical and Convergence Institute, Gachon Gil Medical Center, Incheon 21999, Korea; sicrios912@naver.com
[3] Jeju Marine Research Center, Korea Institute of Ocean Science and Technology (KIOST), Jeju 63349, Korea; sjheo@kiost.ac.kr
[4] Department of Biology, University of Science and Technology (UST), Daejeon 34113, Korea
[5] Lee Gil Ya Cancer and Diabetes Institute, Gachon University, Incheon 21999, Korea
[6] College of Pharmacy, Gachon University, Incheon 21999, Korea
* Correspondence: sunnyday8109@gmail.com (S.-H.C.); hsjun@gachon.ac.kr (H.-S.J.); Tel./Fax: +82-41-660-1550 (S.-H.C.); +82-32-899-6056 (H.-S.J.)

Received: 7 August 2020; Accepted: 15 September 2020; Published: 18 September 2020

Abstract: Non-alcoholic fatty liver disease (NAFLD) is a common cause of chronic liver disease, encompassing a range of conditions caused by lipid deposition within liver cells, and is also associated with obesity and metabolic diseases. Here, we investigated the protective effects of diphlorethohydroxycarmalol (DPHC), which is a polyphenol isolated from an edible seaweed, *Ishige okamurae*, on palmitate-induced lipotoxicity in the liver. DPHC treatment repressed palmitate-induced cytotoxicity, triglyceride content, and lipid accumulation. DPHC prevented palmitate-induced mRNA and protein expression of SREBP (sterol regulatory element-binding protein) 1, C/EBP (CCAAT-enhancer-binding protein) α, ChREBP (carbohydrate-responsive element-binding protein), and FAS (fatty acid synthase). In addition, palmitate treatment reduced the expression levels of phosphorylated AMP-activated protein kinase (AMPK) and sirtuin (SIRT)1 proteins, and DPHC treatment rescued this reduction. Moreover, DPHC protected palmitate-induced liver toxicity and lipogenesis, as well as inflammation, and enhanced AMPK and SIRT1 signaling in zebrafish. These results suggest that DPHC possesses protective effects against palmitate-induced toxicity in the liver by preventing lipogenesis and inflammation. DPHC could be used as a potential therapeutic or preventive agent for fatty liver diseases.

Keywords: hepatic steatosis; lipogenesis; seaweed; polyphenol

1. Introduction

Nonalcoholic fatty liver disease (NAFLD) is one of the most common causes of chronic liver diseases worldwide and is characterized by fat deposition in the hepatocytes of patients without history of excessive alcohol consumption. NAFLD is also associated with metabolic complications, including obesity, type 2 diabetes, hyperlipidemia, hypertension and metabolic syndrome [1,2]. Although simple fatty liver itself may be considered a benign disorder, it can progress to hepatitis, fibrosis, and eventually lead to irreversible end-stage liver diseases such as cirrhosis and liver cancer. To control the onset and progression of fatty liver, it is important to inhibit lipogenesis in hepatocytes. Increasing evidence indicates that a large number of polyphenols naturally present in fruits and vegetables may be potential candidates for the treatment of NAFLD [3,4].

Free fatty acids (FFAs) contribute to the liver triglyceride (TG) pool, and the primary sources of FFAs are serum FFAs from adipose tissue and dietary fatty acids [5]. Serum FFA levels are elevated in obese subjects [6], and a previous study reported that serum FFA levels are also elevated in patients with NAFLD [7]. Palmitate, a saturated FFA, is the most common circulating FFA. It has been reported that saturated fatty acids induce hepatocyte lipoapoptosis, and palmitate is more toxic than other saturated and unsaturated fatty acids [8]. TG synthesis caused by FFA accumulation results in severe hepatic injury and fibrosis [9]. Therefore, FFAs are considered to be one of the most important factors that play a crucial role in the pathogenesis of NAFLD [10]. However, it remains unclear how palmitate contributes to inflammation and fibrosis in the liver, and what molecular mechanisms are involved in the pathogenesis of NAFLD and in the progression to inflammation and fibrosis.

Diphlorethohydroxycarmalol (DPHC) is a polyphenolic compound from the edible seaweed *Ishige okamurae*. Several studies have shown various biological functions of DPHC, including antioxidant activity [11–13], anti-adipogenic activity [14], anti-inflammatory activity [15], and cytoprotective effects in vitro [14,16–20] and in animal models [21]. Although these diverse effects of DPHC have been investigated, no studies have reported its effects on hepatic steatosis. In this study, we investigated the possible protective effect of DPHC against palmitate-induced lipogenesis and inflammation in the liver in vitro and in a zebrafish model.

2. Results

2.1. DPHC Protects against Palmitate-Induced Lipotoxicity in HepG2 Cells

In order to determine whether DPHC has a protective effect against palmitate-induced toxicity in human hepatocytes, we treated HepG2 cells, a human hepatoma cell line, with palmitate. DPHC alone did not exhibit any toxicity in the cells (Figure 1a). Cytotoxicity was observed in palmitate-treated cells in a dose-dependent manner (Figure 1b). Pretreatment with 40 µM DPHC significantly blocked the cytotoxic effect of palmitate (Figure 1c). To confirm whether DPHC attenuates lipotoxicity, a DNA damage assay was performed, which demonstrated that palmitate induced cellular damage and was protected against by pretreatment of DPHC (Figure 1c), indicating that DPHC possesses a protective effect against palmitate-induced toxicity in HepG2 cells.

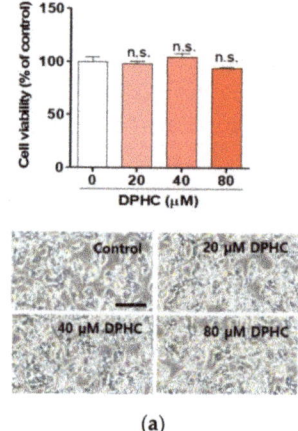

(a)

Figure 1. *Cont.*

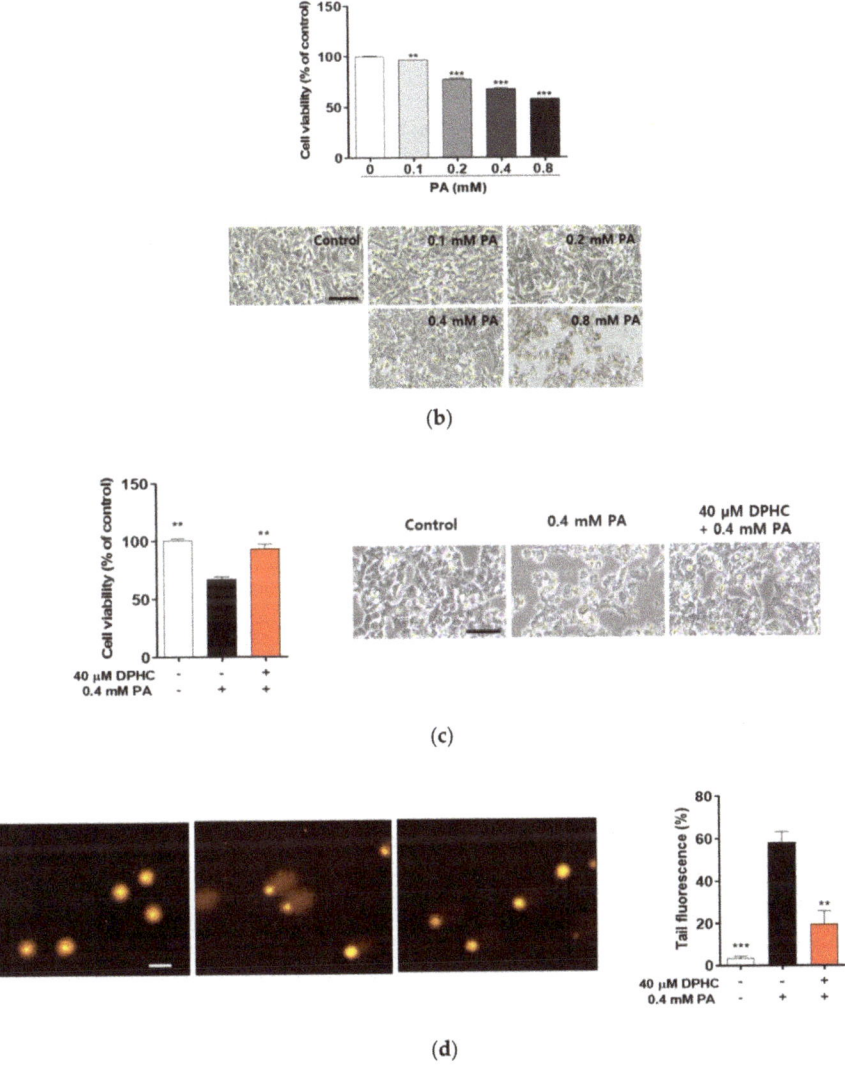

Figure 1. Diphlorethohydroxycarmalol (DPHC) protects against palmitate-induced lipotoxicity in HepG2 cells. (**a**) HepG2 cells were incubated with the indicated concentrations of DPHC for 24 h. (**b**) HepG2 cells were incubated with the indicated concentrations of palmitate (PA) for 24 h. (**c**) HepG2 cells were incubated with and without 40 μM DPHC for 1 h, and then further incubated with or without 0.4 mM palmitate for 24 h. Images were captured at the end of incubation, and CCK-8 assays were subsequently performed. Scale bar indicates 400 μm. (**d**) HepG2 cells were incubated with and without 40 μM DPHC for 1 h, and then further incubated with or without 0.4 mM palmitate for 24 h. DNA damage migration was captured by a fluorescence microscope, and the intensity was measured using Image J. Scale bar indicates 50 μm. Experiments were performed in triplicate. ** $p < 0.01$, *** $p < 0.001$, n.s. indicates no statistical significance.

2.2. DPHC Prevents Palmitate-Induced Lipid Accumulation in HepG2 Cells

FFAs may play a major role in the development of NAFLD, which is associated with TG accumulation in the liver [22,23]. Therefore, we determined whether DPHC can attenuate the production of palmitate-induced TG accumulation in HepG2 cells. As expected, TG production was significantly increased by palmitate treatment, whereas pretreatment with DPHC significantly reduced palmitate-induced TG accumulation (Figure 2a). In addition, intracellular neutral lipid Oil Red O staining was increased by palmitate treatment, whereas DPHC pretreatment of the cells reduced this lipid droplet accumulation (Figure 2b). These results suggest that DPHC ameliorates palmitate-induced lipogenesis in HepG2 cells.

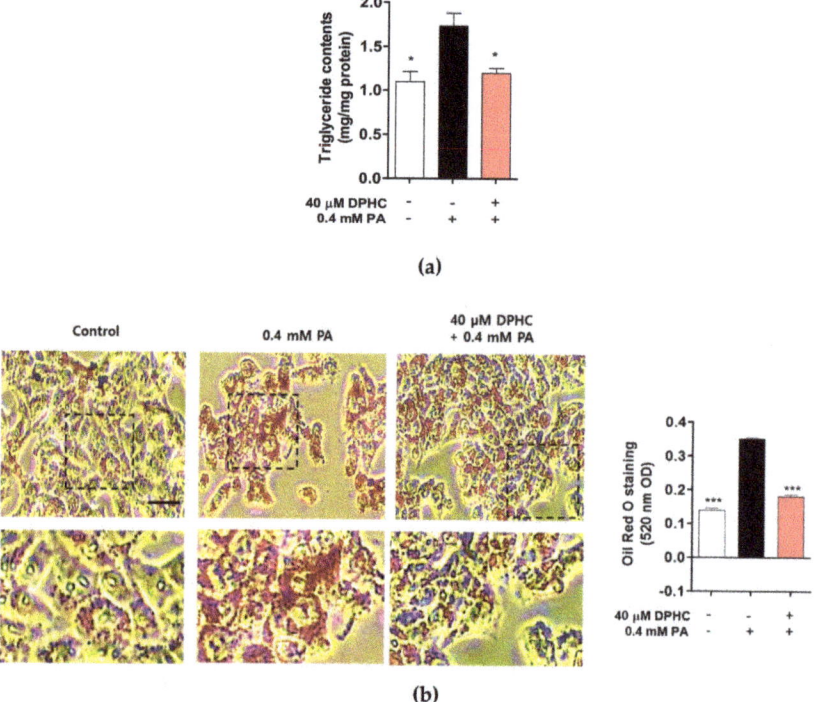

Figure 2. DPHC prevents palmitate-induced lipid accumulation in HepG2 cells. HepG2 cells were incubated with and without 40 µM DPHC for 1 h, and then further incubated with or without 0.4 mM palmitate (PA) for 24 h. (a) Triglyceride content. (b) Oil Red O staining. Scale bar indicates 50 µm. Experiments were performed in triplicate. * $p < 0.05$, *** $p < 0.001$.

2.3. DPHC Inhibits Palmitate-Induced Lipogenesis-Related Gene Expression in HepG2 Cells

To examine whether DPHC prevents lipogenesis in HepG2 cells, we examined the mRNA and protein expression of lipogenesis-related genes. We found that the mRNA expression of sterol regulatory element-binding protein (SREBP)1c, CCAAT-enhancer-binding protein (C/EBP)α, carbohydrate-responsive element-binding protein (ChREBP), and fatty acid synthase (FAS) were increased by palmitate exposure, whereas increases in levels of these mRNAs were suppressed, similar to control levels (Figure 3a–d). In addition, protein expression levels of SREBP1, C/EBPβ, ChREBP, and FAS were also increased by palmitate treatment, and this increase was abolished by DPHC pretreatment prior to palmitate treatment (Figure 3e). These results suggest that DPHC may prevent lipid accumulation by inhibiting the expression of lipogenesis-related genes induced by palmitate in HepG2 cells.

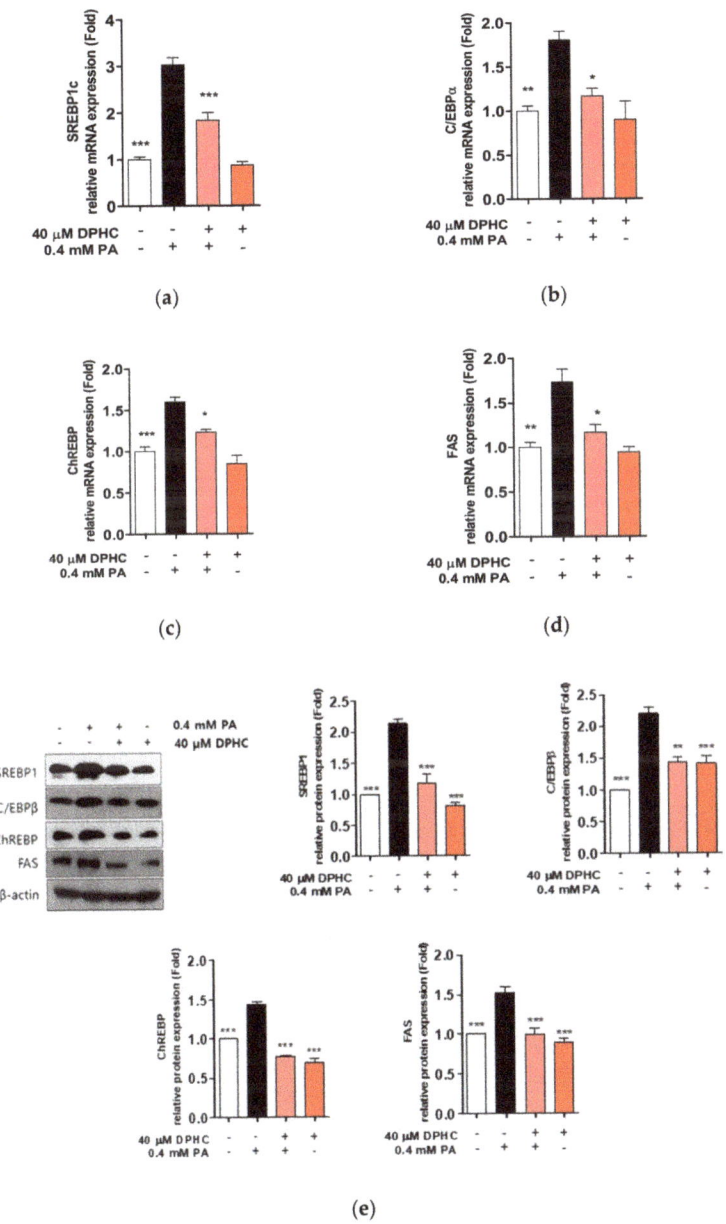

Figure 3. DPHC prevents palmitate-induced lipogenesis in HepG2 cells. Cells were incubated with and without 40 μM DPHC for 1 h, and then further incubated with or without 0.4 mM palmitate (PA) for 24 h. Lipogenesis-related genes (**a**) *SREBP1c*, (**b**) *C/EBPβ*, (**c**) *ChREBP*, and (**d**) *FAS* mRNA expression levels were identified by RT-qPCR. (**e**) Lipogenesis-related protein expression detection was performed by western blot. Experiments were performed in triplicate. * $p < 0.05$, ** $p < 0.01$, *** $p < 0.001$.

2.4. DPHC Rescues Palmitate-Induced Reduction of Phosphorylated AMP-Activated Protein Kinase (AMPK) and Sirtuin (SIRT)1 in HepG2 Cells

AMPK plays a central role in the regulation of lipid metabolism by switching on inhibition of lipid synthesis [24,25], and may be a therapeutic target for treating fatty liver disease. Therefore, we determined whether DPHC stimulates the AMPK signaling pathway. We found that the protein level of phosphorylated AMPK was significantly decreased by palmitate treatment, and this decrease was rescued with DPHC pretreatment of cells (Figure 4a), suggesting that DPHC may upregulate the phosphorylation of AMPK.

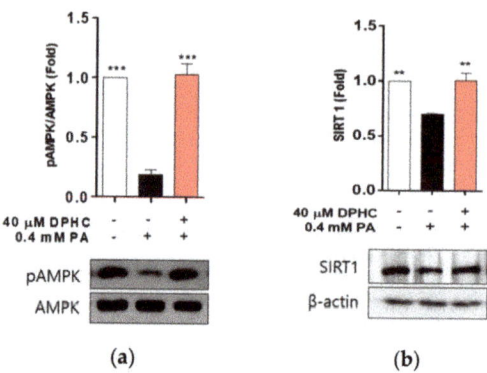

Figure 4. DPHC improves protein expression levels of phosphorylated AMP-activated protein kinase (AMPK) and AMP-activated protein kinase (SIRT)1 against palmitate in HepG2 cells. The cells were incubated with and without 40 µM DPHC for 1 h, and then further incubated with or without 0.4 mM palmitate (PA) for 24 h. (a) AMPK and (b) SIRT1 protein expression levels were determined by western blotting. Experiments were performed in triplicate. ** $p < 0.01$, *** $p < 0.001$.

The nicotine adenine dinucleotide (NAD($^+$))-dependent protein deacetylase activation of SIRT1 is positively associated with the protection of hepatocytes against palmitate-induced lipotoxicity [26], and is currently emerging as a potential therapeutic target for treating fatty liver disease [27,28]. Thus, we determined whether DPHC activates SIRT1, and found that the protein expression level of SIRT1 was decreased by palmitate treatment, and this decrease was rescued by DPHC pretreatment (Figure 4b). These results suggest that DPHC may induce SIRT1 expression, contributing to the prevention of lipotoxicity.

2.5. DPHC Protects against Palmitate-Induced Liver Lipogenesis in Zebrafish

To determine whether DPHC directly protects against liver damage in vivo, we used transgenic zebrafish (*Danio rerio*) expressing enhanced green fluorescent protein (EGFP) under the control of the liver fatty acid-binding protein promoter. Zebrafish embryos were preincubated in 40 µM DPHC for 1 h and then further incubated with 1 mM palmitate for 72 h. EGFP expression in the liver was observed to be reduced by palmitate treatment, whereas higher expression of EGFP was observed in DPHC-pretreated embryos (Figure 5a).

Next, we determined whether DPHC can attenuate palmitate-induced lipogenesis-related gene expression in zebrafish embryos. Hepatocytes expression in zebrafish liver was also reduced in palmitate embryos, whereas it was protected against by DPHC pretreatment. As expected, mRNA expression levels of SREBP1c, C/EBP1α, and FAS were significantly increased by palmitate treatment, whereas these increases were reduced by DPHC pretreatment (Figure 5c–e). These results suggest that DPHC may ameliorate palmitate-induced lipogenesis in the liver of zebrafish.

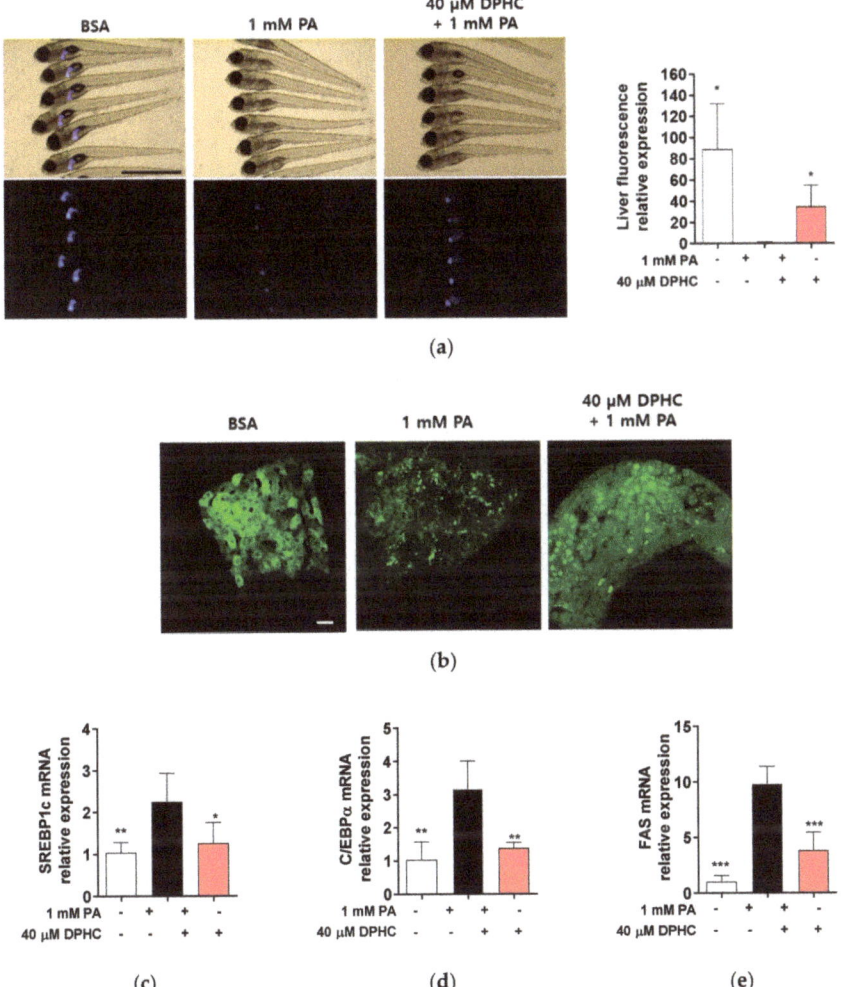

Figure 5. DPHC protects against palmitate-induced liver lipogenesis in zebrafish. At 3 days post-fertilization, zebrafish were incubated with and without 40 μM DPHC for 1 h, and then further incubated with or without 1 mM palmitate (PA) for 72 h. (**a**) Representative phase contrast images of zebrafish and fluorescence microscopy images of the zebrafish liver. Fluorescence relative value was calculated by ImageJ. Scale bar indicates 700 μm. (**b**) Representative confocal microscopy images of the isolated zebrafish liver. Scale bar indicates 10 μm. Total RNA was extracted from zebrafish liver and mRNA expression levels of (**c**) *SREBP1c*, (**d**) *C/EBPβ*, and (**e**) *FAS* were analyzed by RT-qPCR. $n = 12$–15 embryos. * $p < 0.05$, ** $p < 0.01$, *** $p < 0.001$ versus PA-treated group.

2.6. DPHC Protects against Palmitate-Induced Liver Inflammation in Zebrafish

Accumulation of FFAs induces inflammation and causes lipotoxic effects in the liver [6]. Because fatty acid metabolism plays a role in the inflammatory response, we determined whether DPHC attenuates palmitate-induced inflammation in the liver of zebrafish. We identified that mRNA expression levels of interleukin (IL)-1β, tumor necrosis factor (TNF)-α, and cyclooxygenase (COX)-2a were increased by palmitate treatment, whereas these increases were reduced in embryos pretreated with DPHC (Figure 6a–c), suggesting that DPHC may protect against pro-inflammatory cytokine overexpression.

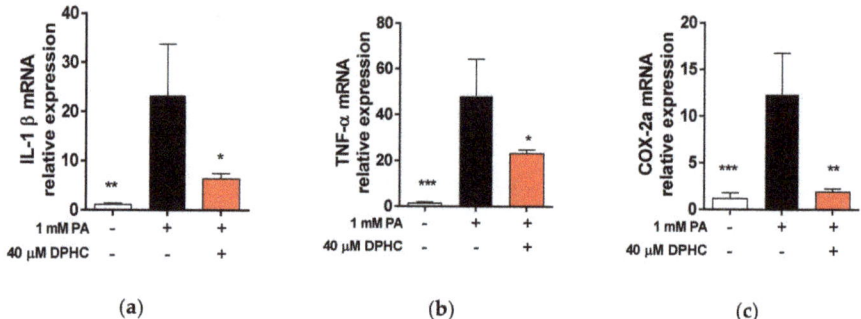

(a) (b) (c)

Figure 6. DPHC protects against palmitate-induced liver inflammation in zebrafish. At 3 days post-fertilization, zebrafish were incubated with and without 40 µM DPHC for 1 h, and then further incubated with or without 1 mM palmitate (PA) for 72 h. Total RNA was extracted from zebrafish liver, and mRNA expression levels of (a) IL-1β, (b) TNF-α, and (c) COX-2a were analyzed by RT-qPCR. PA: palmitic acid. $n = 12$–15 embryos. * $p < 0.05$, ** $p < 0.01$, *** $p < 0.001$.

2.7. DPHC Protects against Palmitate-Induced Reduction of Phosphorylated AMP-Activated Protein Kinase (AMPK) and Sirtuin (SIRT)1 in Zebrafish

We determined whether DPHC stimulates the AMPK and SIRT1 signaling pathway in zebrafish. We found that the protein level of phosphorylated AMPK and SIRT1 was significantly decreased by palmitate treatment, and this decrease was rescued with DPHC pretreatment of zebrafish (Figure 7), suggesting that DPHC may upregulate the phosphorylation of AMPK and SIRT1 in in vivo zebrafish. These results suggest that DPHC may induce AMPK and SIRT1 expression, contributing to the prevention of lipotoxicity in zebrafish liver.

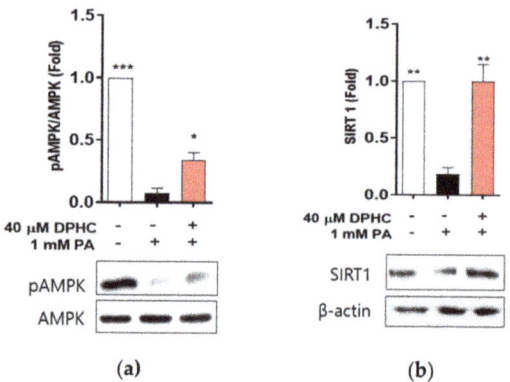

(a) (b)

Figure 7. DPHC improves protein expression levels of phosphorylated AMPK and SIRT1 against palmitate in zebrafish liver. Zebrafish embryos were incubated with and without 40 µM DPHC for 1 h, and then further incubated with or without 1 mM palmitate (PA) for 24 h. (a) AMPK and (b) SIRT1 protein expression levels were determined by western blotting. Experiments were performed in triplicate. * $p < 0.05$, ** $p < 0.01$, *** $p < 0.001$.

3. Discussion

NAFLD is recognized as a global health problem and as a common cause of chronic liver disease. To date, there are two major strategies in NAFLD therapy: (1) lifestyle modification, including dietary modification and physical exercise, and (2) pharmaceutical therapies. Lifestyle modifications with diet and exercise have been recommended as the initial management. However, these changes are difficult to achieve and sustain over time. Therefore, attention has been focused on finding pharmacologic agents for the treatment and/or prevention of NAFLD. Although several drugs to treat NAFLD are currently available, satisfactory outcomes have not been achieved. Therefore, natural products have been considered as alternative treatments to prevent NAFLD, or to stop its progression through several mechanisms, such as the downregulation of pro-inflammatory cytokines, antioxidant effects, or by anti-dyslipidemic properties [29–31]. Recently, constituents of seaweed origin have emerged in studies seeking improvements in NAFLD [32,33].

Polyphenolics are a type of flavonoid, which represents the most common group of dietary components, and have been suggested to be consistently associated with a reduced risk of developing chronic diseases, including diabetes mellitus, cardiovascular disease, and inflammation, as well as NAFLD [34–36].

Polyphenolic compounds, which are known to exhibit various biological activities, such as antioxidant, anti-inflammatory, and anti-glycation effects, are found in the edible seaweed *Ishige okamurae* [37–39]. However, it is not known whether DHPC, one polyphenolic compound from *I. okamurae*, might ameliorate palmitate-induced NAFLD. In the present study, we investigated the effects of DPHC on palmitate-induced lipogenesis, as well as inflammation, in HepG2 cells and zebrafish. Our study demonstrated that palmitate treatment caused hepatic toxicity, increased lipogenesis-related gene expression, and increased levels of pro-inflammatory cytokines. All of these effects were significantly attenuated by pretreatment with DPHC.

FFA is a prominent causative factor of NAFLD [40], and increased FFA levels have been observed in patients with NAFLD [41,42]. FFA induces excessive TG accumulation in hepatocytes, and this alters lipid metabolism in the liver [43]. SREBP-1c is a master transcriptional regulator of lipogenesis, and is highly expressed in the liver [44]. ChREBP is a transcription factor, which is activated by carbohydrate, and induces both glycolysis and lipogenesis [45]. In addition, C/EBPβ is a transcription factor, which is known to be an important regulator in fatty liver disease [46]. We found that palmitate treatment induced fat accumulation and elevated the mRNA and protein levels of SREBP-1c, ChREBP, and C/EBPβ; however, DPHC treatment inhibited these increases in HepG2 cells. Consistent with these results, the expression of *FAS*, a target gene of SREBP-1c and ChREBP, was increased by palmitate treatment, and DPHC pretreatment inhibited this increase. These results indicated that DPHC might have an ameliorating effect on fatty liver through the inhibition of the expression of lipogenic genes.

SIRT1 is a protein belonging to the sirtuin family, which widely affects lipid metabolism with AMPK signaling [47]. SIRT1-AMPK signaling in several metabolic tissues, including the liver, has been reported to increase rates of fatty acid oxidation, and to repress lipogenesis, largely by modulating SREBP-1 [48,49]. Thus, the SIRT1-AMPK axis has emerged as a major signaling system in regulating the lipid-lowering action in tissues, including the liver. The major therapeutic effect of polyphenol supplementation in NAFLD is reported to be mediated by the activation of AMPK [50,51]. The results obtained in this study were comparable, which allowed us to draw the following conclusions: DPHC pretreatment increases AMPK phosphorylation, which entails the downregulation of SREBP-1 expression levels [50]. Furthermore, a number of investigations have revealed that polyphenolic compounds significantly affect lipid metabolism [52], decrease plasma TG [53], and reduce lipid peroxidation [54]. Therefore, we suggest that DPHC, as used in this study, may also regulate lipid metabolism. In addition, the activation of AMPK and SIRT1 by polyphenols [55–57] inhibits inflammation [58], as well as suppresses the development of NAFLD [59–61]. These reports suggest that polyphenolic compounds have a prominent NAFLD development-alleviating effect.

It is widely acknowledged that hepatocyte inflammatory responses are associated with obesity and involve liver lipid accumulation, subsequently progressing to hepatic steatosis in the course of NAFLD. Lipid accumulation is one of the causative factors for inflammation, and accelerates the progress of NAFLD [62]. Some polyphenols significantly inhibit pro-inflammatory cytokines and transcription factors, including *IL-1*, *IL-6*, *TNF-α*, *NF-kB*, and *COX-2*, in the liver [63,64], DPHC is reported to possess anti-inflammatory effects in keratinocytes [15]. Therefore, we determined whether DPHC affects the expression of pro-inflammatory cytokines in the liver of zebrafish. In this study, we observed that DPHC can significantly reduce the expression of pro-inflammatory cytokines in the liver of zebrafish, suggesting that DPHC possesses anti-inflammation functions in NAFLD.

In summary, we demonstrated that DPHC reduced hepatic toxicity, diminished the expression of *SREBP-1*, *C/EBPβ*, *ChREBP*, and *FAS*, and enhanced *AMPK* and *SIRT1* expression, as well as reduced hepatic inflammation induced by palmitate. These results suggested that the activation of the AMPK signaling pathway may play a critical role in the suppressive effect of DPHC on lipogenesis, as well as in the promoting effect of DPHC on SIRT1. These findings may provide molecular evidence for the use of DPHC as a therapeutic agent in the management of NAFLD. However, although DPHC showed an excellent hepatic protective effect against PA in the in vivo zebrafish model in this study, it is necessary to confirm whether it is safe in both healthy and in hyperglycemia or obesity state when taking DPHC for a long time as pharmaceutical agent.

4. Materials and Methods

4.1. Preparation of DPHC from Ishige okamurae

The DPHC isolated from the seaweed *Ishige okamurae* was used. The preparation procedure of DPHC was described in our previous study [40].

4.2. Cell Culture

The human liver hepatocellular cell line HepG2 was obtained from the American Type Culture Collection (ATCC, Manassas, VA, USA). The cells were cultured in DMEM (Dulbecco Modified Eagle Medium, Welgene, Kyungsangbuk-do, Korea) supplemented with 10% FBS (Fetal Bovine Serum, Welgene), 100 U/mL penicillin, and 100 µg/mL streptomycin (Welgene), and were maintained in a humidified incubator with 5% CO_2.

4.3. Assessment of Cell Viability

Cell viability was estimated using a cell counting kit (D-Plus™ CCK; Dongin LS, Kyunggi-do, Korea) that measures water-soluble tetrazolium. For the CCK assay, HepG2 cells (2×10^4 cells/well) were seeded into 96-well plates. After 16 h, the cells were treated with DPHC and/or palmitate (Sigma, St. Louis, MO, USA) at 37 °C. D-Plus™ CCK solution was then added to the wells for a total reaction volume of 110 µL. After 2 h of incubation, optical absorbance was measured at a wavelength of 450 nm. The optical density of the formazan generated in control cells was considered to represent 100% viability.

4.4. Triglyceride Content Determination

HepG2 cells (2×10^5 cells/well) were seeded into 12-well plates. After 16 h, the cells were treated with DPHC and/or palmitate (Sigma) at 37 °C. TG levels were estimated using a TG quantification kit (BioVision, Milpitas, CA, USA) according to the manufacturer's protocol. Briefly, cells were dissolved in 5% NP-40–H_2O, and glycerol converted from TGs was measured.

4.5. Oil Red O Staining

The total intracellular lipid content was evaluated by Oil Red O staining. Briefly, cells were fixed in 4% paraformaldehyde in PBS (phosphate buffered saline, Welgene) for 30 min, stained with freshly prepared 0.28% Oil Red O for 30 min at room temperature, and then rinsed with water. Cell images were captured by photomicroscopy (Nikon Eclipse Ts2, Tokyo, Japan) equipped with eXcope XCAM 1080 (DIXI Science, Daejeon, Korea). For quantitative analysis of cellular lipids, 1 mL of isopropanol was added to the stained cells. The extracted dye was removed immediately by gentle pipetting, and its absorbance was read using a spectrophotometer at 510 nm. Data are represented as percentages of control cells.

4.6. RT-qPCR

Total RNA was extracted from HepG2 cells and zebrafish liver using RNAiso plus (Takara Bio Inc., Kusatsusi, Japan), and cDNA was prepared using a PrimeScript™ cDNA synthesis kit (Takara Bio Inc.) according to the manufacturer's instructions. cDNA samples were analyzed using SYBR® Premix Taq™, ROX plus (Takara Bio Inc.) on a Bio-Rad cycler (Hercules, CA, USA). Gene expression was normalized to that of the endogenous housekeeping control gene β-actin, which was not influenced by palmitate. Relative expression was calculated for each gene using the $\Delta\Delta C_T$ method (where C_T is the threshold cycle). The primer sequences used are listed in Table 1.

Table 1. Primer sequences.

Gene name		Sequence 5'-3'
SREBP1c (HepG2 cells)	Forward	TCGCGGAGCCATGGATT
	Reverse	GGAAGTCACTGTCTTGGTTGTTGA
C/EBPα (HepG2 cells)	Forward	GACACGCTGCGGGGCATCT
	Reverse	CTGCTCCCCTTCCTTCTCTCA
ChREBP (HepG2 cells)	Forward	GTCTGCAGGCTCGGAACAG
	Reverse	AAGGAGGAAATCAGAACTCAGGAA
FAS (HepG2 cells)	Forward	GCAAATTCGACCTTTCTCAGAA
	Reverse	GTAGGACCCCGTGGAATGTC
Cyclophilin (HepG2 cells)	Forward	TGCCATCGCCAAGGAGTAG
	Reverse	TGCACAGACGGTCACTCAAA
IL-1β (Zebrafish)	Forward	TCAAACCCCAATCCACAGAG
	Reverse	TCACTTCACGCTCTTGGATG
TNF-α (Zebrafish)	Forward	AGAAGGAGAGTTGCCTTTACCGCT'
	Reverse	AACACCCTCCATACACCCGACTTT
COX-2 (Zebrafish)	Forward	AGCCCTACTCATCCTTTGAGG
	Reverse	TCAACCTTGTCTACGTGACCATA
FAS (Zebrafish)	Forward	GCACCGGTACTAAGGTTGGA
	Reverse	CAGACGCCATGTTCAAGAGA
β-actin (Zebrafish)	Forward	AATCTTGCGGTATCCACGAGACCA
	Reverse	TCTCCTTCTGCATCCTGTCAGCAA

SREBP1c: sterol regulatory element-binding protein 1; C/EBP: CCAAT-enhancer-binding protein; ChREBP: carbohydrate-responsive element-binding protein; FAS: fatty acid synthase; IL-1: interleukin 1; TNF: tumor necrosis factor; COX: cyclooxygenase.

4.7. Western Blotting

HepG2 cells (1×10^5 cells/well) were seeded into six-well plates, and the cells were incubated with vehicle (control) or 40 μM DPHC for 1 h, and then further incubated with or without 0.4 mM palmitate for 24 h. The cells were lysed using 1% Triton X-100-PBS and protease inhibitor cocktail (GenDEPOT, Barker, TX, USA) for 20 min, on ice. The lysates were fractionated by centrifugation at 12,000 rpm for 20 min at 4 °C, and the pellets were used for western blotting. Protein concentrations were measured using a DC protein assay kit (Bio-Rad, Hercules, CA, USA). The lysates were separated by SDS-PAGE and transferred to PVDF (polyvinylidene fluoride) membranes (Millipore, Billerica, MA, USA). Membranes were incubated with 5% skimmed milk for 1 h at room temperature, and then incubated with primary antibodies overnight at 4 °C. After washing extensively, membranes were incubated with horseradish peroxidase-conjugated secondary antibody (Jackson ImmunoResearch, West Grove, PA, USA). Signals were detected using WESTSAVE (Ab Frontier, Seoul, Korea) and an enhanced chemiluminescence system. ImageJ software was used to quantify the band intensities of western blots. The primary antibodies used were anti-SREBP1, anti-C/EBPβ, anti-ChREBP, anti-FAS, and anti-β-actin. All primary antibodies were purchased from Santa Cruz Biotechnology (Santa Cruz, CA, USA).

4.8. Zebrafish Experiments

The zebrafish embryo procedures used in the present study were conducted according to the guidelines established by the Gachon University Ethics Review Committee for Animal Experiments.

Transgenic zebrafish embryos expressing EGFP under the control of the liver fatty acid-binding protein promoter Tg(lfabp-egfp) were obtained from the Korean Zebrafish Organogenesis Mutant Bank. At 3 days post-fertilization (dpf), embryos were arrayed in 12-well plates for experiments. At 3 dpf, embryos ($n = 12–15$) were transferred to 12-well plates and maintained in 1 mL of embryo media (0.003% sea salt, 0.0075% calcium sulfate). Embryos were preincubated with 40 µM DPHC for 1 h, and then further incubated in the presence of 1 mM palmitate for 72 h. Thereafter, the embryos were rinsed in embryo media and anaesthetized using 2-phenoxy ethanol (Sigma) before experiments. The zebrafish were imaged using a stereo fluorescence microscope (M165FC, Leica, Wetzlar, Germany) and confocal microscope (LSM710, Zeiss, Oberkochen, Germany). After isolation of the liver, mRNA expression levels of specific genes were determined.

4.9. Statistical Analysis

Significant differences were compared using one-way analysis with subsequent multiple comparison test (Tukey) of variance using GraphPad prism version 6.0 (GraphPad software, San Diego, CA, USA). Data are presented as means ± SEM. Differences were considered significant at $p < 0.05$ versus the PA-treated group.

Author Contributions: S.-H.C. participated in the experimental design, carried out all assays for the cells and zebrafish, performed the statistical analysis, and participated in drafting the manuscript. Y.H. carried out RT-qPCR and performed the statistical analysis. S.-J.H. isolated DPHC. H.-S.J. conceived the study, participated in its design and coordination, and prepared the manuscript. All authors have read and agreed to the published version of the manuscript.

Funding: This research was funded by grants from the Korea Health Technology RnD project through the Ministry of Health and Welfare (HI14C1135), the Korea Institute of Ocean Science and Technology (grant number PE99822), and the Basic Science Research Program through the National Research Foundation of Korea (NRF) funded by the Ministry of Science, ICT, & Future Planning (grant number 2020R1C1C1007712).

Conflicts of Interest: The authors declare no conflict of interest.

References

1. Marchesini, G.; Bugianesi, E.; Forlani, G.; Cerrelli, F.; Lenzi, M.; Manini, R.; Natale, S.; Vanni, E.; Villanova, N.; Melchionda, N.; et al. Nonalcoholic fatty liver, steatohepatitis, and the metabolic syndrome. *Hepatology* **2003**, *37*, 917–923. [CrossRef] [PubMed]
2. Chalasani, N.; Younossi, Z.; Lavine, J.E.; Diehl, A.M.; Brunt, E.M.; Cusi, K.; Charlton, M.; Sanyal, A.J. The diagnosis and management of non-alcoholic fatty liver disease: Practice Guideline by the American Association for the Study of Liver Diseases, American College of Gastroenterology, and the American Gastroenterological Association. *Hepatology* **2012**, *55*, 2005–2023. [CrossRef] [PubMed]
3. Abenavoli, L.; Milic, N.; Luzza, F.; Boccuto, L.; De Lorenzo, A. Polyphenols Treatment in Patients with Nonalcoholic Fatty Liver Disease. *J. Transl. Intern. Med.* **2017**, *5*, 144–147. [CrossRef] [PubMed]
4. Gan, L.; Meng, Z.J.; Xiong, R.B.; Guo, J.Q.; Lu, X.C.; Zheng, Z.W.; Deng, Y.P.; Luo, B.D.; Zou, F.; Li, H. Green tea polyphenol epigallocatechin-3-gallate ameliorates insulin resistance in non-alcoholic fatty liver disease mice. *Acta Pharmacol. Sin.* **2015**, *36*, 597–605. [CrossRef]
5. Machado, M.V.; Diehl, A.M. Pathogenesis of Nonalcoholic Steatohepatitis. *Gastroenterology* **2016**, *150*, 1769–1777. [CrossRef]
6. Boden, G. Obesity and free fatty acids. *Endocrinology Metab. Clin. N. Am.* **2008**, *37*, 635–646. [CrossRef]

7. Fujita, K.; Nozaki, Y.; Wada, K.; Yoneda, M.; Fujimoto, Y.; Fujitake, M.; Endo, H.; Takahashi, H.; Inamori, M.; Kobayashi, N.; et al. Dysfunctional very-low-density lipoprotein synthesis and release is a key factor in nonalcoholic steatohepatitis pathogenesis. *Hepatology* **2009**, *50*, 772–780. [CrossRef]
8. Malhi, H.; Bronk, S.F.; Werneburg, N.W.; Gores, G.J. Free Fatty Acids Induce JNK-dependent Hepatocyte Lipoapoptosis. *J. Biol. Chem.* **2006**, *281*, 12093–12101. [CrossRef]
9. Yamaguchi, K.; Yang, L.; McCall, S.; Huang, J.; Yu, X.X.; Pandey, S.K.; Bhanot, S.; Monia, B.P.; Li, Y.X.; Diehl, A.M. Inhibiting triglyceride synthesis improves hepatic steatosis but exacerbates liver damage and fibrosis in obese mice with nonalcoholic steatohepatitis. *Hepatology* **2007**, *45*, 1366–1374. [CrossRef]
10. Tilg, H.; Moschen, A.R. Evolution of inflammation in nonalcoholic fatty liver disease: The multiple parallel hits hypothesis. *Hepatology* **2010**, *52*, 1836–1846. [CrossRef]
11. Heo, S.J.; Hwang, J.Y.; Choi, J.I.; Lee, S.H.; Park, P.J.; Kang, H.; Oh, C.; Kim, D.W.; Han, J.S.; Jeon, Y.J.; et al. Protective effect of diphlorethohydroxycarmalol isolated from *Ishige okamurae* against high glucose-induced-oxidative stress in human umbilical vein endothelial cells. *Food Chem. Toxicol.* **2010**, *48*, 1448–1454. [CrossRef] [PubMed]
12. Lee, S.H.; Choi, J.I.; Heo, S.J.; Park, M.H.; Park, P.J.; Jeon, B.T.; Kim, S.K.; Han, J.S.; Jeon, Y.J. Diphlorethohydroxycarmalol isolated from Pae (*Ishige okamurae*) protects high glucose-induced damage in RINm5F pancreatic β cells via its antioxidant effects. *Food Sci. Biotechnol.* **2012**, *21*, 239–246. [CrossRef]
13. Piao, M.J.; Kang, K.A.; Kim, K.C.; Chae, S.; Kim, G.O.; Shin, T.; Kim, H.S.; Hyun, J.W. Diphlorethohydroxycarmalol attenuated cell damage against UVB radiation via enhancing antioxidant effects and absorbing UVB ray in human HaCaT keratinocytes. *Environ. Toxicol. Pharmacol.* **2013**, *36*, 680–688. [CrossRef] [PubMed]
14. Park, M.H.; Han, J.S.; Jeon, Y.-J.; Kim, H.-J. Effect of Diphlorethohydroxycarmalol Isolated from *Ishige okamurae* on Apoptosis in 3 t3-L1 Preadipocytes. *Phytotherapy Res.* **2012**, *27*, 931–936. [CrossRef]
15. Kang, G.J.; Han, S.C.; Koh, Y.S.; Kang, H.K.; Jeon, Y.J.; Yoo, E.S. Diphlorethohydroxycarmalol, Isolated from *Ishige okamurae*, Increases Prostaglandin E2 through the Expression of Cyclooxygenase-1 and -2 in HaCaT Human Keratinocytes. *Biomol. Ther.* **2012**, *20*, 520–525. [CrossRef]
16. Piao, M.J.; Kumara, M.H.S.R.; Kim, K.C.; Kang, K.A.; Kang, H.K.; Lee, N.H.; Hyun, J.W. Diphlorethohydroxycarmalol Suppresses Ultraviolet B-Induced Matrix Metalloproteinases via Inhibition of JNK and ERK Signaling in Human Keratinocytes. *Biomol. Ther.* **2015**, *23*, 557–563. [CrossRef]
17. Piao, M.J.; Hewage, S.R.K.M.; Han, X.; Kang, K.A.; Kang, H.-K.; Lee, N.H.; Hyun, J.W. Protective Effect of Diphlorethohydroxycarmalol against Ultraviolet B Radiation-Induced DNA Damage by Inducing the Nucleotide Excision Repair System in HaCaT Human Keratinocytes. *Mar. Drugs* **2015**, *13*, 5629–5641. [CrossRef]
18. Kang, N.J.; Han, S.C.; Kang, G.J.; Koo, D.H.; Koh, Y.S.; Hyun, J.W.; Lee, N.H.; Ko, M.H.; Kang, H.K.; Yoo, E.S. Diphlorethohydroxycarmalol Inhibits Interleukin-6 Production by Regulating NF-κB, STAT5 and SOCS1 in Lipopolysaccharide-Stimulated RAW264.7 Cells. *Mar. Drugs* **2015**, *13*, 2141–2157. [CrossRef]
19. Kang, M.C.; Cha, S.H.; Wijesinghe, W.; Kang, S.M.; Lee, S.H.; Kim, E.A.; Song, C.B.; Jeon, Y.J. Protective effect of marine algae phlorotannins against AAPH-induced oxidative stress in zebrafish embryo. *Food Chem.* **2013**, *138*, 950–955. [CrossRef]
20. Heo, S.J.; Cha, S.H.; Kim, K.N.; Lee, S.H.; Ahn, G.; Kang, H.; Oh, C.; Choi, Y.U.; Affan, A.; Kim, D.; et al. Neuroprotective Effect of Phlorotannin Isolated from *Ishige okamurae* Against H_2O_2-Induced Oxidative Stress in Murine Hippocampal Neuronal Cells, HT22. *Appl. Biochem. Biotechnol.* **2012**, *166*, 1520–1532. [CrossRef]
21. Ahn, M.; Moon, C.; Yang, W.; Ko, E.J.; Hyun, J.W.; Joo, H.G.; Jee, Y.; Lee, N.H.; Park, J.W.; Ko, R.K.; et al. Diphlorethohydroxycarmalol, isolated from the brown algae *Ishige okamurae*, protects against radiation-induced cell damage in mice. *Food Chem. Toxicol.* **2011**, *49*, 864–870. [CrossRef] [PubMed]
22. Wree, A.; Broderick, L.; Canbay, A.; Hoffman, H.M.; Feldstein, A.E. From NAFLD to NASH to cirrhosis—New insights into disease mechanisms. *Nat. Rev. Gastroenterol. Hepatol.* **2013**, *10*, 627–636. [CrossRef] [PubMed]
23. Puri, P.; Baillie, R.; Wiest, M.M.; Mirshahi, F.; Choudhury, J.; Cheung, O.; Sargeant, C.; Contos, M.J.; Sanyal, A.J. A lipidomic analysis of nonalcoholic fatty liver disease. *Hepatology* **2007**, *46*, 1081–1090. [CrossRef]
24. O'Neill, H.M.; Holloway, G.P.; Steinberg, G.R. AMPK regulation of fatty acid metabolism and mitochondrial biogenesis: Implications for obesity. *Mol. Cell. Endocrinol.* **2013**, *366*, 135–151. [CrossRef] [PubMed]
25. Day, E.A.; Ford, R.J.; Steinberg, G.R. AMPK as a Therapeutic Target for Treating Metabolic Diseases. *Trends Endocrinol. Metab.* **2017**, *28*, 545–560. [CrossRef]

26. Shen, C.; Dou, X.; Ma, Y.; Ma, W.; Li, S.; Song, Z. Nicotinamide protects hepatocytes against palmitate-induced lipotoxicity via SIRT1-dependent autophagy induction. *Nutr. Res.* **2017**, *40*, 40–47. [CrossRef]
27. Ding, R.B.; Bao, J.; Deng, C.X. Emerging roles of SIRT1 in fatty liver diseases. *Int. J. Biol. Sci.* **2017**, *13*, 852–867. [CrossRef]
28. Colak, Y.; Ozturk, O.; Senates, E.; Tuncer, I.; Yorulmaz, E.; Adali, G.; Doganay, L.; Enc, F.Y. SIRT1 as a potential therapeutic target for treatment of nonalcoholic fatty liver disease. *Med. Sci. Monit.* **2011**, *17*, HY5–HY9. [CrossRef]
29. Hu, X.Q.; Wang, Y.; Wang, J.; Xue, Y.; Li, Z.; Nagao, K.; Yanagita, T.; Xue, C. Dietary saponins of sea cucumber alleviate orotic acid-induced fatty liver in rats via PPARα and SREBP-1c signaling. *Lipids Health Dis.* **2010**, *9*, 25. [CrossRef]
30. Aghazadeh, S.; Amini, R.; Yazdanparast, R.; Ghaffari, S.H.; Seyed, H.G. Anti-apoptotic and anti-inflammatory effects of Silybum marianum in treatment of experimental steatohepatitis. *Exp. Toxicol. Pathol.* **2011**, *63*, 569–574. [CrossRef]
31. Xu, J.Y.; Zhang, L.; Li, Z.P.; Ji, G. Natural Products on Nonalcoholic Fatty Liver Disease. *Curr. Drug Targets* **2015**, *16*, 1347–1355. [CrossRef] [PubMed]
32. Park, E.Y.; Choi, H.; Yoon, J.Y.; Lee, I.Y.; Seo, Y.; Moon, H.S.; Hwang, J.H.; Jun, H.S. Polyphenol-Rich Fraction of Ecklonia cava Improves Nonalcoholic Fatty Liver Disease in High Fat Diet-Fed Mice. *Mar. Drugs* **2015**, *13*, 6866–6883. [CrossRef] [PubMed]
33. Song, W.; Wang, Z.; Zhang, X.; Li, Y. Ethanol Extract from Ulva prolifera Prevents High-Fat Diet-Induced Insulin Resistance, Oxidative Stress, and Inflammation Response in Mice. *BioMed Res. Int.* **2018**, *2018*, 1–9. [CrossRef] [PubMed]
34. Xiao, J.; Hogger, P. Dietary polyphenols and type 2 diabetes: Current insights and future perspectives. *Curr. Med. Chem.* **2015**, *22*, 23–38. [CrossRef] [PubMed]
35. Tangney, C.C.; Rasmussen, H.E. Polyphenols, inflammation, and cardiovascular disease. *Curr. Atheroscler. Rep.* **2013**, *15*, 324. [CrossRef]
36. Rodriguez-Ramiro, I.; Vauzour, D.; Minihane, A.M. Polyphenols and non-alcoholic fatty liver disease: Impact and mechanisms. *Proc. Nutr. Soc.* **2016**, *75*, 47–60. [CrossRef]
37. Heo, S.J.; Kim, J.P.; Jung, W.K.; Lee, N.H.; Kang, H.S.; Jun, E.M.; Park, S.H.; Kang, S.M.; Lee, Y.J.; Park, P.J.; et al. Identification of chemical structure and free radical scavenging activity of diphlorethohydroxycarmalol isolated from a brown alga, *Ishige okamurae*. *J. Microbiol. Biotechnol.* **2008**, *18*, 676–681.
38. Fernando, I.P.S.; Kim, H.S.; Sanjeewa, K.; Oh, J.Y.; Jeon, Y.J.; Lee, W.W. Inhibition of inflammatory responses elicited by urban fine dust particles in keratinocytes and macrophages by diphlorethohydroxycarmalol isolated from a brown alga *Ishige okamurae*. *ALGAE* **2017**, *32*, 261–273. [CrossRef]
39. Cha, S.H.; Hwang, Y.; Heo, S.J.; Jun, H.S. Diphlorethohydroxycarmalol Attenuates Methylglyoxal-Induced Oxidative Stress and Advanced Glycation End Product Formation in Human Kidney Cells. *Oxid. Med. Cell. Longev.* **2018**, *2018*, 3654095. [CrossRef]
40. Takahara, I.; Akazawa, Y.; Tabuchi, M.; Matsuda, K.; Miyaaki, H.; Kido, Y.; Kanda, Y.; Taura, N.; Ohnita, K.; Takeshima, F.; et al. Toyocamycin attenuates free fatty acid-induced hepatic steatosis and apoptosis in cultured hepatocytes and ameliorates nonalcoholic fatty liver disease in mice. *PLoS ONE* **2017**, *12*, e0170591. [CrossRef]
41. Ogawa, Y.; Imajo, K.; Honda, Y.; Kessoku, T.; Tomeno, W.; Kato, S.; Fujita, K.; Yoneda, M.; Saito, S.; Saigusa, Y.; et al. Palmitate-induced lipotoxicity is crucial for the pathogenesis of nonalcoholic fatty liver disease in cooperation with gut-derived endotoxin. *Sci. Rep.* **2018**, *8*, 11365. [CrossRef] [PubMed]
42. Chen, J.W.; Kong, Z.L.; Tsai, M.L.; Lo, C.Y.; Ho, C.T.; Lai, C.S. Tetrahydrocurcumin ameliorates free fatty acid-induced hepatic steatosis and improves insulin resistance in HepG2 cells. *J. Food Drug Anal.* **2018**, *26*, 1075–1085. [CrossRef] [PubMed]
43. Liu, Q.; Bengmark, S.; Qu, S. The role of hepatic fat accumulation in pathogenesis of non-alcoholic fatty liver disease (NAFLD). *Lipids Health. Dis.* **2010**, *9*, 42. [CrossRef]

44. Shimomura, I.; Bashmakov, Y.; Ikemoto, S.; Horton, J.D.; Brown, M.S.; Goldstein, J.L. Insulin selectively increases SREBP-1c mRNA in the livers of rats with streptozotocin-induced diabetes. *Proc. Natl. Acad. Sci. USA* **1999**, *96*, 13656–13661. [CrossRef] [PubMed]
45. Yu, Y.; Maguire, T.G.; Alwine, J.C. ChREBP, a glucose-responsive transcriptional factor, enhances glucose metabolism to support biosynthesis in human cytomegalovirus-infected cells. *Proc. Natl. Acad. Sci. USA* **2014**, *111*, 1951–1956. [CrossRef]
46. Schroeder-Gloeckler, J.M.; Rahman, S.M.; Janssen, R.C.; Qiao, L.; Shao, J.; Roper, M.; Fischer, S.J.; Lowe, E.; Orlicky, D.J.; McManaman, J.L.; et al. CCAAT/enhancer-binding protein beta deletion reduces adiposity, hepatic steatosis, and diabetes in Lepr(db/db) mice. *J. Biol. Chem.* **2007**, *282*, 15717–15729. [CrossRef]
47. Houtkooper, R.H.; Pirinen, E.; Auwerx, J. Sirtuins as regulators of metabolism and healthspan. *Nat. Rev. Mol. Cell Biol.* **2012**, *13*, 225–238. [CrossRef]
48. Suchankova, G.; Nelson, L.E.; Gerhart-Hines, Z.; Kelly, M.; Gauthier, M.S.; Saha, A.K.; Ido, Y.; Puigserver, P.; Ruderman, N. Concurrent regulation of AMP-activated protein kinase and SIRT1 in mammalian cells. *Biochem. Biophys. Res. Commun.* **2009**, *378*, 836–841. [CrossRef]
49. Canto, C.; Gerhart-Hines, Z.; Feige, J.N.; Lagouge, M.; Noriega, L.; Milne, J.C.; Elliott, P.J.; Puigserver, P.; Auwerx, J.; Noriega, L. AMPK regulates energy expenditure by modulating NAD^+ metabolism and SIRT1 activity. *Nature* **2009**, *458*, 1056–1060. [CrossRef]
50. Choi, Y.J.; Suh, H.-R.; Yoon, Y.; Lee, K.J.; Kim, D.G.; Kim, S.; Lee, B.H. Protective effect of resveratrol derivatives on high-fat diet induced fatty liver by activating AMP-activated protein kinase. *Arch. Pharmacal Res.* **2014**, *37*, 1169–1176. [CrossRef]
51. Ajmo, J.M.; Liang, X.; Rogers, C.Q.; Pennock, B.; You, M. Resveratrol alleviates alcoholic fatty liver in mice. *Am. J. Physiol. Gastrointest. Liver Physiol.* **2008**, *295*, G833–G842. [CrossRef] [PubMed]
52. Jeon, S.M.; Lee, S.A.; Choi, M.S. Antiobesity and Vasoprotective Effects of Resveratrol in ApoE-Deficient Mice. *J. Med. Food* **2014**, *17*, 310–316. [CrossRef] [PubMed]
53. Andrade, J.M.O.; Paraíso, A.F.; de Oliveira, M.V.M.; Martins, A.M.E.D.B.L.; Neto, J.F.; Guimarães, A.L.S.; de Paula, A.M.; Qureshi, M.; Santos, S.H.S. Resveratrol attenuates hepatic steatosis in high-fat fed mice by decreasing lipogenesis and inflammation. *Nutrition* **2014**, *30*, 915–919. [CrossRef] [PubMed]
54. Li, L.; Hai, J.; Li, Z.; Zhang, Y.; Peng, H.; Li, K.; Weng, X. Resveratrol modulates autophagy and NF-κB activity in a murine model for treating non-alcoholic fatty liver disease. *Food Chem. Toxicol.* **2014**, *63*, 166–173. [CrossRef] [PubMed]
55. Deng, X.Q.; Chen, L.L.; Li, N.X. The expression of SIRT1 in nonalcoholic fatty liver disease induced by high-fat diet in rats. *Liver Int.* **2007**, *27*, 708–715. [CrossRef]
56. Baur, J.A.; Pearson, K.J.; Price, N.L.; Jamieson, H.A.; Lerin, C.; Kalra, A.; Prabhu, V.V.; Allard, J.S.; López-Lluch, G.; Lewis, K.; et al. Resveratrol improves health and survival of mice on a high-calorie diet. *Nature* **2006**, *444*, 337–342. [CrossRef]
57. Zygmunt, K.; Faubert, B.; MacNeil, J.; Tsiani, E. Naringenin, a citrus flavonoid, increases muscle cell glucose uptake via AMPK. *Biochem. Biophys. Res. Commun.* **2010**, *398*, 178–183. [CrossRef]
58. Velagapudi, R.; El-Bakoush, A.; Lepiarz, I.; Ogunrinade, F.; Olajide, O.A. AMPK and SIRT1 activation contribute to inhibition of neuroinflammation by thymoquinone in BV2 microglia. *Mol. Cell. Biochem.* **2017**, *435*, 149–162. [CrossRef]
59. Shang, J.; Chen, L.L.; Xiao, F.X.; Sun, H.; Ding, H.C.; Xiao, H. Resveratrol improves non-alcoholic fatty liver disease by activating AMP-activated protein kinase. *Acta Pharmacol. Sin.* **2008**, *29*, 698–706. [CrossRef]
60. Pisonero-Vaquero, S.; González-Gallego, J.; Sánchez-Campos, S.; García-Mediavilla, M.V. Flavonoids and Related Compounds in Non-Alcoholic Fatty Liver Disease Therapy. *Curr. Med. Chem.* **2015**, *22*, 2991–3012. [CrossRef]
61. Van de Wier, B.; Koek, G.H.; Bast, A.; Haenen, G.R.M.M. The potential of flavonoids in the treatment of non-alcoholic fatty liver disease. *Crit. Rev. Food Sci. Nutr.* **2015**, *57*, 834–855. [CrossRef] [PubMed]
62. He, P.P.; He, P.P.; Wen, M.; Zou, J.Q.; Wang, Y.; Yang, J.X.; Hu, L.Z.; Zheng, X.L.; Chen, Y.S.; Su, H.; et al. Nobiletin reduces LPL-mediated lipid accumulation and pro-inflammatory cytokine secretion through upregulation of miR-590 expression. *Biochem. Biophys. Res. Commun.* **2019**, *508*, 97–101. [CrossRef] [PubMed]

63. Yang, Y.; Li, S.; Yang, Q.; Shi, Y.; Zheng, M.; Liu, Y.; Chen, F.; Song, G.; Xu, H.; Wan, T.; et al. Resveratrol Reduces the Proinflammatory Effects and Lipopolysaccharide-Induced Expression of HMGB1 and TLR4 in RAW264.7 Cells. *Cell. Physiol. Biochem.* **2014**, *33*, 1283–1292. [CrossRef] [PubMed]
64. Adibi, P.; Faghihzadeh, F.; Hekmatdoost, A. Resveratrol and liver: A systematic review. *J. Res. Med. Sci.* **2015**, *20*, 797–810. [CrossRef] [PubMed]

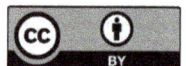 © 2020 by the authors. Licensee MDPI, Basel, Switzerland. This article is an open access article distributed under the terms and conditions of the Creative Commons Attribution (CC BY) license (http://creativecommons.org/licenses/by/4.0/).

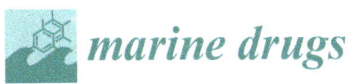

Review

Fucoidan Characterization: Determination of Purity and Physicochemical and Chemical Properties

Ahmed Zayed [1,2], Mona El-Aasr [2], Abdel-Rahim S. Ibrahim [2] and Roland Ulber [1,*]

1. Institute of Bioprocess Engineering, Technical University of Kaiserslautern, Gottlieb-Daimler-Straße 49, 67663 Kaiserslautern, Germany; ahmed.zayed1@pharm.tanta.edu.eg
2. Department of Pharmacognosy, Tanta University, College of Pharmacy, El-Guish Street, Tanta 31527, Egypt; moelaasar@pharm.tanta.edu.eg (M.E.-A.); abdelrahim.ibrahim@pharm.tanta.edu.eg (A.-R.S.I.)
* Correspondence: ulber@mv.uni-kl.de; Tel.: +49-(0)-631-205-4043; Fax: +49-631-205-4312

Received: 27 October 2020; Accepted: 17 November 2020; Published: 19 November 2020

Abstract: Fucoidans are marine sulfated biopolysaccharides that have heterogenous and complicated chemical structures. Various sugar monomers, glycosidic linkages, molecular masses, branching sites, and sulfate ester pattern and content are involved within their backbones. Additionally, sources, downstream processes, and geographical and seasonal factors show potential effects on fucoidan structural characteristics. These characteristics are documented to be highly related to fucoidan potential activities. Therefore, numerous chemical qualitative and quantitative determinations and structural elucidation methods are conducted to characterize fucoidans regarding their physicochemical and chemical features. Characterization of fucoidan polymers is considered a bottleneck for further biological and industrial applications. Consequently, the obtained results may be related to different activities, which could be improved afterward by further functional modifications. The current article highlights the different spectrometric and nonspectrometric methods applied for the characterization of native fucoidans, including degree of purity, sugar monomeric composition, sulfation pattern and content, molecular mass, and glycosidic linkages.

Keywords: fucoidans; fucoidanases; glycosidic linkages; molecular masses; NMR; structure–activity relationships

---

1. Introduction

Marine polysaccharides are classified as sulfated (SPs) and nonsulfated macromolecules that are mainly derived from micro- and macroalgae [1,2]. In particular, macroalgal SPs show more diverse chemical characteristics than nonsulfated analogues, in terms of their molecular weight, monosaccharide composition, and sulfate content and position, which interact with various biological targets at different levels leading to diverse and promising pharmacological activities [2,3]. They are found in different phyla, such as in Phaeophytes or brown algae (e.g., fucoidans), Rhodophytes or red algae (e.g., carrageenan), and Chlorophytes or green algae (e.g., ulvan) [2,4]. Despite brown algae, with 1755 species, not being the most abundant class, their SP fucoidans show more potential applications in different areas than those isolated from ulvan and carrageenan [5–7].

Fucoidans are known as fucose-containing sulfated polysaccharides (FCSPs), where L-fucose always predominates other sugar monomers, such as galactose, mannose, glucose, and uronic acids. L-fucose may exceed 90% of the total sugar composition of fucoidans [8]. Yet, galactose, as in the case of sulfated galactofucans, may possess similar ratios to fucose [9]. Another type of FCSP is isolated from marine invertebrates, called sulfated fucans. In contrast, they are composed of L-fucose only. Hence, the term fucoidans has recently been adopted specifically for the heterogenous marine SPs rich in fucose and derived from the different species of brown algae, including the old names fucoidin and fucoidan, to be consistent with the International Union of Pure and Applied Chemistry

(IUPAC) nomenclature system [10]. They are species-specific and, therefore, they do not have a universal chemical structure. Yet, they represent the major component of cell walls and the extracellular matrix (ECM) along with alginate and cellulose in brown seaweeds [11,12]. The physicochemical and chemical heterogeneity of fucoidans was discussed previously, as well as the way in which it affects their application [13]. In addition, fucoidans are characterized by high molecular weights, up to 950 kDa in the native fucoidan of *Hizikia fusiforme* or *Sargassum fusiforme* [14]. The presence of sulfate ester groups imparts a negative charge on the macromolecule skeleton responsible for the anionic characteristic of fucoidans [15]. Moreover, chain branching increases the complexity of fucoidans compared to sulfated fucans derived from marine invertebrates [16,17]. Therefore, an investigation of these two groups of fucose-containing biopolymers, i.e., sulfated fucans and fucoidans, requires different investigational approaches. Owing to their complicated chemical structures, enzymatic hydrolysis, mild acid hydrolysis, and autohydrolysis of native fucoidans are always involved in the elucidation of their fine structural features. Such pretreatments enable the production of oligomers or simple fractions that are easily interpreted [18].

Various applications of fucoidans in the therapeutic [19], cosmeceutical [20], nutraceutical/ functional foods [21], diagnostic [22], and drug delivery [23] fields have increased awareness concerning their importance, especially in the last few decades. Specifically, the pharmacological activities of fucoidans make them a candidate for the treatment of bleeding disorders [24], inflammation [25], viral infections [26], malignant tumors [27], and immune disorders [28]. Hence, current studies are focusing on pharmacokinetic and tissue distribution investigations after oral and topical administration of fucoidans [29–31]. These studies may help the administration of fucoidans in prospective human clinical trials. Meanwhile, the modification of native fucoidans via chemical or enzymatic treatment may result in an increase in their biological activity [11,32].

The mechanisms involved in the biological interactions of fucoidans with various targets are not only based on charge density, but also fine chemical features [33]. Hence, the major obstacle for the determination of structure–activity relationships is the complex structures of such polysaccharides [34]. These activities are highly correlated with the structural and nonstructural features of fucoidans [35,36], as summarized in Figure 1. Examples include relationships between high molecular weight and anticoagulant activity [37,38], low molecular weight and cancer apoptosis [39], and selective angiogenic activity in tumors as antiangiogenic [40] or in impaired tissues as proangiogenic agents [41]. Moreover, it was reported that the sulfation pattern was an important factor, especially at C-4 for anti-Herpes simplex virus infection [42] or at C-2 and C-3 for anti-coagulant activity [43], as well as the sulfate content (charge density) for cytotoxic and anticancer activity [44–47] or repair potential of injured kidney cells [48], the branching degree for antitumor activity [49], and the monosaccharide composition in terms of uronic acid content for antioxidant activity [50]. Moreover, more than one factor may be involved, such as the sulfate/fucose molar ratio, as shown in the attenuation of oxidative stress-induced cellular cytotoxicity by the crude fucoidan prepared from *Sargassum crassifolium* [51], or the high sulfate and low uronic acid content for significant anticoagulant activity as shown by *Ecklonia cava* fucoidan [11,52].

In addition, the quality and content of fucoidan in commercial products can affect its use. The most well-known example constitutes its cosmeceutical applications, which are improved by the presence of phlorotannins owing to the antioxidant activity of polyphenolics [53]. Hence, the quantitative determination of fucoidans is highly important for the prevention of interferences from coextracted contaminants when investigating the bioactivities and assuring the quality of commercially available products [54,55].

Therefore, the qualitative and quantitative determination of fucoidans and their coextracted contaminants is a must before physicochemical, chemical, and biological characterization. Afterward, the other functional motifs of fucoidan should be well characterized, such as its molecular weight, monomeric composition, sulfate content and pattern, and glycosidic linkage. Lastly, relationships with certain activities may be identified, and the putative mechanisms of action can be constructed to explain such activities. The current article focuses on the possible tests and investigations which help in the full characterization of fucoidans after downstream processing.

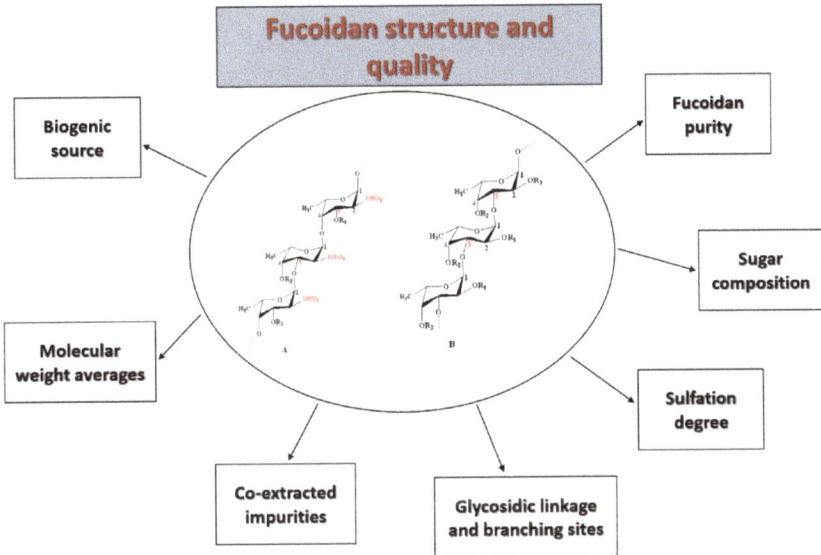

Figure 1. Summary of the different factors affecting the biological behavior of fucoidans. These factors should be characterized for the successful application of fucoidans.

2. Chemistry of Fucoidans

The chemistry of fucoidans is highly variable according to their origin, especially regarding their complexity. For instance, fucoidans derived from seaweeds commonly show a branched and more sulfated skeleton with the presence of numerous sugar monomers in addition to α-L-fucose. However, marine invertebrate fucoidans, such as echinoderms (e.g., sea cucumber) and urchins (e.g., *Strongylocentrotus droebachiensis*), are less complex, consisting of a linear and regular chain of repeating α-L-fucose units [10,16,56–58]. These differences make algal fucoidans a more preferable biogenic resource than those from marine invertebrates, in addition to their multiple and interesting biological activities [59].

In the literature, several structural models for seaweed fucoidans have been suggested to describe their important structural features [6,60–62] depending on their macroalgal biogenic origin, including species, age, geographical origin, and season of harvesting [9,13,63]. Cao et al. presented several representative fucoidan structures isolated from *Fucus evanescens*, *Fucus vesiculosus*, *Sargassum mcclurei*, *Turbinaria ornata*, *Saccharina cichorioides*, and *Undaria pinnatifida* [9].

Nevertheless, the most widely accepted models are those introduced by Cumashi et al. [64] and Ale et al. [35]. They proposed that seaweed fucoidans are highly heterogenous within brown seaweed species, composed of a linear or branched sulfated L-fucopyranoside backbone linked by not only alternating α-(1→3) and α-(1→4) linkages, but also α-(1→4) and α-(1→3) linkages only. Other sugar monomers can also be found, such as β-D-galactose, β-D-mannose, α-D-glucuronic acid, α-D-glucose, and β-D-xylose, but their positions and binding modes are still not understood [64,65]. However, Bilan et al. studied a fucoidan fraction isolated from *Sargassum polycystum* (Fucales) and found 2-linked sulfated α-D-galactopyranose residues [62]. Moreover, the L-fucose unit is mono- or disulfated and may be acetylated. These groups are responsible for the anionic characteristic of fucoidans.

According to the models proposed by Cumashi et al. and Ale et al., the chemical structures of fucoidans are represented on the basis of their origin, as shown in Figure 2. For examples, in Fucales, fucoidans show L-fucopyranoside chains linked with alternating α-(1→4) and α-(1→3) glycosidic linkages. C-2 and/or C-4 (rarely at C-3) are usually substituted with sulfate ester groups (–SO$_3^-$), according to the type of glycosidic linkages [9]. Moreover, side branching was detected at C-4, alternating with sulfate groups in *F. serratus* L. in α-(1→3) L-fucopyranoside units. On the other hand, in Laminariales and Chordariales, fucoidan subunits are mainly linked by α-(1→3) glycosidic linkages. Additionally, at C-2, other sugar monomers can be detected as a side branch, whereas sulfate ester groups are common at C-4. The chemical structures may also vary within the same organism on the basis of the applied extraction methods [66].

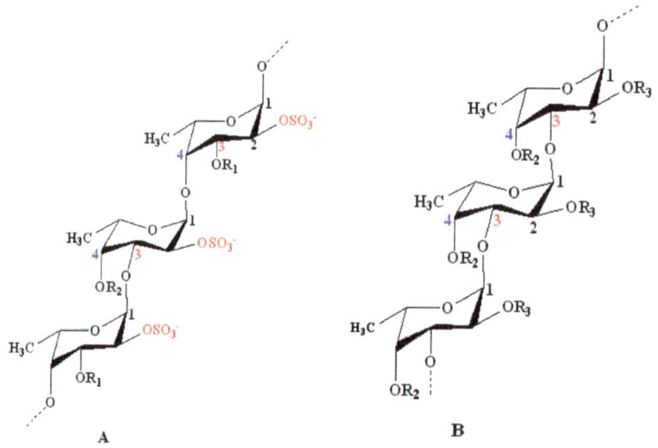

Figure 2. Structural models for the chemical structure of fucoidans derived from some species of seaweeds as proposed by Cumashi et al. and Ale et al. [35,64]. **Model A**: Model representing fucoidans from some species of Fucales. It shows repeating L-fucopyranoside units linked with alternating α-(1→4) and α-(1→3) glycosidic linkages. C-2 is always substituted with a sulfate ester group. Examples include *Fucus vesiculosus* and *Ascophyllum nodosum*: R_1 = SO$_3^-$, R_2 = H; *F. serratus* L.: R_1 = H, R_2 = side chain or SO$_3^-$; and *Fucus evanescens* C. Ag: R_1 = H, R_2 = SO$_3^-$ or H. **Model B**: Model representing some species of Laminariales and Chordariales. Both orders show a repeated α-(1→3)-linked branched L-fucopyranoside backbone at C-2. Sulfate ester groups mainly substitute C-4 and sometimes C-2. Examples include *Laminaria saccharina* (Laminariales): R_2 = OSO$_3^-$, R_3 = H alternating with OSO$_3^-$ and L-fucose; and *Cladosiphon okamuranus* (Chordariales): R_2 = OSO$_3^-$ alternating with H, R_3 = OSO$_3^-$ alternating with H and uronic acid. Other minor sugar units (e.g., mannose and galactose) and acetyl groups occur in fucoidan structures at certain unknown positions [64].

Recently, Usoltseva et al. revealed other models in Laminariales members, i.e., *Saccharina* or *Laminaria cichorioides* and *Laminaria longipes*. They detected unusual fucoidans with α-(1→3) linkages that also contain α-(1→4)- and α-(1→2)-linked fucopyranoside residues [67]. Additionally, Wang et al. showed that α-(1→4) linkages may be present in the fucoidan backbone of *Laminaria japonica* [68]. As a consequence of these complex characteristics and heterogeneity, it is always difficult to characterize the chemical structure of the whole polymer using a single technique. Spectrometric methods (e.g., Fourier-transform infrared (FT-IR), NMR and MS) are used to elucidate the structural features, especially the position of sulfate ester groups and glycosidic bonds. In addition, chromatographic methods, such as gel permeation (GPC) also known as size-exclusion chromatography (SEC), are applied for the determination of molecular-weight parameters or averages. Currently, advanced hyphenated spectrometric techniques, such as HPLC–MS/MS, are applied [69,70]. Furthermore, the application of regio- and stereoselective enzymatic degrading fucoidans isolated from marine bacteria provided new insight into the chemical structure of fucoidan, when combined with spectrometric methods [6,14]. These items are discussed in Section 6.

3. Characterization of Fucoidan Quality

3.1. Fucoidan Characteristics

3.1.1. Sugar Content

The Dubois or phenol–sulfuric acid assay is a simple acid-catalyzed condensation reaction, which is commonly employed for the determination of total sugar concentration in carbohydrates [71]. Fucoidan and 5% (w/v) aqueous phenol solutions are mixed, and then concentrated sulfuric acid is carefully added. Afterward, the sample is mixed vigorously, and the absorbance is recorded at 490 nm. The reaction mechanism is based on color development upon the dehydration of sugars to furfural derivatives with sulfuric acid. The furfural product is then condensed with phenol to produce stable colored compounds.

The Somogyi–Nelson test is also used for the determination of reducing sugars, where copper and fucoidan solutions are mixed carefully and incubated in a boiling water bath. Afterward, the arsenic molybdate reagent is added. The reaction mixture is then incubated at room temperature and analyzed at 500 nm. The mechanism is based on a redox reaction, where reducing sugars are oxidized by the weakly alkaline copper reagent to a sugar acid, while Cu^{2+} is reduced to Cu^{+}. Then, the arsenic molybdate reagent is used to regenerate Cu^{2+} ions, thereby reducing arsenic molybdate and producing a characteristic blue color [72,73].

3.1.2. Fucose Content

The Dische or cysteine–sulfuric acid assay is carried out to quantify L-fucose content in hydrolyzed fucoidan solutions [74]. The test consists of mixing the fucoidan solution with diluted sulfuric acid (1:6). Then, the reaction mixture is incubated at 100 °C for a period, and the reaction is stopped by cooling in an ice bath. Thereafter, an aqueous L-cysteine solution is added, and the absorbance is measured at two wavelengths, namely, 396 and 430 nm. According to the difference of those two measurements, the possible interference of hexoses can be excluded [75]. However, algal polyphenols may interfere to a great extent in colorimetric fucose determination. Alternatively, as fucose is a neutral sugar, it can be determined using more sensitive methods, such as HPLC and GC after derivatization [28]. Details are provided in Section 4.3 with regard to the investigation of fucoidan monomeric composition.

3.1.3. Fucoidan Content

The usual problem in the quantitative determination of fucoidan content is the absence of an appropriate standard. Commercial preparations may be insufficiently purified and may be structurally different from analytical samples. Nevertheless, on the basis of the anionic characteristic of fucoidans, thiazine dyes, such as in the toluidine blue (TB) assay according to Hahn et al. [76] and the Heparin Red® Ultra assay according to Warttinger et al. [77,78], can be applied. The TB assay is based on the formation of a charge-transfer complex between the thiazine dye and the polysaccharide [79]. It consists of mixing fucoidan-containing solutions with TB at pH 1 for better reaction sensitivity. The absorbance is then measured at 632 nm using an aqueous solution of commercially purified fucoidan as a reference standard in a concentration range of 0–2.5 g·L^{-1}. The color changes are demonstrated in Figure 3, whereby Figure 3A shows the metachromatic effect of fucoidan on the polycationic thiazine dye toluidine blue. A hypochromic effect is shown with a hypsochromic shift of the toluidine blue ultraviolet/visible light (UV/Vis) spectrum following the addition of polyanionic molecules (e.g., fucoidan). On the other hand, the Heparin Red® Ultra assay is based on the fluorescence-quenching ability of fucoidans after incubation with Heparin Red® reagent, as depicted in Figure 3C. It may be carried out using excitation and emission wavelengths of 570 and 605 nm, respectively. The reaction shows potential selectivity for fucoidan even in the presence of sodium alginate salt, as demonstrated in Figure 3D [78]. The Heparin Red® Ultra assay also demonstrates great sensitivity in a linear range of 0.0–8.0 µg·mL^{-1}. The results of such investigations indicate the relative quality of fucoidans and their degree of purity.

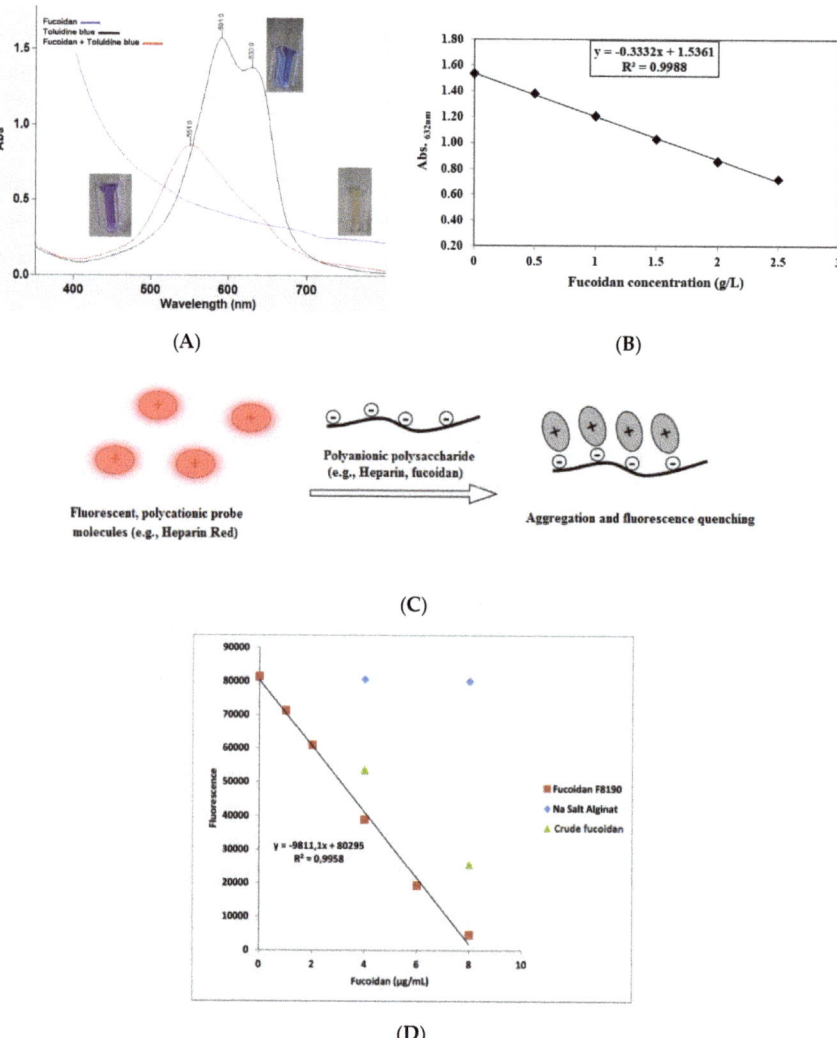

Figure 3. (**A**) Metachromatic effect of fucoidan on the polycationic thiazine dye toluidine blue (TB). A hypsochromic shift and hypochromic effect are observed after the reaction of TB with fucoidans. (**B**) Calibration curve of TB assay showing the reaction linearity in a specified fucoidan concentration, i.e., 0–2.5 g·L^{-1}. (**C**) Representation of polyanionic polysaccharide reaction with fluorescent perylene diimide molecules (e.g., Heparin Red®). The reaction electrostatically produces aggregates, followed by fluorescence quenching (modified according to [80]). (**D**) Calibration curve of Heparin Red® assay showing crude fucoidan samples deviating from the linear range of the reference sample with no interference from alginate [81]. The ultraviolet/visible light (UV/Vis) measurement was conducted using a UV/Vis spectrometer (Cary 60 UV/Vis, Agilent Technologies, USA), while the fluorescence was recorded using a spectrofluorometer (FP-8300, JASCO Deutschland GmbH, Germany).

The principle behind the reaction of fucoidans with basic or cationic dyes was successfully applied using Alcian blue stain for the detection of fucoidans and its fragments after degradation experiments with fucoidanases in carbohydrate polyacrylamide gel electrophoresis (C-PAGE) [82]. Moreover, other similar anionic polysaccharides from carrageenan could be detected using the same principle [83]. Currently, several commercial highly purified fucoidans are marketed by well-known companies, such as Sigma-Aldrich® and Marinova®, derived from *F. vesiculosus* and other brown algae species [17,84].

A more sensitive and selective electrochemical method for the detection of fucoidan was developed by Kim et al. in biological fluids and nutritional supplements. The method is based on potentiometric sensors using polyion-sensitive membrane electrodes. Examples of compounds acting as ion exchangers were tridodecyl methylammonium (TDMA) and dinonylnaphthalene sulfonate (DNNS) [17,85].

3.1.4. Sulfate Content

As developed by Dodgson and Price, sulfate content can be analyzed on the basis of barium sulfate ($BaSO_4$) precipitation after the addition of barium chloride ($BaCl_2$) in gelatin using sodium sulfate (Na_2SO_4) or potassium sulfate (K_2SO_4) [86,87]. The sulfate amount is determined by turbidimetry at 500 nm [88]. Since sulfate ester groups are susceptible to hydrolysis, turbidimetric analysis requires preliminary liberation of the sulfate groups via acid hydrolysis using 4 M HCl at 100 °C for 6 h [89] or 2 M trifluoroacetic acid (TFA) at 100 °C for 8 h [90].

Using inductively coupled plasma mass spectrometry (ICP-MS), the sulfate content of fucoidan isolated from *L. hyperborean* was determined. Sulfur contents were determined by dissolving the dried fucoidan (70 °C for 90 min) in 1 M HNO_3. The sulfation degree was determined by utilizing a mass balance equation, assuming that every sulfate group was associated with a sodium counterion [91].

3.1.5. Uronic Acid Content

A colorimetric determination of uronic acids is usually performed using *meta*-phenylphenol according to the procedures presented by Filisetti-Cozzi and Carpita [15,92] or Blumenkrantz and Asboe-Hansen [93]. The same principle can be applied with *m*-phenylphenol to form a colored condensation product, where the sugar is firstly dehydrated by heating with sulfuric acid before the addition of *m*-phenylphenol and incubation at room temperature. The absorbance is then recorded at 525 nm. A modified uronic acid carbazole reaction is sometimes also applied [84,94].

Moreover, specific HPLC techniques based on monomer derivatization were reported. They include high-performance anion-exchange chromatography (HPAEC) coupled with pulsed amperometry detection (PAD). This method is commonly known as Dionex HPAEC–PAD, i.e., implementing a Dionex ICS-2500 system equipped with CarboPac™ PA20 analytical and guard columns. It depends on the fact that uronic acids are weak acids that can be derivatized to oxyanions at alkaline pH values [95,96].

In Section 3.2.3, alginate is discussed as a potential contaminant of fucoidans, leading to an increase in uronic acid content in fucoidan products if not properly removed. Hence, the identification of uronic acids is necessary to distinguish the components of fucoidan from the components of alginic acids. The uronic acids of fucoidans mainly constitute α-D-glucuronic acid [97,98], while those in alginate constitute α-L-guluronic acid (G-block) and β-D-mannuronic acid (M-block) linked via α-(1→4) bonds [99], as shown in Figure 4. These blocks produce a characteristic NMR pattern, from which the M/G ratio can be calculated [100,101].

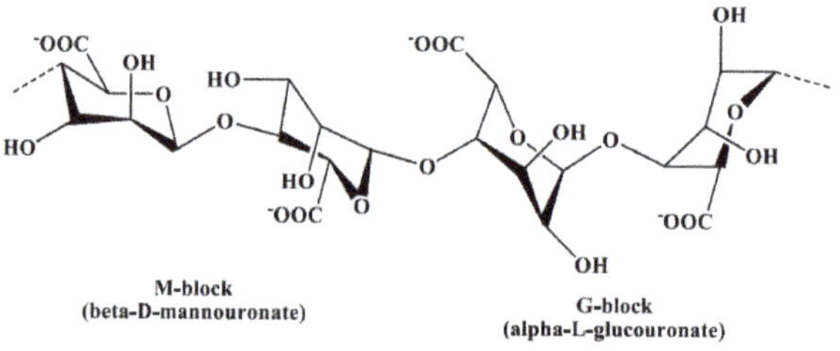

Figure 4. Chemical structure of alginate composed of α-L-guluronic acid (G-block) and β-D-mannuronic acid (M-block) linked via α-(1→4) glycosidic bonds.

3.2. Potential Coextracted Impurities

Since fucoidans are found in a highly complicated cell-wall matrix in addition to other polymers, such as cellulose, alginate, and protein, as well as polyphenols [102], several investigations should be carried out to detect and quantify such components. Moreover, other components may be also coextracted and present in crude fucoidans such as laminaran, mannitol, lipids, and pigments [59,103,104]. Hence, comprehensive downstream processes should be applied to remove all of these compounds as best as possible [54]. However, for reproducible and trusted biological activities, potential contaminants, such as proteins, alginate, laminaran, and total phenolic content should be quantified to determine the quality grade of fucoidans.

3.2.1. Protein

The Folin–phenol [105] and Bradford assays are applied to determine protein content in fucoidan products, using bovine serum albumin as a reference standard for calibration [15,106]. The Lowry and Bradford assays are based on colorimetric determination, where they produce colored solutions recorded at 750 and 595 nm, respectively, in response to protein and/or amino acids. The Folin–phenol reagent consists of phosphomolybdic–phosphotungstic acid, which is reduced to a blue-colored solution by protein in an alkaline Cu^{2+} tartrate solution [105,107], whereas the color in the Bradford assay is formed due to complex formation between the protein and the Coomassie blue G-250 dye. Under acidic conditions, the protonated red dye is transformed to an anionic blue form through a dye–protein electrostatic and hydrophobic interaction [108,109].

Both assays show variable results, due to variations in protein composition, pH, and sample concentration [107], whereby only the tyrosine, tryptophan, and cysteine amino acids can react [110]. In addition, the Lowry method is not specific enough since the results are highly affected by the presence of interfering compounds that can also chelate Cu^{2+} (e.g., nitrogenous and phenolic compounds) [110,111].

3.2.2. Phenolic Compounds

Phenolic compounds in brown algae vary structurally from simple molecules (e.g., hydroxybenzoic acid derivatives, such as gallic, phenolic, and cinnamic acids) or flavonoids (e.g., flavan-3-ol derivatives, such as epicatechin or epigallocatechin) to more complex phlorotannin polymeric structures (e.g., phlorethols, fuhalols, fucols, fucophlorethols, and eckol) [112].

As previously discussed, polyphenols are tightly noncovalently bound to fucoidans in the cell wall, which contribute along with fucoxanthin to the brown color of the crude fucoidan extract [54]. The total phenolic content can be quantified using the Folin–Ciocalteu method, especially for crude fucoidan products [113,114]. Additionally, the 2,4-dimethoxybenzaldehyde (DMBA) assay may be applied for phlorotannin content [115]. The Folin–Ciocalteu method is similar to the Folin–phenol applied for protein determination; however, the absorbance is recorded at 620 nm [114]. Nonetheless, interference from sugar monomers is common and may lead to false results. Gallic acid is commonly used as a reference standard and, therefore, the results are expressed as gallic acid equivalents [116].

3.2.3. Alginate

Precipitation of alginate by divalent ions (e.g., Ca^{2+} or Ba^{2+}) is a common pretreatment step during fucoidan extraction [35,117]. An acidic medium, i.e., below the pKa of carboxylic groups, also helps in the precipitation of alginate as alginic acid [118]. Therefore, for the efficient removal of alginate during fucoidan extraction, both conditions are usually applied [38]. Nevertheless, traces of alginate are frequently detected in crude fucoidan extracts from brown algae [96]. Even the application of enzyme-assisted extraction employing an alginate lyase from Sphingomonas sp. (SALy) resulted in the crude fucoidan product containing substantial alginate, thus requiring a further purification step [119,120].

Since alginate is composed of β-D-mannuronic (M-block) and α-L-guluronic (G-block) acids as building blocks [121], it may interfere with the determination of uronic acids during fucoidan chemical characterization. Therefore, alginate can instead be determined as a function of the metachromatic change induced upon binding to cationic dyes, such as 1,9-dimethyl methylene blue (DMMB) [122], or using the TB assay. However, due to the different pKa values of the sulfate ester group in fucoidans and carboxylic group in alginate, the different measurements at pH 1.0 and pH 7.0 can be used to quantify alginate content, where, at pH 1.0, fucoidan is ionized and interacts only with TB, while, at pH 7.0, both are ionized and induce color changes [76]. Dionex HPAEC–PAD can potentially be applied for the specific determination of alginate building blocks, thereby excluding interference from the uronic acids of fucoidans [96].

3.2.4. Laminaran

Laminaran is a neutral water-soluble glucan found in brown algae functioning as a reserve food [103,104]. Its presence in crude fucoidan preparations is highly possible, owing to its precipitation with fucoidan after the addition of high volumes of ethanol (e.g., 70% v/v). Enzyme-assisted fucoidan extraction conducted using commercial enzyme mixtures, i.e., carbohydrase mixtures, can target the degradation of laminarin, leading to its removal [119]. Fortunately, laminarin cannot interact with cationic dyes during the determination of fucoidan content using TB and perylene diimide derivative (PDD) assays. The same principle is applied in the purification of fucoidan using anion exchange chromatography (e.g., DEAE–cellulose) in the presence of laminaran [54]. Therefore, laminaran is easily separated from fucoidan after the first step of purification.

4. Physicochemical Characteristics and Structural Features

4.1. Elemental Analysis

Elemental analysis is very important for comparative studies, which may be used to compare different fucoidan fractions as a tool to justify the purification process. A decrease in nitrogen content (%) and an increase in sulfur content (%) are critical elements for fucoidan quality, which may be interpreted as the removal/absence of proteins and an improvement in the sugar monomer–sulfate ratio, respectively [38,117,123]. Hence, protein content can be estimated by multiplying the percentage of N by 6.25. Similarly, the content of sulfate groups (as $-SO_3^-Na^+$) can be calculated on the basis of the percentage of S [21,44,113]. Moreover, for the determination of sulfation degree in fucoidans, a number of equations were developed, as shown in Equations (1) and (2) [44].

$$NSS = \frac{C\%/12}{S\%/32} / 6 \qquad (1)$$

$$\text{Degree of sulfation} = 1/NSS \qquad (2)$$

where NSS is the number of sulfate esters per monosaccharide, 12 and 32 are the atomic weights of carbon and sulfur, respectively, and 6 is the number of carbon atoms in a sugar monomer assuming that all monomers in the polymer are hexoses.

4.2. Molecular Weight Averages

The molar mass, molecular size distribution, and chain conformation of polymers are among the important parameters affecting fucoidan applications. The molecular size of fucoidans ranges from 13 to 950 kDa. They can be classified, according to their molecular weight, into three classes: low-molecular-weight fucoidans (LMWFs) with a polymer size <10 kDa, medium-molecular-weight fucoidans (MMWFs) (10–10,000 kDa), and high-molecular-weight fucoidans (HMWFs) (>10,000 kDa) [124]. Chromatographic methods, i.e., gel filtration and anion exchange, are mostly used, whether separately or in combination, for the molecular mass determination of fucoidans. Examples of columns used include diethylaminoethyl (DEAE) Sepharose, Zorbax GF-450, OH-PAK SB-806 HQ, Sephadex G-50, Sephadex G-100, DEAE Toyopearl 650 M, Superdex 75 HR, and DEAE cellulose. The column should be firstly calibrated with polysaccharides of definite molecular sizes such as dextrans, pullulans, carrageenans, or heparins. However, the results show a range of molecular sizes instead of an exact value. Moreover, a polyacrylamide gel system, i.e., C-PAGE, can be used, where the polysaccharides are stained with a combination of Alcian blue and silver nitrate. C-PAGE can only be used to separate LMWFs in contrast to native unhydrolyzed polymers which are retained at the top of the gel [14,38,82].

Recently, with the aid of gel permeation or size-exclusion chromatography (GPC/SEC) coupled with multi-angle static light scattering, quasi-elastic light scattering and refractive index detection system (i.e., SEC–MALS–QELS–RI analysis), important structural characteristics could be estimated, in the context of Mw, Mn, Mp, PDI, and size (root-mean-square (rms) radius, R_h) [125]. The number-average molecular weight or molar mass (Mn) indicates the average molecular weight of all polymer chains, while the weight-average molecular weight (Mw) considers the molecular weight of chains contributing to the molecular weight average. On the other hand, the molecular weight of the highest peak (Mp) determines the mode of molecular weight distribution. In addition, the polydispersity index (PDI) measures the broadness of the molecular weight distribution of polymers, where a larger PDI denotes a broader molecular weight distribution [126]. Equations (3)–(5) are applied for measurement of the above parameters, and they are now an integral part of many applications or as as add-on used in GPC/SEC techniques, such as the GPC Extension from Clarity Chromatography Station (starting from version 2.3).

$$Mn = \frac{\sum N_i M_i}{\sum N_i} \quad (3)$$

$$Mw = \frac{\sum N_i M_i^2}{\sum N_i M_i} \quad (4)$$

$$PDI = \frac{Mw}{Mn} \quad (5)$$

where Mi is the molecular weight of a chain, and Ni is the number of chains of that molecular weight.

Natural polymers such as proteins are usually monodisperse, with a PDI of approximately 1. However, polysaccharides are quite different, exhibiting PDIs greater than 1 [127]. The production of fucoidans with different molecular weight averages is possible through fractionation methods, such as via precipitation with increasing volumes of acetone, ethanol, or isopropanol, filtration membranes of a defined molecular weight cutoff (MWCO) [84], and gradient elution using NaCl during the elution step of ion-exchange chromatography purification, where a higher NaCl molarity elutes fucoidan fractions characterized by higher polarity, i.e., a higher sulfation degree and higher molecular weight [38,128].

4.3. Monomeric Composition

The detection of sugar monomers in polysaccharides is conducted after the step of acid hydrolysis [129], e.g., heating at 90–121 °C for 2–4 h with 4 M trifluoroacetic acid (TFA), applied for the isolation of sulfated galactofucan from the sporophyll of *U. pinnatifida* [130], 2 M HCl, applied for the commercial fucoidans of *F. vesiculosus* [88], and the two-step sulfuric acid treatment for 60 min with 72% H_2SO_4 at 30 °C followed by hydrolysis for 60 min in 4% H_2SO_4, applied for the crude fucoidans isolated from *Saccharina latissima* and *Laminaria digitata* [129,131]. Afterward, the hydrolysate is neutralized, filtered, and subjected to a liquid chromatography (HPLC) step, using different reference sugar monomers, such as arabinose, fructose, fucose, galactose, glucose, glucosamine, mannose, and xylose. The lead form Aminex HPX-87P column (Bio-Rad, Hercules, CA, USA) is widely used for carbohydrate analysis, operated at 80 °C and coupled with a refractive index (RI) detector [97,131]. A MetaCarb 67H column (Agilent Technologies, Santa Clara, CA, USA) operated at 45 °C may also be applied [132].

Moreover, the analysis of neutral and amino-containing monomers can be achieved via derivatization. The conversion of monomers to alditol acetate derivatives is more reliable, with subsequent separation using organic volatile solvents (e.g., dichloromethane), followed by analysis performed using GC/ESI-MS [8,133]. The reaction cascade consists of an initial reduction in alkaline medium followed by acetylation using acetic anhydride in the presence of 1-methylimidazole [84].

Recently, a comprehensive and fast method was developed by Rühmann et al. as function of monomer derivatization by 1-phenyl-3-methyl-5-pyrazolone (PMP) using liquid chromatography equipped with different detectors, such as UV and MS detectors or both (LC–UV–ESI-MS/MS) [134], which was successfully applied for the characterization of fucoidan isolated from *F. vesiculosus* [38].

4.4. Glycosidic Linkage

Methylation using the CH_3I/NaOH method for deacetylated and desulfated fucoidans, followed by hydrolysis, reduction, and acetylation as before, enables sugar derivatization to alditol acetates that can be determined using GC/MS [135]. The scheme of reactions is summarized in Figure 5. Complete methylation can be confirmed upon disappearance of the OH band (3200–3700 cm^{-1}) in the IR spectrum [136]. This method is commonly performed to determine glycosidic linkages and, consequently, branching sites in polysaccharides.

The desulfation step can be carried out enzymatically using sulfoesterase or chemically. Despite the regioselectivity of the enzymatic reaction, chemical desulfation is frequently conducted [60]. The chemical reaction involves a solvolytic desulfation, which consists of firstly passing the fucoidan solution through a cationic exchange resin, i.e., Amberlite CG-120 column (H^+-form). Then, the main desulfation step is conducted via incubation of the pyridinium salt of fucoidan in dimethyl sulfoxide (DMSO) at 100 °C for 3–10 h [137–139]. In addition, the incubation of equal volumes of desulfated fucoidan with concentrated aqueous NH_3 overnight at elevated temperature, i.e., 37 °C, resulted in the deacetylation of fucoidans [33,139].

Alternatively, periodate oxidation/Smith degradation can be applied for the analysis of fucoidan glycosidic linkages. The fucoidan is oxidized with $NaOI_4$ and then reduced with $NaBH_4$. Afterward, the product is hydrolyzed using acid and analyzed via GC [140,141]. However, it is worth mentioning that the (1→3) linkages between fucose residues and the high degree of substitution of hydroxyls make fucoidans resistant to Smith degradation [33]. The analysis of glycosidic linkages can also be achieved using NMR, as further discussed in Section 5.2.

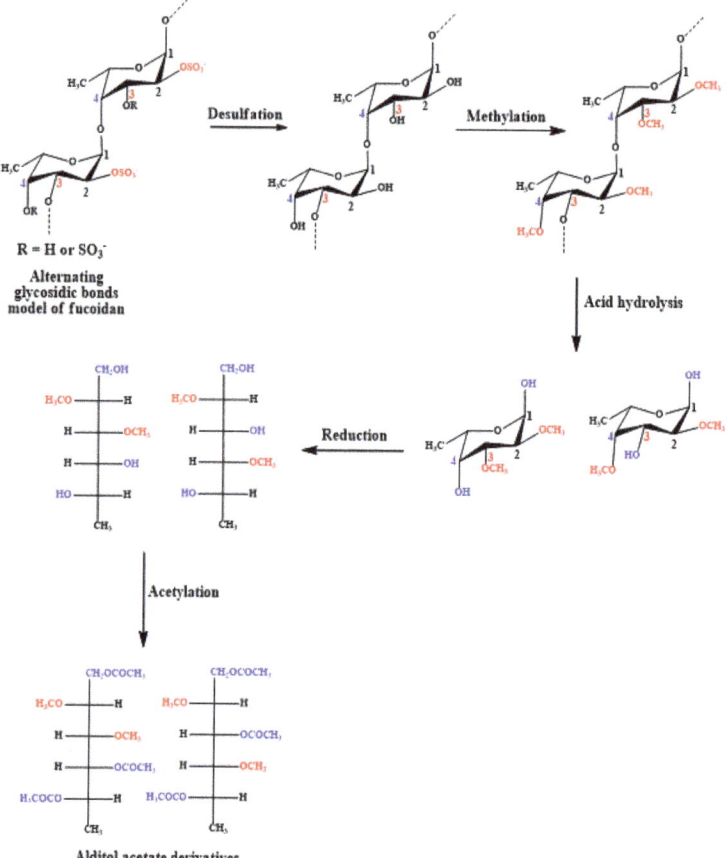

Figure 5. Derivatization of desulfated and deacetylated fucoidan monomers to volatile alditol acetates, which may be subsequently analyzed using GC/MS.

4.5. Others

Other characteristics, such as solubility and optical activity, should also be investigated [38]. It is well known that fucoidans are polar compounds and freely soluble in water. Hence, turbidity may indicate the presence of impurities, such as proteins and the Ca salt of alginate. In addition to water, fucoidans are highly soluble in solvents with high dielectric constants [59], as well as with acidic and alkaline pH values. However, to guard against polymer hydrolysis, their stability was investigated, showing that solutions prepared in a pH range from 5.8 to 9.5 were stable [142]. In contrast, fucoidans are practically insoluble in ethanol or cetyltrimethylammonium bromide (CTAB) and, therefore, both solvents can be applied for fucoidan precipitation and isolation form algal crude extracts [37,54].

Due to the predominance of L-(−)fucose in fucoidan backbones, fucoidans are optically active molecules, with fucoidan solutions showing a levorotatory characteristic when exposed to plane-polarized light [6]. Moreover, researches of fucoidan chemistry always try to link its chemical properties, i.e., molecular weight, polydispersity, branching, sulfate content, and uronic acid content, with its physical rheological properties [133]. Fucoidan aqueous solutions generally possess low viscosity. Nevertheless, the degree of viscosity mainly depends on the temperature, pH, molecular weight, concentration, sulfate content, and degree of branching [142–145]. One example is fucoidan isolated from *L. japonica*, which has a molecular weight of 10.5 kDa and a high content of fucose and sulfate. Increasing the fucoidan concentration resulted in an increase in solution viscosity. Meanwhile, increasing fucoidan concentration led to a decrease in solution pH [146]. In addition, the aqueous solutions of fucoidan isolated from *L. religiosa* and *U. pinnatifida* showed low viscosity, characterized by a pseudoplastic rheological behavior [144]. Furthermore, Monsur et al. investigated several fucoidan fractions isolated from *Turbinaria turbinata*. They were Newtonian fluids regarding the direct relationship between shear stress and shear rate, as well as in the context of solution concentration. Concurrently, they found that the fraction with the highest molecular weight, sulfate content, and polydispersity exhibited the lowest viscosity [133].

Furthermore, the type of algal species and the presence of ions can affect the viscosity of fucoidan solutions [146]. The highest viscosity of a fucoidan aqueous solution was reported for fucoidan isolated from *F. vesiculosus* algae species [147], while the viscosity of fucoidan solutions obtained from *Cladosiphom okamuranus* increased linearly with increasing polymer concentration up to 2% (w/v), as well as after the addition of salts such as NaCl or $CaCl_2$. However, viscosity may reflect the amount of contaminating alginate left in the fucoidan extract, since the viscosity of alginate is very high [148,149].

Interestingly, fucoidans differ from other polysaccharides, as they do not possess the ability to form a gel alone, where mixing with other positively charged polymers is needed to produce gel, owing to ionic interactions [145,146]. The thermal degradation of fucoidans, including their melting points, was studied [38,133]. For further information on other physical parameters such as the consistency, flow behavior, and rheological properties of fucoidans, as well as the ways in which these properties affect fucoidan applications in the pharmaceutical industry, including drug delivery, interested readers may refer to [146,150], where the design of fucoidan-based nanosystems and other nanocarriers encapsulating fucoidan was shown to depend on the physiochemical behavior of fucoidans, e.g., physical appearance, chemical features, molecular weight (Mw), solubility, pH, and melting point [146,151].

5. Spectrometry and Chemical Characterization

Due to their complex chemical structures, several spectrometric methods (e.g., FT-IR, NMR, and MS) have been used to elucidate the structural features of fucoidans, including the position of sulfate groups and glycosidic bonds, and the molecular weight. Furthermore, the application of regio- and stereoselective fucoidan-degrading enzymes isolated from marine bacteria provided new insights into the chemical structure of fucoidan [43,74].

5.1. FT-IR

The preliminary identification of fucoidan functional groups is always performed by scanning samples using FT-IR between 400 and 4000 cm^{-1} [152,153]. Fucoidans show characteristic and typical IR bands for their functional structural building blocks (e.g., the O–H group of monomeric monosaccharides, C–H, asymmetric stretching of S=O and C–O–S of sulfate ester groups, and O–C–O and C–O–C of glycosidic and intramolecular linkages at 3421, 2940, 1221, 827, 1634, and 1010 cm^{-1}, respectively) [123,153]. Moreover, peaks between 1650 and 1800 cm^{-1} for C=O groups indicate whether fucoidans are acetylated and contain uronic acid residues [133,154,155].

Other important information may be extracted from the IR spectra, such as the axial position of the sulfate ester group at C-4 [21,156]. A complex pattern between 840 and 800 cm^{-1} is commonly shown, indicating the different substitutions of sulfate ester groups at the most abundant C-4 and C-2/C-3 positions, showing a peak and a shoulder for the axial 4-position of C–O–S and equatorial 2/3-position of C–O–S, respectively [157]. To exclude the bending vibration of the C–H group of sugars, IR results should be compared with NMR data after sulfate ester alkali hydrolysis and methylation analysis to determine the exact sulfate position [6,158]. In addition, IR bands at 622 and 583 cm^{-1} result from the asymmetric and symmetric O=S=O deformation of sulfates [159].

Anomeric C–H deformation may be also identified in IR spectra, where the β-anomeric type is represented by a small peak at 890 cm^{-1}, while the α-analogue appears theoretically at around 860 cm^{-1}, which may be overlapped by stronger sulfate bands in the same range [8,140].

However, the structural information provided in FT-IR spectra may not be very valuable, especially for the determination of secondary sulfate ester groups. Signals describing the positions of secondary sulfate groups depend on the real conformation of monosaccharide units, which may be considerably distorted in branched and heavily sulfated chains by neighboring substituents [160].

5.2. NMR

Previously published articles have shown the valuable information presented by NMR for structural elucidation and the numerous structural features of different fucoidans from different origins. One- and two-dimensional (1D and 2D) NMR experiments of fucoidans, including ^{1}H- and ^{13}C-NMR, demonstrate relatively well-interpreted spectra related to the sulfation pattern and glycosidic linkages. Two approaches are usually applied in NMR experiments for obtaining valuable structure information, i.e., careful fractionation of crude fucoidan and/or specific chemical modification, such as desulfation. Such treatments are aimed at producing regular or masked regular backbones, resulting in NMR spectra that can be interpreted [161]. An example of successful fractionation of a crude algal fucoidan to obtain a fucoidan fraction having regular structure, which was elucidated using NMR spectra, was described by Bilan et al., where they obtained a regular fucoidan from the brown seaweed *Fucus distichus* [162]. Fractionation is commonly conducted during the elution of purified fucoidan from the anion-exchange column via the salting out mechanism using different molar concentrations of NaCl, i.e., gradient elution. A relationship was identified between NaCl concentration and the molecular weight and sulfate content of the obtained fucoidan fraction, thereby facilitating the structural elucidation of various relatively simple fractions [38,119]. Moreover, fractionation may also carried out through dialysis membranes of different molecular weight cutoff (MWCO), such as the fractionation of crude fucoidan into LMWFs and HMWFs [28]. For further information on such treatments, interested readers can refer to the recently published review discussing the different downstream processes applied in fucoidan production by Zayed et al. [54]. The production of oligomer fractions or fragments is considered a potential tool for polymer simplification, i.e., enzymatic depolymerization, prior to NMR experiments. This step can be performed by enzymatic treatment of the native fucoidan with fucoidan-degrading enzymes, i.e., fucoidanases [161,163]. In addition, the application of fucoidanases on desulfated or deacetylated fucoidans may result in more valuable structural information [34]. The desulfation and deacetylation of fucoidans is applied to produce simpler compounds, allowing a comparison of the chemical shifts (δ, ppm) with standard sugars or the native polymer, especially because sulfate ester groups cause deshielding of neighboring protons and carbons, consequently appearing downfield in the NMR spectra [8,139,163,164]. Some examples of fucoidans or sulfated fucans elucidated by 1D and 2D NMR are discussed below in detail.

5.2.1. 1D NMR

Fucoidans from *F. vesiculosus* and *Ascophyllum nodosum* (Fucales) are the simplest form of algal fucoidans. They are polymers of alternating α-(1→3)- and α-(1→4)-linked L-fucopyranoside repeating units ([→4)-α-L-Fucp-(1→3)-α-L-Fucp-(1→4)-α-L-Fucp-(1→3)-α-L-Fucp(1→]) [35,43], where some structural features can be elucidated from NMR spectra. In the ^{1}H-NMR spectrum, singlet peaks of the shielded protons at around 1.2 ppm are assigned to the –CH$_3$ groups (H-6) of the L-fucose monomer. Other peaks appearing slightly shifted between 3.8 and 4.5 ppm can be assigned to H-2, H-3, H-4, and H-5. Moreover, the anomeric proton H-1 can be observed deshielded at 5.2 ppm, confirming the α-linked sugar monomers. The presence of other sugars such as galactose, mannose, and xylose can be deduced from signals in regions lower than 3.7 ppm, as reported in the fucoidan isolated from *S. polycystum* [165]. The NMR analysis of these fucoidans was recorded for their native forms, which produced low-resolution spectra.

Additionally, in the ^{13}C-NMR spectrum of a fucoidan fraction isolated from *S. mcclurei* (Fucales) of a galactofucan nature, major intense peaks could be easily elucidated. They included the –CH$_3$ group (C-6) appearing in an upfield region, i.e., 15–17 ppm, and the anomeric carbon at C-1 in a downfield region, i.e., 96–100 ppm. Other peaks showed several degrees of multiplicity owing to the presence of various glycosidic linkages and sulfation patterns [138]. These peaks are typical for an α-fucopyranoside backbone [166]. Acetylated moieties in the fucoidan structure can also be easily detected in ^{13}C-NMR spectra, where methyl (–CH$_3$) and carbonyl (C=O) groups of the O-acetyl group appear in upfield (i.e., 21–22 ppm) and downfield (i.e., 170–180 ppm) regions, respectively. Examples include fucoidans isolated from *S. japonica* and *U. pinnatifida* [167,168].

Furthermore, the effect of the sulfate ester group (–OSO$_3^-$) on the chemical shifts (δ, ppm) of attached C and accompanied Hs is among the features that can be revealed by NMR. This helps the elucidation of sulfation pattern with fucoidan backbones. An example includes the structural characterization of fucoidans isolated from *S. myriocystum*. The presence of a downfield signal at 4.84 ppm in ^{1}H-NMR indicated a sulfate group at position C-4, while the chemical shifts of other hydrogen atoms C-2, C-3, and C-5 appeared at 4.80, 4.22, and 4.77, respectively. These data were confirmed in the ^{13}C-NMR spectrum, where C-4 appeared at 81.33 ppm, while the C-3 position was confirmed by the signal at 76.39 ppm [169]. Similarly, *Nemacystus decipiens* fucoidan showed sulfation substitution at C-4 and, consequently, H-4 appeared more deshielded at 4.9 ppm than the other protons [170]. Furthermore, fucoidan, i.e., xylogalactofucan, isolated from *Sphacelaria indica*, showed 4-O-sulfated residues at C-4 according to the presence of a peak in the ^{1}H-NMR spectrum at 4.4 ppm, which was assigned to H-4 and confirmed by IR analysis [171]. In other cases, the sulfation pattern was demonstrated and confirmed at mainly C-2 and partially C-4 in fucoidan isolated from *F. evanescens* C.Ag by NMR data [166]. However, other studies preferred analyzing desulfated and deacetylated fucoidan residues for simpler and more easily interpreted spectra [172].

The main L-fucopyranose backbone of fucoidan isolated from *S. binderi* was determined by comparing the ^{1}H-NMR and attached proton test (APT) NMR spectra with commercial food-grade fucoidan and an α-L-fucose standard. The positions of the sulfate groups were determined through the difference in proton and ^{13}C-NMR chemical shifts with respect to the α-L-fucose standard. The downfield proton and C chemical shifts at H-2 (0.90 ppm difference) and C-2 (14.97 ppm difference) compared with the peaks of α-L-fucose were due to the presence of a sulfate group at C-2 [173].

5.2.2. 2D NMR

Homonuclear (e.g., correlation spectroscopy (COSY), total correlated spectroscopy (TOCSY), nuclear Overhauser effect spectroscopy (NOESY), and rotating frame Overhauser effect spectroscopy (ROESY)) and heteronuclear (e.g., heteronuclear multiple bond correlation (HMBC) and heteronuclear single quantum coherence (HSCQ)) 2d NMR techniques have been used to further reveal the potential structural secrets of numerous fucoidans (e.g., *F. serratus*, *S. latissimi*, *Chorda filum*, and *F. evanescens*) [139,167,172,174].

It is valuable to study the desulfated product of native fucoidans to identify the glycosidic linkages of their backbone, as in the case of fucan sulfate isolated from the *Holothuria albiventer* sea cucumber [174]. The correlation between H-1 and H-3 of polymer residues was identified in the ROESY spectrum, confirming the presence of (1→3) linkages. Furthermore, the sequences of the repeating units were also determined as a function of the long-range scalar HMBC correlations. For estimation of the configurations at the glycosidic linkages, the direct coupling constant ($^1J_{C-H}$) of C-1 for each monosaccharide residue was also obtained from the 2D ^{13}C/^{1}H HMBC spectrum. The large values of 170–175 Hz for these fucose residues indicated that the protons are equatorially positioned [175]. Moreover, taking account of the vicinal coupling constant ($^3J_{1H-2H}$) of 3 Hz for fucose residues, the configuration at C-1 of these residues was determined as the α-form [174].

Other highly regular homogeneous sulfated fucans were isolated from sea cucumbers *Holothuria fuscopunctata*, *Thelenota ananas*, and *Stichopus horrens*. Their glycosidic linkage sequences were obtained from the selected ROESY and HMBC cross-signals. The correlation between H-1 and H-4 of both H. fuscopunctata and T. ananas fucan sulfates was identified in the ROESY and HMBC spectra, whereas, for the S. horrens fucan sulfate, correlation between H-1 and H-3 was observed, confirming the presence of α-(1→4) glycosidic bonds in both H. fuscopunctata and T. ananas fucan sulfates. The structural sequences of the three fucoidans from H. fuscopunctata, T. ananas, and S. horrens were →4-α-L-Fucp-(3SO$_3^-$)-1→, →4-α-L-Fucp-(2SO$_3^-$)-1→, and →3-α-L-Fucp-(2SO$_3^-$)-1→, respectively [176].

5.3. Mass Spectrometry

Mass spectrometry (MS) is widely used to provide valuable structural information, especially if the fucoidans vary in terms of their glycosidic linkages and/or sulfation patterns [138]. However, it is difficult to be applied to fucoidans with high molecular weights or a high degree of sulfation [163], since depolymerization or autohydrolysis of the polymer should firstly be carried out [177,178]. In addition, the labile nature of sulfate ester groups in high-molecular-weight fucoidans results in the polymers exhibiting desulfation rather than ionization [179]. Thus, the ions generated from desulfation dominate the mass spectra, limiting the obtained structural data of native fucoidans [125,180].

Therefore, prior to the mass spectrometric measurement, pretreatments are applied, including fucoidan depolymerization, leading to the generation of oligomers. In addition, structural modifications, including desulfation and deacetylation, are applied. Such pretreatments result in more easily interpreted spectra compared to the native high-molecular-weight sulfated forms. The polymer can be chemically depolymerized via partial acid hydrolysis using 0.2 N TFA at 60 °C or 0.75 mM H$_2$SO$_4$ at 60 °C following the solvolytic desulfation step [179]. In contrast with autohydrolysis, enzymatic depolymerization by fucoidanses was reported, albeit not widely [181]. Nevertheless, the role of fucoidan-degrading enzymes or fucoidanses is discussed in Section 6 regarding their enzymatic modifications of fucoidans as a potential prerequisite for conducting spectrometric analysis.

The analysis of oligomers can be performed using negative ion tandem electrospray ionization (ESI-MS) and matrix-assisted laser desorption/ionization (MALDI-TOF) mass spectrometers [135]. The reasonable interpretation of fragmentation patterns can reveal many structural features in the produced oligomers useful in understanding the structure of the whole polymer. The MALDI-TOF analyzer is more convenient for the analysis of fucoidan fragments, i.e., fucooligosaccharides, adding more sensitivity and accuracy with respect to classical MS and NMR methods which detect minor constituents, as in the case of fucoidan isolated from F. evanescens [179,182]. The systematic nomenclature developed by Domon et al. is still approved for carbohydrate fragmentations in the MS/MS spectra of glycoconjugates [183].

Anastyuk et al. reported an optimization protocol for the application of tandem MS techniques, including ESI-MS and MALDI-TOF-MS in the structural elucidation of fucoidans isolated from different brown algal species. The protocol also reported the common fragments of S. cichorioides fucoidan detected in MS spectra using both techniques in a comparative approach following autohydrolysis. Fragment ions at m/z 97 and 225 were always detected, representing the sulfate anion and [FucSO$_3$–H$_2$O], respectively. In addition, the m/z peaks at 243.02 and 389.08 corresponded to the [FucSO$_3$]$^-$ and [Fuc$_2$SO$_3$]$^-$ fragment ions [179]. However, other characteristic fragments were detected at different m/z, due to differences related to ionization mode, including the inclusion of Na with the produced fragments, i.e., [Fuc$_3$(SO$_3$)$_3$]$^{3-}$ and [Fuc$_3$(SO$_3$Na)$_3$–Na]$^-$ at m/z 231.01 and 739.1 in ESI-MS and MALDI-TOF-MS spectra, respectively. The interpretation of such spectra confirmed the presence of 3-linked 2,4-disulfated α-L-fucan as the main backbone of S. cichorioides and F. evanescens fucoidans [179]. Cuong et al. elucidated the chemical structure of Sargassum henslowianum on the basis of MS data. The ESI-MS results demonstrated a major signal at m/z 243 corresponding to [M − H]$^-$ of the monosulfated fucose [FucSO$_3$]$^-$ ion. Other signals indicated α-(1→3)-linked L-fucopyranose as the fucoidan backbone, whereas the sulfate positions varied, but were mostly located at positions C-2 (m/z 139), C-3 (m/z 169), and C-4 (m/z 183) of the fucose residues. These results depicted the sulfation pattern of this fucoidan to be mostly at C-2 and C-4 and sometimes at the C-3 position of fucose residues [90], according to the previous findings of Tissot et al. [184]. They showed that the three isomers have different fragmentation patterns. While the 3-O-sulfated fucose lost a hydrogenosulfate anion, the other isomers, i.e., 2-O-, and 4-O-sulfated fucose, exhibited cross-ring fragmentation, producing ^{0,2}X and ^{0,2}A daughter ions, respectively [184].

Sample preparation is also important, whereby the sample should be mixed with 0.5 M 2,5-dihydroxy benzoic acid (DHB) in MeOH for positive-ion experiments or 0.5 M arabinoosazone matrix for negative-ion experiments in acetone. The negative-ion experiment requires a further 10-fold dilution of the sample in water [185].

Galmero et al. recently established a new fast method for carbohydrate glycosidic linkage determination. The developed method employed ultrahigh-performance liquid chromatography coupled with triple-quadrupole mass spectrometry (UHPLC/QqQ-MS) analysis performed in multiple reaction monitoring (MRM) mode, using a library of 22 glycosidic linkages built from commercial oligosaccharide standards. Permethylation and hydrolysis conditions alongside LC–MS/MS parameters were optimized, resulting in a workflow requiring only 50 µg of substrate for analysis [91]. This method can be used in the future for the determination of fucoidan glycosidic linkages.

6. Role of Fucoidan-Degrading Enzymes in Structural Elucidation

Fucoidan-degrading enzymes can be applied for the production of chemically defined bioactive oligosaccharides by hydrolyzing the sulfated fucans and fucoidans [14,186,187]. They include fucoidanases and sulfatases, which play very critical roles in the structural elucidation of fucoidan macromolecules in combination with spectrometric methods [188–190]. They are characterized using mild conditions, as a function of regio- and stereoselectivity, to determine the exact pattern of sulfation and glycosidic linkages compared with toxic (e.g., pyridine used in solvolytic desulfation), nonselective, and tedious chemical or physical modifications [139,167,191,192]. Moreover, fucoidanases preserve the sulfation pattern, which is among the major factors implicated in various biological activities [130]. Such enzymes are mainly isolated from symbionts (e.g., Proteobacteria and Bacteroidetes) associated with brown algae or marine invertebrates [193]. Interestingly, Ohshiro et al. detected both activities, i.e., fucoidan desulfation and depolymerization, using degrading enzymes isolated from the *Flavobacterium* sp. F-31. These enzymes worked on the fucoidan isolated from *Cladosiphon okamuranus* as a carbon source. Nevertheless, the desulfation activity of such enzymes was notably detected following the enzymatic degradation step of native fucoidan, i.e., depolymerized fractions [194].

Fucoidanases were first described in 1967 by Thanassi and Nakada after their isolation from the hepatopancreas *Haliotus* sp. [34,195]. They are among glycosidases (EC3.2.1.-GH 107) that catalyze the hydrolysis of glycosidic bonds between sulfated fucose residues in fucoidans [9,195]. On the basis of their mode of action, they were previously classified according to the types of glycosidic linkages they act on and further subclassified as *endo-* or *exo-*hydrolyases. Therefore, they were recently classified as *endo-*fucoidanases or α-L-fucoidan endohydrolases (EC3.2.1.44 or EC3.2.1.211 and EC3.2.1.212), as defined in Expasy, where EC 3.2.1.211 is believed to cleave *endo-*α-(1→3) L-fucoside linkages, while EC 3.2.1.212 likely cleaves α-(1→4) L-fucoside linkages, in addition to the *exo-*type, including EC 3.2.1.B47, without affecting the sulfate ester groups in the fucoidan backbone. In contrast, there are fucosidases which catalyze the cleavage of nonsulfated fucose residues from other fucose-containing compounds [195,196]. Moreover, fucoglucoronnomannan lyases were first shown to cleave linkages between mannose and glucuronic acids in a lyase manner by Takayama et al. in 2002 [197] and Sakai et al. in 2003 [198]. Later, they were analyzed on different fucoidan substrates by Cao et al. in 2018 [9] and suggested to cleave α-(1→4) linkages. They include the *endo-*fucoglucuronomannan lyases FdlA (GenBank accession number: AAO00510.1) and FdlB (GenBank accession number: AAO00511.1) [9].

In contrast, not many sequences of sulfatases acting on fucoidans have yet been found [199], as fucoidan sulfatases or sulfoesterases have not yet been well explored. Scarce studies have involved their putative mechanisms in the investigation of fucoidan sulfation pattern. They include enzymes isolated from the marine bacterium *Wenyingzhuangia fucanilytica* named SWF1 (GenBank accession number: WP_068825883.1) and SWF4 (GenBank accession number: WP_068828765.1) belonging to the family of formylglycine-dependent enzymes (SulfAtlas), i.e., *exo*-2O- and -3O-fucoidan sulfatase) [190] and *Pecten maximus*, i.e., 2O- fucoidan sulfatase [137].

Marine bacteria and mollusks have been reported to be the major sources of fucoidanases [9]. Among frequently used fucoidanases is FcnA (GenBank accession number: CAI47003.1) and its C-terminal truncated version named FcnA2. FcnA was produced by recombinant DNA technology via cloning its encoding gene from the marine bacterium *Mariniflexile fucanivorans* SW5T. FcnA2 showed *endo* α-(1→4) cleavage activity on *Pelvetia canaliculate* fucoidan [200]. Hence, the recent production of modified stabilized fucoidanases, i.e., FcnA2, via C-terminal target truncation helped the enzymatic production of more defined fucoidan fractions from different fucoidans [9]. In addition, Fda1 (GenBank accession number: AAO00508.1) and Fda2 (GenBank accession number: AAO00509.1) produced by *Alteromonas* sp. SN-1009 were α-(1→3)-specific, catalyzing the cleavage of the fucoidan isolated from *Kjellmaniella crassifolia* or *Saccharina sculpera* [197]. Moreover, the marine bacterium *Formosa algae* (KMM 3553T) produced FFA1 (GenBank accession number: WP_057784217.1) and FFA2 (GenBank accession number: WP_057784219.1). They demonstrated *endo* α-(1→4) cleavage activity on fucoidan isolated from *F. evanescens* [161]. FcnA, Fda1, Fda2, FFA1, and FFA2 all belong to the glycoside hydrolase family GH107 in CAZy [16,196,201]. Recently, a novel *endo*-fucoidanse was characterized and recognized as the first member of the GH168 family in CAZy. It was isolated from the marine bacterium *W. fucanilytica* CZ1127^T and encoded by the gene *funA*. Heterologous expression of the gene resulted in the production of FunA that specifically cleaved the α-(1→3) glycosidic linkage between the 2-O-sulfated and nonsulfated fucose residues of the sea cucumber *Isostichopus badionotus* sulfated fucan [202].

In the last few years, several sulfated fucan hydrolases were isolated. However, most studies were aimed at characterizing enzyme specificity and decreasing the molecular weight of fucoidans for modification of their activities and easy handling, whereas only few studies produced fragments which were structurally defined by spectrometric analysis. Examples include fucoidanases isolated from *Luteolibacter Algae* H18 and *Flavibacterium* sp. F-31 catalyzing the hydrolysis of *C. okamuranus* fucoidans [194,203,204], the gut contents of the sea cucumber *Sticopus japonicus* (Strain, SI-1234) catalyzing *C. okamuranus* and *A. nodosum* fucoidans [198], *Sphingomona spaucimobilis* PF-1 (FNase S) catalyzing *U. pinnatifida* fucoidans [130], Alteromonadaceae (Strain SN-1009) catalyzing *Kjellmaniella crassifolia* fucoidans [205], *Dendryphiellaarenaria* TM94 catalyzing *F. vesiculosus* fucoidans [206], and *Pseudoalteromonas citrea* KMM 3296 and *Littorina kurila* catalyzing *F. evanescens* fucoidans [207]. In addition, a novel α-L-fucosidase was isolated from the marine bacterium *Wenyingzhuangia fucanilytica* CZ1127^T that acts on the α-(1→4)-fucosidic linkage of *Thelenotaananas* (wild sea cucumber) fucoidans [208]. Table 1 summarizes the previously characterized fucoidanases and fucoidan sulfatases that produced well-defined fucoidan fragments.

Table 1. Examples of different fucoidanases and fucoidan sulfatases, including the source of catalyzed fucoidans and their mode of cleavage action.

Enzyme Source and Accession Number in GenBank *	Enzyme Substrate (Fucoidan Source)	Mode of Cleaving Actions EC Number *	Degradation Product and Structural Features	Ref.
Fucoidanases				
Flavobacteriaceae strain, i.e., *Mariniflexilefucanivorans* SW5^T - FcnA: CAI47003.1 - FdlA: AAO00510.1 - FdlB: AAO00511.1	*Pelvetia canaliculata*	- endo α-(1→4) - (EC 3.2.1.212)	→3)-α-L-Fucp, 2-OSO$_3^-$ -(1→4)-α-L-Fucp-2,3-OSO$_3^-$	[82,200,209]
Formosa algae (FFA1) - WP_057784217.1	*Sargassum horneri*	- endo α-(1→4) - (EC 3.2.1.212)	→3)-α-L-Fucp, 2-OSO$_3^-$ -(1→4)-α-L-Fucp-2,3-OSO$_3^-$ -(1→ fragment, with insertion of →3)-α-L-Fucp, 2,4-OSO3$^-$ -(1→	[16]
	F. evanescens		→3)-α-L-Fucp, 2,4-OSO$_3^-$ -(1→4)-α-L-Fucp-2,4-OSO$_3^-$ -(1→4) -α-L-Fucp, 2-OSO$_3^-$ -(1→	[161]
Formosa algae KMM 3553^T (FFA2) - WP_057784219.1	*F. evanescens*	- endo α-(1→4) - (EC 3.2.1.212)	→3)-α-L-Fucp, 2,4-OSO$_3^-$ -(1→4)-α-L-Fucp, 2-OSO$_3^-$ -(1→ and →3)-α-L-Fucp, 2-OSO$_3^-$ -(1→4)-α-L-Fucp-2-OSO$_3^-$ -(1→ α-L-Fucp-2-OSO$_3^-$ (1→3)-α-L-Fucp-2-OSO$_3^-$ and α-L-Fucp-2,3-OSO$_3^-$ (1→3)-α-L-Fucp,2-OSO$_3^-$	[196] [34]
Fucobacter marina SA-0082	*Kjellmaniella crassifolia* (sulfated fucoglucuronomanna)	- endo-α-D-mannosidase - (EC 3.2.1.130)	Trisaccharides composed of - Δ^{4,5}GlcpUA-(1→2)-α-L-Fucp, 3-OSO$_3^-$ -(1→3)-α-D-Manp, - Δ^{4,5}GlcpUA-(1→2)-α-L-Fucp, 3- OSO$_3^-$ -(1→3)-α-D-Manp, 6-OSO$_3^-$, and - Δ^{4,5}GlcpUA-(1→2)-α-L-Fucp, 2,4-OSO$_3^-$ -(1→3)-α-D-Manp, 6-OSO$_3^-$	[210]
Pseudoalteromonas citrea, KMM 3296, KMM 3297, and KMM 3298 strains	*L. cichorioides* (20–40 kD)	- endo α-(1→3) - (EC 3.2.1.211)	Sulfated α-L-fucoolygosaccharides of 1.7–5.0 kDa and 1.3–5.0 kDa by KMM 3296 and KMM 3298 strains, respectively	[211]
Littorina kurila	*F. distichus*	- endo α-(1→3) - (EC 3.2.1.211)	→3)-α-L-Fucp-2,4-OSO$_3^-$ -(1→4)-α-L-Fucp-2-OSO$_3^-$ -(1→	[212]
Wenyingzhuangia fucanilytica CZ1127^T - ANW96115.1 - ANW96116.1 - ANW96098.1 - ANW96097.1	*Isostichopus badionotus*	- endo α-(1→3) - (EC 3.2.1.211)	α-L-Fucp-(1→3)-α-L-Fucp(2,4-OSO$_3^-$)-(1→3)- α-L-Fucp(2-OSO$_3^-$)-(1→3)-α-L-Fucp(2-OSO$_3^-$)	[202]

Table 1. Cont.

		Sulfatases or sulfoesterases	
Wenyingzhuangia fucanilytica CZ1127ᵀ - SWF1: WP_068825883.1 - SWF4: WP_068828765.1	F. evanescens and S. horneri	exo-2O and -3O-fucoidan sulfatase - (EC 3.1.6.B2)	[190]
Pecten maximus	A. nodosum	2O-fucoidan sulfatase - (EC 3.1.6.B2)	[137]

* whenever available.

7. Conclusions and Future Perspectives

Fucoidans are multifunctional macromolecules, in which several structural motifs participate in and affect their wide spectrum of applications. Therefore, numerous characteristics should be assigned (e.g., sulfation pattern and content, monomeric composition, degree of purity, molecular weight distribution, and glycosidic linkage) before their further applications, especially as there are several marketed fucoidan products. Hence, single analytical methods are not able to answer all the questions regarding the various fucoidan features. It is also beneficial if the fucoidan characteristics can be related to the required activities. This may help researchers to understand and reveal some of fucoidan's secrets. Somewhat old techniques are still applied; however, recently, other novel techniques were developed to more easily obtain and confirm results. These include advanced spectrometric (i.e., NMR and MS) and chromatographic coupled to spectrometric (GC/MS) methods. Moreover, fucoidan-degrading enzymes play a potential role prior to further analyses with advanced spectrometric methods, and they possess several advantages compared with chemical modification methods.

Therefore, the outlook in the field of fucoidan characterization and structural elucidation should focus on the metagenomic analysis of genes encoding such enzymes, where their overexpression and characterization may be a more effective tool in combination with spectrometric techniques. This will enable an understanding of the fucoidan mechanism of action and its exact interaction with different human targets.

Author Contributions: A.Z. planned the article's topics. A.Z. and M.E.-A. wrote the manuscript. A.-R.S.I. and R.U. participated in data collection and revised the final draft. All authors have read and agreed to the published version of the manuscript.

Funding: This research was funded by the Deutsche Forschungsgemeinschaft (DFG, German Research Foundation), grant number 172116086-SFB 926.

Acknowledgments: The authors would like to specially thank Hannah Niehuis and Emilie Marie Ulber for harvesting the *F. vesiculosus* algae during our research on fucoidan.

Conflicts of Interest: The authors declare no conflict of interest.

References

1. Ruocco, N.; Costantini, S.; Guariniello, S.; Costantini, M. Polysaccharides from the marine environment with pharmacological, cosmeceutical and nutraceutical potential. *Molecules* **2016**, *21*, 551. [CrossRef] [PubMed]
2. de Jesus Raposo, M.F.; de Morais, A.M.; de Morais, R.M. Marine polysaccharides from algae with potential biomedical applications. *Mar. Drugs* **2015**, *13*, 2967–3028. [CrossRef] [PubMed]
3. Garcia-Vaquero, M.; Rajauria, G.; O'Doherty, J.V.; Sweeney, T. Polysaccharides from macroalgae: Recent advances, innovative technologies and challenges in extraction and purification. *Food Res. Int.* **2017**, *99*, 1011–1020. [CrossRef] [PubMed]
4. Venkatesan, J.; Anil, S.; Rao, S.; Bhatnagar, I.; Kim, S.K. Sulfated polysaccharides from macroalgae for bone tissue regeneration. *Curr. Pharm. Des.* **2019**, *25*, 1200–1209. [CrossRef]
5. Li, J.; Cai, C.; Yang, C.; Li, J.; Sun, T.; Yu, G. Recent advances in pharmaceutical potential of brown algal polysaccharides and their derivatives. *Curr. Pharm. Des.* **2019**, *25*, 1290–1311. [CrossRef]
6. Li, B.; Lu, F.; Wei, X.; Zhao, R. Fucoidan: Structure and bioactivity. *Molecules* **2008**, *13*, 1671–1695. [CrossRef]
7. Hamid, S.S.; Wakayama, M.; Ichihara, K.; Sakurai, K.; Ashino, Y.; Kadowaki, R.; Soga, T.; Tomita, M. Metabolome profiling of various seaweed species discriminates between brown, red, and green algae. *Planta* **2019**, *249*, 1921–1947. [CrossRef]
8. Kopplin, G.; Rokstad, A.M.; Mélida, H.; Bulone, V.; Skjåk-Bræk, G.; Aachmann, F.L. Structural characterization of fucoidan from Laminaria hyperborea: Assessment of coagulation and inflammatory properties and their structure-function relationship. *ACS Appl. Bio Mater.* **2018**, *1*, 1880–1892. [CrossRef]
9. Cao, H.T.T.; Mikkelsen, M.D.; Lezyk, M.J.; Bui, L.M.; Tran, V.T.T.; Silchenko, A.S.; Kusaykin, M.I.; Pham, T.D.; Truong, B.H.; Holck, J.; et al. Novel enzyme actions for sulphated galactofucan depolymerisation and a new engineering strategy for molecular stabilisation of fucoidan degrading enzymes. *Mar. Drugs* **2018**, *16*, 422. [CrossRef]

10. Deniaud-Bouët, E.; Hardouin, K.; Potin, P.; Kloareg, B.; Hervé, C. A review about brown algal cell walls and fucose-containing sulfated polysaccharides: Cell wall context, biomedical properties and key research challenges. *Carbohydr. Polym.* **2017**, *175*, 395–408. [CrossRef]
11. Wang, Y.; Xing, M.; Cao, Q.; Ji, A.; Liang, H.; Song, S. Biological activities of fucoidan and the factors mediating its therapeutic effects: A review of recent studies. *Mar. Drugs* **2019**, *17*, 183. [CrossRef] [PubMed]
12. Michel, G.; Tonon, T.; Scornet, D.; Cock, J.M.; Kloareg, B. The cell wall polysaccharide metabolism of the brown alga Ectocarpus siliculosus. Insights into the evolution of extracellular matrix polysaccharides in eukaryotes. *New Phytol.* **2010**, *188*, 82–97. [CrossRef]
13. Zayed, A.; Ulber, R. Fucoidan Production: Approval Key Challenges and Opportunities. *Carbohydr. Polym.* **2019**, *211*, 289–297. [CrossRef]
14. Holtkamp, A.D.; Kelly, S.; Ulber, R.; Lang, S. Fucoidans and fucoidanases-focus on techniques for molecular structure elucidation and modification of marine polysaccharides. *Appl. Microbiol. Biotechnol.* **2009**, *82*, 1–11. [CrossRef] [PubMed]
15. Borazjani, N.J.; Tabarsa, M.; You, S.; Rezaei, M. Improved immunomodulatory and antioxidant properties of unrefined fucoidans from Sargassum angustifolium by hydrolysis. *J. Food. Sci. Technol.* **2017**, *54*, 4016–4025. [CrossRef] [PubMed]
16. Silchenko, A.S.; Rasin, A.B.; Kusaykin, M.I.; Kalinovsky, A.I.; Miansong, Z.; Changheng, L.; Malyarenko, O.S.; Zueva, A.O.; Zvyagintseva, T.N.; Ermakova, S.P. Structure, enzymatic transformation, anticancer activity of fucoidan and sulphated fucooligosaccharides from Sargassum horneri. *Carbohydr. Polym.* **2017**, *175*, 654–660. [CrossRef]
17. Fitton, J.H.; Stringer, D.N.; Karpiniec, S.S. Therapies from fucoidan: An update. *Mar. Drugs* **2015**, *13*, 5920–5946. [CrossRef]
18. Menshova, R.V.; Shevchenko, N.M.; Imbs, T.I.; Zvyagintseva, T.N.; Malyarenko, O.S.; Zaporoshets, T.S.; Besednova, N.N.; Ermakova, S.P. Fucoidans from brown alga Fucus evanescens: Structure and biological activity. *Front. Mar. Sci.* **2016**, *3*, 129. [CrossRef]
19. Fitton, J.H.; Stringer, D.S.; Park, A.Y.; Karpiniec, S.N. Therapies from fucoidan: New developments. *Mar. Drugs* **2019**, *17*, 571. [CrossRef]
20. Fitton, J.H.; Dell'Acqua, G.; Gardiner, V.-A.; Karpiniec, S.S.; Stringer, D.N.; Davis, E. Topical benefits of two fucoidan-rich extracts from marine macroalgae. *Cosmetics* **2015**, *2*, 66–81. [CrossRef]
21. Zhao, Y.; Zheng, Y.; Wang, J.; Ma, S.; Yu, Y.; White, W.L.; Yang, S.; Yang, F.; Lu, J. Fucoidan extracted from Undaria pinnatifida: Source for nutraceuticals/functional foods. *Mar. Drugs* **2018**, *16*, 321. [CrossRef] [PubMed]
22. Chauvierre, C.; Aid-Launais, R.; Aerts, J.; Chaubet, F.; Maire, M.; Chollet, L.; Rolland, L.; Bonafé, R.; Rossi, S.; Bussi, S.; et al. Pharmaceutical development and safety evaluation of a GMP-grade fucoidan for molecular diagnosis of cardiovascular diseases. *Mar. Drugs* **2019**, *17*, 699. [CrossRef] [PubMed]
23. Venkatesan, J.; Anil, S.; Kim, S.-K.; Shim, M.S. Seaweed polysaccharide-based nanoparticles: Preparation and applications for drug delivery. *Polymers* **2016**, *8*, 30. [CrossRef] [PubMed]
24. Zhang, Z.; Till, S.; Knappe, S.; Quinn, C.; Catarello, J.; Ray, G.J.; Scheiflinger, F.; Szabo, C.M.; Dockal, M. Screening of complex fucoidans from four brown algae species as procoagulant agents. *Carbohydr. Polym.* **2015**, *115*, 677–685. [CrossRef] [PubMed]
25. Park, H.Y.; Han, M.H.; Park, C.; Jin, C.Y.; Kim, G.Y.; Choi, I.W.; Kim, N.D.; Nam, T.J.; Kwon, T.K.; Choi, Y.H. Anti-inflammatory effects of fucoidan through inhibition of NF-κB, MAPK and Akt activation in lipopolysaccharide-induced BV2 microglia cells. *Food Chem. Toxicol.* **2011**, *49*, 1745–1752. [CrossRef]
26. Prokofjeva, M.M.; Imbs, T.a.I.; Shevchenko, N.M.; Spirin, P.V.; Horn, S.; Fehse, B.; Zvyagintseva, T.N.; Prassolov, V.S. Fucoidans as potential inhibitors of HIV-1. *Mar. Drugs* **2013**, *11*, 3000–3014. [CrossRef]
27. Atashrazm, F.; Lowenthal, R.M.; Woods, G.M.; Holloway, A.F.; Dickinson, J.L. Fucoidan and cancer: A multifunctional molecule with anti-tumor potential. *Mar. Drugs* **2015**, *13*, 2327–2346. [CrossRef]
28. Yoo, H.J.; You, D.-J.; Lee, K.-W. Characterization and immunomodulatory effects of high Molecular weight fucoidan Fraction from the sporophyll of Undaria pinnatifida in cyclophosphamide-induced immunosuppressed mice. *Mar. Drugs* **2019**, *17*, 447. [CrossRef]
29. Pozharitskaya, O.N.; Shikov, A.N.; Obluchinskaya, E.D.; Vuorela, H. The pharmacokinetics of fucoidan after topical application to rats. *Mar. Drugs* **2019**, *17*, 687. [CrossRef]

30. Zhan, E.; Chu, F.; Zhao, T.; Chai, Y.; Liang, H.; Song, S.; Ji, A. Determination of fucoidan in rat plasma by HPLC and its application in pharmacokinetics. *Pak. J. Pharm. Sci.* **2020**, *33*, 1–9.
31. Bai, X.; Zhang, E.; Hu, B.; Liang, H.; Song, S.; Ji, A. Study on absorption mechanism and tissue distribution of fucoidan. *Molecules* **2020**, *25*, 1087. [CrossRef] [PubMed]
32. Krylova, N.V.; Ermakova, S.P.; Lavrov, V.F.; Leneva, I.A.; Kompanets, G.G.; Iunikhina, O.V.; Nosik, M.N.; Ebralidze, L.K.; Falynskova, I.N.; Silchenko, A.S.; et al. The comparative analysis of antiviral activity of native and modified fucoidans from brown algae Fucus evanescens in vitro and in vivo. *Mar. Drugs* **2020**, *18*, 224. [CrossRef] [PubMed]
33. Bilan, M.I.; Usov, A.I. Structural analysis of fucoidans. *Nat. Prod. Commun.* **2008**, *3*, 1639–1648. [CrossRef]
34. Silchenko, A.S.; Kusaykin, M.I.; Kurilenko, V.V.; Zakharenko, A.M.; Isakov, V.V.; Zaporozhets, T.S.; Gazha, A.K.; Zvyagintseva, T.N. Hydrolysis of fucoidan by fucoidanase isolated from the marine bacterium, Formosa algae. *Mar. Drugs* **2013**, *11*, 2413–2430. [CrossRef]
35. Ale, M.T.; Mikkelsen, J.D.; Meyer, A.S. Important determinants for fucoidan bioactivity: A critical review of structure-function relations and extraction methods for fucose-containing sulfated polysaccharides from brown seaweeds. *Mar. Drugs* **2011**, *9*, 2106–2130. [CrossRef]
36. Morya, V.K.; Kim, J.; Kim, E.-K. Algal fucoidan: Structural and size-dependent bioactivities and their perspectives. *Appl. Microbiol. Biotechnol.* **2012**, *93*, 71–82. [CrossRef]
37. Ustyuzhanina, N.E.; Ushakova, N.A.; Zyuzina, K.A.; Bilan, M.I.; Elizarova, A.L.; Somonova, O.V.; Madzhuga, A.V.; Krylov, V.B.; Preobrazhenskaya, M.E.; Usov, A.I.; et al. Influence of fucoidans on hemostatic system. *Mar. Drugs* **2013**, *11*, 2444–2458. [CrossRef]
38. Zayed, A.; Muffler, K.; Hahn, T.; Rupp, S.; Finkelmeier, D.; Burger-Kentischer, A.; Ulber, R. Physicochemical and biological characterization of fucoidan from Fucus vesiculosus purified by dye affinity chromatography. *Mar. Drugs* **2016**, *14*, 79. [CrossRef]
39. Lu, J.; Shi, K.K.; Chen, S.; Wang, J.; Hassouna, A.; White, L.N.; Merien, F.; Xie, M.; Kong, Q.; Li, J.; et al. Fucoidan extracted from the New Zealand Undaria pinnatifida-physicochemical comparison against five other fucoidans: Unique low molecular weight fraction bioactivity in breast cancer cell lines. *Mar. Drugs* **2018**, *16*, 461. [CrossRef]
40. Chen, M.C.; Hsu, W.L.; Hwang, P.A.; Chou, T.C. Low molecular weight fucoidan inhibits tumor angiogenesis through downregulation of HIF-1/VEGF signaling under hypoxia. *Mar. Drugs* **2015**, *13*, 4436–4451. [CrossRef]
41. Bouvard, C.; Galy-Fauroux, I.; Grelac, F.; Carpentier, W.; Lokajczyk, A.; Gandrille, S.; Colliec-Jouault, S.; Fischer, A.M.; Helley, D. Low-molecular-weight fucoidan induces endothelial cell migration via the PI3K/AKT pathway and modulates the transcription of genes involved in angiogenesis. *Mar. Drugs* **2015**, *13*, 7446–7462. [CrossRef] [PubMed]
42. Mandal, P.; Mateu, C.G.; Chattopadhyay, K.; Pujol, C.A.; Damonte, E.B.; Ray, B. Structural features and antiviral activity of sulphated fucans from the brown seaweed Cystoseira indica. *Antivir. Chem. Chemother.* **2007**, *18*, 153–162. [CrossRef] [PubMed]
43. Chevolot, L.; Mulloy, B.; Ratiskol, J.; Foucault, A.; Colliec-Jouault, S. A disaccharide repeat unit is the major structure in fucoidans from two species of brown algae. *Carbohydr. Res.* **2001**, *330*, 529–635. [CrossRef]
44. Zayed, A.; Hahn, T.; Finkelmeier, D.; Burger-Kentischer, A.; Rupp, S.; Krämer, R.; Ulber, R. Phenomenological investigation of the cytotoxic activity of fucoidan isolated from Fucus vesiculosus. *Process Biochem.* **2019**, *81*, 182–187. [CrossRef]
45. Wei, X.; Cai, L.; Liu, H.; Tu, H.; Xu, X.; Zhou, F.; Zhang, L. Chain conformation and biological activities of hyperbranched fucoidan derived from brown algae and its desulfated derivative. *Carbohydr. Polym.* **2019**, *208*, 86–96. [CrossRef]
46. Ale, M.T.; Maruyama, H.; Tamauchi, H.; Mikkelsen, J.D.; Meyer, A.S. Fucose-containing sulfated polysaccharides from brown seaweeds inhibit proliferation of melanoma cells and induce apoptosis by activation of caspase-3 in vitro. *Mar. Drugs* **2011**, *9*, 2605–2621. [CrossRef]
47. Cho, M.L.; Lee, B.-Y.; You, S. Relationship between oversulfation and conformation of low and high molecular weight fucoidans and evaluation of their in vitro anticancer activity. *Molecules* **2010**, *16*, 291–297. [CrossRef]
48. Ma, X.-T.; Sun, X.-Y.; Yu, K.; Gui, B.-S.; Gui, Q.; Ouyang, J.-M. Effect of content of sulfate groups in seaweed polysaccharides on antioxidant activity and repair effect of subcellular organelles in injured HK-2 cells. *Oxid. Med. Cell. Longev.* **2017**, *2017*, 2542950. [CrossRef]

49. Oliveira, C.; Ferreira, A.S.; Novoa-Carballal, R.; Nunes, C.; Pashkuleva, I.; Neves, N.M.; Coimbra, M.A.; Reis, R.L.; Martins, A.; Silva, T.H. The Key Role of Sulfation and Branching on Fucoidan Antitumor Activity. *Macromol. Biosci.* **2017**, *17*, 1600340. [CrossRef]
50. Zhou, J.; Hu, N.; Wu, Y.L.; Pan, Y.J.; Sun, C.R. Preliminary studies on the chemical characterization and antioxidant properties of acidic polysaccharides from Sargassum fusiforme. *J. Zhejiang Univ. Sci. B* **2008**, *9*, 721–727. [CrossRef]
51. Yang, W.-N.; Chen, P.-W.; Huang, C.-Y. Compositional characteristics and in vitro evaluations of antioxidant and neuroprotective properties of crude extracts of fucoidan prepared from compressional puffing-pretreated Sargassum crassifolium. *Mar. Drugs* **2017**, *15*, 183. [CrossRef] [PubMed]
52. Athukorala, Y.; Jung, W.-K.; Vasanthan, T.; Jeon, Y.-J. An anticoagulative polysaccharide from an enzymatic hydrolysate of Ecklonia cava. *Carbohydr. Polym.* **2006**, *66*, 184–191. [CrossRef]
53. Jesumani, V.; Du, H.; Pei, P.; Aslam, M.; Huang, N. Comparative study on skin protection activity of polyphenol-rich extract and polysaccharide-rich extract from Sargassum vachellianum. *PLoS ONE* **2020**, *15*, e0227308. [CrossRef] [PubMed]
54. Zayed, A.; Ulber, R. Fucoidans: Downstream processes and recent applications. *Mar. Drugs* **2020**, *18*, 170. [CrossRef]
55. Ehrig, K.; Alban, S. Sulfated galactofucan from the brown alga Saccharina latissima—Variability of yield, structural composition and bioactivity. *Mar. Drugs* **2014**, *13*, 76–101. [CrossRef]
56. Mourão, P.A.; Pereira, M.S. Searching for alternatives to heparin: Sulfated fucans from marine invertebrates. *Trends Cardiovasc. Med.* **1999**, *9*, 225–232. [CrossRef]
57. Vilela-Silva, A.C.; Castro, M.O.; Valente, A.P.; Biermann, C.H.; Mourao, P.A. Sulfated fucans from the egg jellies of the closely related sea urchins Strongylocentrotus droebachiensis and Strongylocentrotus pallidus ensure species-specific fertilization. *J. Biol. Chem.* **2002**, *277*, 379–387. [CrossRef]
58. Vilela-Silva, A.C.; Alves, A.P.; Valente, A.P.; Vacquier, V.D.; Mourão, P.A. Structure of the sulfated alpha-L-fucan from the egg jelly coat of the sea urchin Strongylocentrotus franciscanus: Patterns of preferential 2-O- and 4-O-sulfation determine sperm cell recognition. *Glycobiology* **1999**, *9*, 927–933. [CrossRef]
59. Hahn, T.; Lang, S.; Ulber, R.; Muffler, K. Novel procedures for the extraction of fucoidan from brown algae. *Process Biochem.* **2012**, *47*, 1691–1698. [CrossRef]
60. Jiao, G.; Yu, G.; Zhang, J.; Ewart, H.S. Chemical Structures and Bioactivities of Sulfated Polysaccharides from Marine Algae. *Mar. Drugs* **2011**, *9*, 196–223. [CrossRef]
61. Patankar, M.S.; Oehninger, S.; Barnett, T.; Williams, R.L.; Clark, G.F. A revised structure for fucoidan may explain some of its biological activities. *J. Biol. Chem.* **1993**, *268*, 21770–21776. [PubMed]
62. Bilan, M.I.; Grachev, A.A.; Shashkov, A.S.; Thuy, T.T.T.; Van, T.T.T.; Ly, B.M.; Nifantiev, N.E.; Usov, A.I. Preliminary investigation of a highly sulfated galactofucan fraction isolated from the brown alga Sargassum polycystum. *Carbohydr. Res.* **2013**, *377*, 48–57. [CrossRef] [PubMed]
63. Fletcher, H.R.; Biller, P.; Ross, A.B.; Adams, J.M.M. The seasonal variation of fucoidan within three species of brown macroalgae. *Algal Res.* **2017**, *22*, 79–86. [CrossRef]
64. Cumashi, A.; Ushakova, N.A.; Preobrazhenskaya, M.E.; D'Incecco, A.; Piccoli, A.; Totani, L.; Tinari, N.; Morozevich, G.E.; Berman, A.E.; Bilan, M.I.; et al. A comparative study of the anti-inflammatory, anticoagulant, antiangiogenic, and antiadhesive activities of nine different fucoidans from brown seaweeds. *Glycobiology* **2007**, *17*, 541–552. [CrossRef] [PubMed]
65. Duarte, M.E.; Cardoso, M.A.; Noseda, M.D.; Cerezo, A.S. Structural studies on fucoidans from the brown seaweed Sargassum stenophyllum. *Carbohydr. Res.* **2001**, *333*, 281–293. [CrossRef]
66. Ale, M.T.; Meyer, A.S. Fucoidans from brown seaweeds: An update on structures, extraction techniques and use of enzymes as tools for structural elucidation. *RSC Adv.* **2013**, *3*, 8131–8141. [CrossRef]
67. Usoltseva, R.V.; Shevchenko, N.M.; Malyarenko, O.S.; Anastyuk, S.D.; Kasprik, A.E.; Zvyagintsev, N.V.; Ermakova, S.P. Fucoidans from brown algae Laminaria longipes and Saccharina cichorioides: Structural characteristics, anticancer and radiosensitizing activity in vitro. *Carbohydr. Polym.* **2019**, *221*, 157–165. [CrossRef]
68. Wang, J.; Zhang, Q.; Zhang, Z.; Zhang, H.; Niu, X. Structural studies on a novel fucogalactan sulfate extracted from the brown seaweed Laminaria japonica. *Int. J. Biol. Macromol.* **2010**, *47*, 126–131. [CrossRef]

69. Zhu, Z.; Zhu, B.; Ai, C.; Lu, J.; Wu, S.L.; Liu, Y.; Wang, L.; Yang, J.; Song, S.; Liu, X. Development and application of a HPLC-MS/MS method for quantitation of fucosylated chondroitin sulfate and fucoidan in sea cucumbers. *Carbohydr. Res.* **2018**, *466*, 11–17. [CrossRef]
70. Yu, L.; Xue, C.; Chang, Y.; Xu, X.; Ge, L.; Liu, G.; Wang, Y. Structure elucidation of fucoidan composed of a novel tetrafucose repeating unit from sea cucumber Thelenota ananas. *Food Chem.* **2014**, *146*, 113–119. [CrossRef]
71. Dubois, M.; Gilles, K.; Hamilton, J.K.; Rebers, P.A.; Smith, F. A colorimetric method for the determination of sugars. *Nature* **1951**, *168*, 167. [CrossRef] [PubMed]
72. Smogyi, M. Notes on sugar determination. *J. Biol. Chem.* **1952**, *195*, 19–23. [PubMed]
73. Shao, Y.; Lin, A.H. Improvement in the quantification of reducing sugars by miniaturizing the Somogyi-Nelson assay using a microtiter plate. *Food Chem.* **2018**, *240*, 898–903. [CrossRef] [PubMed]
74. Dische, Z.; Shettles, L.B. A specific color reaction of methylpentoses and a spectrophotometric micromethod for their determination. *J. Biol. Chem.* **1948**, *175*, 595–603. [PubMed]
75. Djurdjić, V.; Mandić, L. A spectrophotometric method for simultaneous determination of protein-bound hexoses and fucose with a mixture of L-cysteine and phenol. *Anal. Biochem.* **1990**, *188*, 222–227. [CrossRef]
76. Hahn, T.; Schulz, M.; Stadtmüller, R.; Zayed, A.; Muffler, K.; Lang, S.; Ulber, R. Cationic dye for the specific determination of sulfated polysaccharides. *Anal. Lett.* **2016**, *49*, 1948–1962. [CrossRef]
77. Warttinger, U.; Giese, C.; Harenberg, J.; Krämer, R. Direct quantification of brown algae-derived fucoidans in human plasma by a fluorescent probe assay. *arXiv* **2016**, arXiv:1608.00108.
78. Zayed, A.; Dienemann, C.; Giese, C.; Krämer, R.; Ulber, R. An immobilized perylene diimide derivative for fucoidan purification from a crude brown algae extract. *Process Biochem.* **2018**, *65*, 233–238. [CrossRef]
79. Jiao, Q.; Liu, Q. Simple spectrophotometric method for the estimation of algal polysaccharide concentrations. *J. Agric. Food Chem.* **1999**, *47*, 996–998. [CrossRef]
80. Rappold, M.; Warttinger, U.; Krämer, R. A Fluorescent probe for glycosaminoglycans applied to the detection of dermatan sulfate by a mix-and-read assay. *Molecules* **2017**, *22*, 768. [CrossRef]
81. Zayed, A. *Bioactive Compounds from Marine Sources*; TU Kaiserslautern: Kaiserslautern, Germany, 2018.
82. Descamps, V.; Colin, S.; Lahaye, M.; Jam, M.; Richard, C.; Potin, P.; Barbeyron, T.; Yvin, J.C.; Kloareg, B. Isolation and culture of a marine bacterium degrading the sulfated fucans from marine brown algae. *Mar. Biotechnol.* **2006**, *8*, 27–39. [CrossRef] [PubMed]
83. Ziółkowska, D.; Kaniewska, A.; Lamkiewicz, J.; Shyichuk, A. Determination of carrageenan by means of photometric titration with methylene blue and toluidine blue dyes. *Carbohydr. Polym.* **2017**, *165*, 1–6. [CrossRef] [PubMed]
84. Mak, W.; Wang, S.K.; Liu, T.; Hamid, N.; Li, Y.; Lu, J.; White, W.L. Anti-proliferation potential and content of fucoidan extracted from sporophyll of New Zealand Undaria pinnatifida. *Front. Nutr.* **2014**, *1*, 9. [CrossRef] [PubMed]
85. Kim, J.M.; Nguyen, L.; Barr, M.F.; Morabito, M.; Stringer, D.; Fitton, J.H.; Mowery, K.A. Quantitative determination of fucoidan using polyion-sensitive membrane electrodes. *Anal. Chim. Acta* **2015**, *877*, 1–8. [CrossRef]
86. Dodgson, K.S.; Price, R.G. A note on the determination of the ester sulphate content of sulphated polysaccharides. *Biochem. J.* **1962**, *84*, 106–110. [CrossRef]
87. Dodgson, K.S. Determination of inorganic sulphate in studies on the enzymic and non-enzymic hydrolysis of carbohydrate and other sulphate esters. *Biochem. J.* **1961**, *78*, 312–319. [CrossRef]
88. Oliveira, R.M.; Câmara, R.B.G.; Monte, J.F.S.; Viana, R.L.S.; Melo, K.R.T.; Queiroz, M.F.; Filgueira, L.G.A.; Oyama, L.M.; Rocha, H.A.O. Commercial fucoidans from Fucus vesiculosus can be grouped into antiadipogenic and adipogenic agents. *Mar. Drugs* **2018**, *16*, 193. [CrossRef]
89. Camara, R.B.G.; Costa, L.S.; Fidelis, G.P.; Nobre, L.T.D.B.; Dantas-Santos, N.; Cordeiro, S.L.; Costa, M.S.S.P.; Alves, L.G.; Rocha, H.A.O. Heterofucans from the brown seaweed Canistrocarpus cervicornis with anticoagulant and antioxidant activities. *Mar. Drugs* **2011**, *9*, 124–138. [CrossRef]
90. Cuong, H.D.; Thuy, T.T.T.; Huong, T.T.; Ly, B.M.; Van, T.T.T. Structure and hypolipidaemic activity of fucoidan extracted from brown seaweed Sargassum henslowianum. *Nat. Prod. Res.* **2015**, *29*, 411–415. [CrossRef]
91. Galermo, A.G.; Nandita, E.; Barboza, M.; Amicucci, M.J.; Vo, T.-T.T.; Lebrilla, C.B. Liquid chromatography-tandem mass spectrometry approach for determining glycosidic linkages. *Anal. Chem.* **2018**, *90*, 13073–13080. [CrossRef]

92. Filisetti-Cozzi, T.M.C.C.; Carpita, N.C. Measurement of uronic acids without interference from neutral sugars. *Anal. Biochem.* **1991**, *197*, 157–162. [CrossRef]
93. Blumenkrantz, N.; Asboe-Hansen, G. New method for quantitative determination of uronic acids. *Anal. Biochem.* **1973**, *54*, 484–489. [CrossRef]
94. Bitter, T.; Muir, H.M. A modified uronic acid carbazole reaction. *Anal. Biochem.* **1962**, *4*, 330–334. [CrossRef]
95. Corradini, C.; Cavazza, A.; Bignardi, C. High-performance anion-exchange chromatography coupled with pulsed electrochemical detection as a powerful tool to evaluate carbohydrates of food interest: Principles and applications. *Int. J. Carbohydr. Chem.* **2012**, *2012*, 487564. [CrossRef]
96. Zhang, Z.; Khan, N.M.; Nunez, K.M.; Chess, E.K.; Szabo, C.M. Complete monosaccharide analysis by high-performance anion-exchange chromatography with pulsed amperometric detection. *Anal. Chem.* **2012**, *84*, 4104–4110. [CrossRef]
97. Balboa, E.M.; Rivas, S.; Moure, A.; Dominguez, H.; Parajo, J.C. Simultaneous extraction and depolymerization of fucoidan from Sargassum muticum in aqueous media. *Mar. Drugs* **2013**, *11*, 4612–4627. [CrossRef]
98. Flórez-Fernández, N.; Balboa, E.M.; Domínguez, H. Extraction and purification of fucoidan from marine sources. In *Encyclopedia of Marine Biotechnology*; Kim, S.K., Ed.; John Wiley & Sons Ltd.: Hoboken, NJ, USA, 2020; pp. 1093–1125. [CrossRef]
99. Spadari, C.d.C.; Lopes, L.B.; Ishida, K. Potential use of alginate-based carriers as antifungal delivery system. *Front. Microbiol.* **2017**, *8*, 97. [CrossRef]
100. Bouissil, S.; El Alaoui-Talibi, Z.; Pierre, G.; Michaud, P.; El Modafar, C.; Delattre, C. Use of alginate extracted from Moroccan brown algae to stimulate natural defense in date palm roots. *Molecules* **2020**, *25*, 720. [CrossRef]
101. Belattmania, Z.; Kaidi, S.; El Atouani, S.; Katif, C.; Bentiss, F.; Jama, C.; Reani, A.; Sabour, B.; Vasconcelos, V. Isolation and FTIR-ATR and 1H NMR characterization of alginates from the main alginophyte species of the Atlantic Coast of Morocco. *Molecules* **2020**, *25*, 4335. [CrossRef]
102. Deniaud-Bouët, E.; Kervarec, N.; Michel, G.; Tonon, T.; Kloareg, B.; Hervé, C. Chemical and enzymatic fractionation of cell walls from Fucales: Insights into the structure of the extracellular matrix of brown algae. *Ann. Bot.* **2014**, *114*, 1203–1216. [CrossRef]
103. Malyarenko, O.S.; Usoltseva, R.V.; Zvyagintseva, T.N.; Ermakova, S.P. Laminaran from brown alga Dictyota dichotoma and its sulfated derivative as radioprotectors and radiosensitizers in melanoma therapy. *Carbohydr. Polym.* **2019**, *206*, 539–547. [CrossRef] [PubMed]
104. Takei, M.N.; Kuda, T.; Taniguchi, M.; Nakamura, S.; Hajime, T.; Kimura, B. Detection and isolation of low molecular weight alginate- and laminaran-susceptible gut indigenous bacteria from ICR mice. *Carbohydr. Polym.* **2020**, *238*, 116205. [CrossRef] [PubMed]
105. Lowry, O.H.; Rosebrough, N.J.; Farr, A.L.; Randall, R.J. Protein measurement with the Folin phenol reagent. *J. Biol. Chem.* **1951**, *193*, 265–275. [PubMed]
106. Wu, Q.; Ma, S.; Xiao, H.; Zhang, M.; Cai, J. Purification and the secondary structure of fucoidanase from Fusarium sp. LD8. *Evid. Based Complement. Altern. Med.* **2011**, *2011*, 196190. [CrossRef]
107. Lu, T.-S.; Yiao, S.-Y.; Lim, K.; Jensen, R.V.; Hsiao, L.-L. Interpretation of biological and mechanical variations between the Lowry versus Bradford method for protein quantification. *N. Am. J. Med. Sci.* **2010**, *2*, 325–328. [CrossRef] [PubMed]
108. Brady, P.N.; Macnaughtan, M.A. Evaluation of colorimetric assays for analyzing reductively methylated proteins: Biases and mechanistic insights. *Anal. Biochem.* **2015**, *491*, 43–51. [CrossRef]
109. Bradford, M.M. A rapid and sensitive method for the quantitation of microgram quantities of protein utilizing the principle of protein-dye binding. *Anal. Biochem.* **1976**, *72*, 248–254. [CrossRef]
110. Matsushita, S.; Iwami, N.; Nitta, Y. Colorimetric estimation of amino acids and peptides with the Folin phenol reagent. *Anal. Biochem.* **1966**, *16*, 365–371. [CrossRef]
111. Peterson, G.L. Review of the folin phenol protein quantitation method of lowry, rosebrough, farr and randall. *Anal. Biochem.* **1979**, *100*, 201–220. [CrossRef]
112. Santos, S.A.O.; Félix, R.; Pais, A.C.S.; Rocha, S.M.; Silvestre, A.J.D. The quest for phenolic compounds from macroalgae: A review of extraction and identification methodologies. *Biomolecules* **2019**, *9*, 847. [CrossRef]
113. Rohwer, K.; Neupane, S.; Bittkau, K.S.; Galarza Pérez, M.; Dörschmann, P.; Roider, J.; Alban, S.; Klettner, A. Effects of crude Fucus distichus subspecies evanescens fucoidan extract on retinal pigment epithelium cells-implications for use in age-related macular degeneration. *Mar. Drugs* **2019**, *17*, 538. [CrossRef] [PubMed]

114. Chale-Dzul, J.; Moo-Puc, R.; Robledo, D.; Freile-Pelegrín, Y. Hepatoprotective effect of the fucoidan from the brown seaweed Turbinaria tricostata. *J. Appl. Phycol.* **2015**, *27*, 2123–2135. [CrossRef]
115. Ferreira, R.M.; Ramalho Ribeiro, A.; Patinha, C.; Silva, A.M.S.; Cardoso, S.M.; Costa, R. Water extraction einetics of bioactive compounds of Fucus vesiculosus. *Molecules* **2019**, *24*, 3408. [CrossRef] [PubMed]
116. Lee, J.; Jung, Y.; Shin, J.-H.; Kim, H.K.; Moon, B.C.; Ryu, D.H.; Hwang, G.-S. Secondary metabolite profiling of Curcuma species grown at different locations using GC/TOF and UPLC/Q-TOF MS. *Molecules* **2014**, *19*, 9535–9551. [CrossRef] [PubMed]
117. Hahn, T.; Zayed, A.; Kovacheva, M.; Stadtmüller, R.; Lang, S.; Muffler, K.; Ulber, R. Dye affinity chromatography for fast and simple purification of fucoidan from marine brown algae. *Eng. Life Sci.* **2016**, *16*, 78–87. [CrossRef]
118. Szekalska, M.; Sosnowska, K.; Czajkowska-Kośnik, A.; Winnicka, K. Calcium chloride modified alginate microparticles formulated by the spray drying process: A strategy to prolong the release of freely soluble drugs. *Materials* **2018**, *11*, 1522. [CrossRef] [PubMed]
119. Nguyen, T.T.; Mikkelsen, M.D.; Tran, V.H.N.; Trang, V.T.D.; Rhein-Knudsen, N.; Holck, J.; Rasin, A.B.; Cao, H.T.T.; Van, T.T.T.; Meyer, A.S. Enzyme-assisted fucoidan extraction from brown macroalgae Fucus distichus subsp. evanescens and Saccharina latissima. *Mar. Drugs* **2020**, *18*, 296. [CrossRef]
120. Dörschmann, P.; Mikkelsen, M.D.; Thi, T.N.; Roider, J.; Meyer, A.S.; Klettner, A. Effects of a newly developed enzyme-assisted extraction method on the biological activities of fucoidans in ocular cells. *Mar. Drugs* **2020**, *18*, 282. [CrossRef]
121. Catarino, M.D.; Silva, A.M.S.; Cardoso, S.M. Phycochemical constituents and biological activities of Fucus spp. *Mar. Drugs* **2018**, *16*, 249. [CrossRef]
122. Hallé, J.P.; Landry, D.; Fournier, A.; Beaudry, M.; Leblond, F.A. Method for the quantification of alginate in microcapsules. *Cell Transplant.* **1993**, *2*, 429–436. [CrossRef]
123. Abdella, A.A.; Ulber, R.; Zayed, A. Chitosan-toluidine blue beads for purification of fucoidans. *Carbohydr. Polym.* **2020**, *231*, 115686. [CrossRef] [PubMed]
124. van Weelden, G.; Bobiński, M.; Okła, K.; van Weelden, W.J.; Romano, A.; Pijnenborg, J.M.A. Fucoidan Structure and Activity in Relation to Anti-Cancer Mechanisms. *Mar. Drugs* **2019**, *17*, 32. [CrossRef] [PubMed]
125. Neupane, S.; Bittkau, K.S.; Alban, S. Size distribution and chain conformation of six different fucoidans using size-exclusion chromatography with multiple detection. *J. Chromatogr. A* **2020**, *1612*, 460658. [CrossRef] [PubMed]
126. Patkar, S.N.; Panzade, P.D. Fast and efficient method for molecular weight analysis of cellulose pulp, in-process and finished product. *Anal. Methods* **2016**, *8*, 3210–3215. [CrossRef]
127. Scott, D.; Coleman, P.J.; Mason, R.M.; Levick, J.R. Action of polysaccharides of similar average mass but differing molecular volume and charge on fluid drainage through synovial interstitium in rabbit knees. *J. Physiol.* **2000**, *528*, 609–618. [CrossRef]
128. Somasundaram, S.N.; Shanmugam, S.; Subramanian, B.; Jaganathan, R. Cytotoxic effect of fucoidan extracted from Sargassum cinereum on colon cancer cell line HCT-15. *Int. J. Biol. Macromol.* **2016**, *91*, 1215–1223. [CrossRef]
129. Manns, D.; Deutschle, A.L.; Saake, B.; Meyer, A.S. Methodology for quantitative determination of the carbohydrate composition of brown seaweeds (Laminariaceae). *RSC Adv.* **2014**, *4*, 25736–25746. [CrossRef]
130. Kim, W.J.; Park, J.W.; Park, J.K.; Choi, D.J.; Park, Y.I. Purification and Characterization of a Fucoidanase (FNase S) from a Marine Bacterium Sphingomonas paucimobilis PF-1. *Mar. Drugs* **2015**, *13*, 4398–4417. [CrossRef]
131. Bruhn, A.; Janicek, T.; Manns, D.; Nielsen, M.M.; Balsby, T.J.S.; Meyer, A.S.; Rasmussen, M.l.B.; Hou, X.; Saake, B.; Göke, C.; et al. Crude fucoidan content in two North Atlantic kelp species, Saccharina latissima and Laminaria digitata-seasonal variation and impact of environmental factors. *J. Appl. Phycol.* **2017**, *29*, 3121–3137. [CrossRef]
132. Van Vliet, D.M.; Palakawong Na Ayudthaya, S.; Diop, S.; Villanueva, L.; Stams, A.J.M.; Sánchez-Andrea, I. Anaerobic degradation of sulfated polysaccharides by two novel Kiritimatiellales strains isolated from Black Sea sediment. *Front. Microbiol.* **2019**, *10*, 253. [CrossRef]
133. Monsur, H.A.; Jaswir, I.; Simsek, S.; Amid, A.; Alam, Z. Chemical structure of sulfated polysaccharides from brown seaweed (Turbinaria turbinata). *Int. J. Food Prop.* **2017**, *20*, 1457–1469. [CrossRef]

134. Rühmann, B.; Schmid, J.; Sieber, V. Fast carbohydrate analysis via liquid chromatography coupled with ultra violet and electrospray ionization ion trap detection in 96-well format. *J. Chromatogr. A* **2014**, *1350*, 44–50. [CrossRef] [PubMed]
135. Menshova, R.V.; Anastyuk, S.D.; Ermakova, S.P.; Shevchenko, N.M.; Isakov, V.I.; Zvyagintseva, T.N. Structure and anticancer activity in vitro of sulfated galactofucan from brown alga Alaria angusta. *Carbohydr. Polym.* **2015**, *132*, 118–125. [CrossRef] [PubMed]
136. Zhang, B.W.; Xu, J.L.; Zhang, H.; Zhang, Q.; Lu, J.; Wang, J.H. Structure elucidation of a polysaccharide from Umbilicaria esculenta and its Immunostimulatory activity. *PLoS ONE* **2016**, *11*, e0168472. [CrossRef] [PubMed]
137. Daniel, R.; Berteau, O.; Chevolot, L.; Varenne, A.; Gareil, P.; Goasdoue, N. Regioselective desulfation of sulfated L-fucopyranoside by a new sulfoesterase from the marine mollusk Pecten maximus: Application to the structural study of algal fucoidan (Ascophyllum nodosum). *Eur. J. Biochem.* **2001**, *268*, 5617–5626. [CrossRef]
138. Thinh, P.D.; Menshova, R.V.; Ermakova, S.P.; Anastyuk, S.D.; Ly, B.M.; Zvyagintseva, T.N. Structural characteristics and anticancer activity of fucoidan from the brown alga Sargassum mcclurei. *Mar. Drugs* **2013**, *11*, 1456–1476. [CrossRef]
139. Chizhov, A.O.; Dell, A.; Morris, H.R.; Haslam, S.M.; McDowell, R.A.; Shashkov, A.S.; Nifant'ev, N.E.; Khatuntseva, E.A.; Usov, A.I. A study of fucoidan from the brown seaweed Chorda filum. *Carbohydr. Res.* **1999**, *320*, 108–119. [CrossRef]
140. Luo, D.; Wang, Z.; Nie, K. Structural characterization of a novel polysaccharide from Sargassum thunbergii and its antioxidant and anti-inflammation effects. *PLoS ONE* **2019**, *14*, e0223198. [CrossRef]
141. Luo, D.; Wang, Z.; Li, Z.; Yu, X.-Q. Structure of an entangled heteropolysaccharide from Pholidota chinensis Lindl and its antioxidant and anti-cancer properties. *Int. J. Biol. Macromol.* **2018**, *112*, 921–928. [CrossRef]
142. Tako, M. Rheological characteristics of fucoidan isolated from commercially cultured Cladosiphon okamuranus. *Bot. Mar.* **2003**, *46*, 461–465. [CrossRef]
143. Cho, M.; Choi, W.S.; You, S. Steady and dynamic shear rheology of fucoidan-buckwheat starch mixtures. *Starch-Stärke* **2009**, *61*, 282–290. [CrossRef]
144. KOO, J.-G.; JO, K.-S.; PARK, J.-H. Rheological properties of fucoidans from Laminaria religiosa, sporophylls of Undaria pinnatifida, Hizikia fusiforme and Sagassum fulvellum in Korea. *Korean J. Fish. Aquat. Sci.* **1997**, *30*, 329–333.
145. Sezer, A.D.; Cevher, E. Fucoidan: A versatile biopolymer for biomedical applications. In *Active Implants and Scaffolds for Tissue Regeneration*; Springer: Berlin/Heidelberg, Germany, 2011; pp. 377–406.
146. Citkowska, A.; Szekalska, M.; Winnicka, K. Possibilities of fucoidan utilization in the development of pharmaceutical dosage forms. *Mar. Drugs* **2019**, *17*, 458. [CrossRef]
147. Rioux, L.E.; Turgeon, S.L.; Beaulieu, M. Rheological characterisation of polysaccharides extracted from brown seaweeds. *J. Sci. Food Agric.* **2007**, *87*, 1630–1638. [CrossRef]
148. Lee, K.Y.; Mooney, D.J. Alginate: Properties and biomedical applications. *Prog. Polym. Sci.* **2012**, *37*, 106–126. [CrossRef]
149. Dobrinčić, A.; Balbino, S.; Zorić, Z.; Pedisić, S.; Bursać Kovačević, D.; Elez Garofulić, I.; Dragović-Uzelac, V. Advanced technologies for the extraction of marine brown algal polysaccharides. *Mar. Drugs* **2020**, *18*, 168. [CrossRef] [PubMed]
150. Cunha, L.; Grenha, A. Sulfated seaweed polysaccharides as multifunctional materials in drug delivery applications. *Mar. Drugs* **2016**, *14*, 42. [CrossRef]
151. Chollet, L.; Saboural, P.; Chauvierre, C.; Villemin, J.N.; Letourneur, D.; Chaubet, F. Fucoidans in nanomedicine. *Mar. Drugs* **2016**, *14*, 145. [CrossRef]
152. Yuan, Y.; Macquarrie, D. Microwave assisted extraction of sulfated polysaccharides (fucoidan) from Ascophyllum nodosum and its antioxidant activity. *Carbohydr. Polym.* **2015**, *129*, 101–107. [CrossRef]
153. Huang, C.-Y.; Kuo, C.-H.; Chen, P.-W. Compressional-puffing pretreatment enhances neuroprotective effects of fucoidans from the brown seaweed Sargassum hemiphyllum on 6-hydroxydopamine-induced apoptosis in SH-SY5Y cells. *Molecules* **2017**, *23*, 78. [CrossRef]
154. Saboural, P.; Chaubet, F.; Rouzet, F.; Al-Shoukr, F.; Azzouna, R.B.; Bouchemal, N.; Picton, L.; Louedec, L.; Maire, M.; Rolland, L.; et al. Purification of a low molecular weight fucoidan for SPECT molecular imaging of myocardial infarction. *Mar. Drugs* **2014**, *12*, 4851–4867. [CrossRef] [PubMed]

155. Marinval, N.; Saboural, P.; Haddad, O.; Maire, M.; Bassand, K.; Geinguenaud, F.; Djaker, N.; Ben Akrout, K.; Lamy de la Chapelle, M.; Robert, R.; et al. Identification of a pro-angiogenic potential and cellular uptake mechanism of a LMW highly sulfated fraction of fucoidan from Ascophyllum nodosum. *Mar. Drugs* **2016**, *14*, 185. [CrossRef] [PubMed]

156. Hifney, A.F.; Fawzy, M.A.; Abdel-Gawad, K.M.; Gomaa, M. Industrial optimization of fucoidan extraction from Sargassum sp. and its potential antioxidant and emulsifying activities. *Food Hydrocoll.* **2016**, *54*, 77–88. [CrossRef]

157. Rodriguez-Jasso, R.M.; Mussatto, S.I.; Pastrana, L.; Aguilar, C.N.; Teixeira, J.A. Microwave-assisted extraction of sulfated polysaccharides (fucoidan) from brown seaweed. *Carbohydr. Polym.* **2011**, *86*, 1137–1144. [CrossRef]

158. Pavlenko, A.F.; Belogortseva, N.I.; Kalinovskii, A.I.; Ovodov, Y.S. Determination of the positions of the sulfate groups in sulfated polysaccharides. *Chem. Nat. Compd.* **1976**, *12*, 515–518. [CrossRef]

159. Synytsya, A.; Kim, W.-J.; Kim, S.-M.; Pohl, R.; Synytsya, A.; Kvasnička, F.; Čopíková, J.; Park, Y. Structure and antitumour activity of fucoidan isolated from sporophyll of Korean brown seaweed Undaria pinnatifida. *Carbohydr. Polym.* **2010**, *81*, 41–48. [CrossRef]

160. Bilan, M.I.; Shashkov, A.S.; Usov, A.I. Structure of a sulfated xylofucan from the brown alga Punctaria plantaginea. *Carbohydr. Res.* **2014**, *393*, 1–8. [CrossRef]

161. Silchenko, A.S.; Rasin, A.B.; Kusaykin, M.I.; Malyarenko, O.S.; Shevchenko, N.M.; Zueva, A.O.; Kalinovsky, A.I.; Zvyagintseva, T.N.; Ermakova, S.P. Modification of Native Fucoidan from Fucus Evanescens by Recombinant Fucoidanase from Marine Bacteria Formosa Algae. *Carbohydr. Polym.* **2018**, *193*, 189–195. [CrossRef]

162. Bilan, M.I.; Grachev, A.A.; Ustuzhanina, N.E.; Shashkov, A.S.; Nifantiev, N.E.; Usov, A.I. A highly regular fraction of a fucoidan from the brown seaweed Fucus distichus L. *Carbohydr. Res.* **2004**, *339*, 511–517. [CrossRef]

163. Rasin, A.B.; Silchenko, A.S.; Kusaykin, M.I.; Malyarenko, O.S.; Zueva, A.O.; Kalinovsky, A.I.; Airong, J.; Surits, V.V.; Ermakova, S.P. Enzymatic transformation and anti-tumor activity of Sargassum horneri fucoidan. *Carbohydr. Polym.* **2020**, *246*, 116635. [CrossRef]

164. Bezerra, F.; Pomin, V. Structural mechanisms involved in mild-acid hydrolysis of a defined tetrasaccharide-repeating sulfate fucan. In *Enzymatic Technologies for Marine Polysaccharides*, 1st ed.; Trincone, A., Ed.; Taylor & Francis Group: Boca Raton, FL, USA, 2019; pp. 111–128. [CrossRef]

165. Palanisamy, S.; Vinosha, M.; Marudhupandi, T.; Rajasekar, P.; Prabhu, N.M. Isolation of fucoidan from Sargassum polycystum brown algae: Structural characterization, in vitro antioxidant and anticancer activity. *Int. J. Biol. Macromol.* **2017**, *102*, 405–412. [CrossRef] [PubMed]

166. Bilan, M.I.; Grachev, A.A.; Ustuzhanina, N.E.; Shashkov, A.S.; Nifantiev, N.E.; Usov, A.I. Structure of a fucoidan from the brown seaweed Fucus evanescens C.Ag. *Carbohydr. Res.* **2002**, *337*, 719–730. [CrossRef]

167. Bilan, M.I.; Grachev, A.A.; Shashkov, A.S.; Nifantiev, N.E.; Usov, A.I. Structure of a fucoidan from the brown seaweed Fucus serratus L. *Carbohydr. Res.* **2006**, *341*, 238–245. [CrossRef] [PubMed]

168. Vishchuk, O.S.; Ermakova, S.P.; Zvyagintseva, T.N. Sulfated polysaccharides from brown seaweeds Saccharina japonica and Undaria pinnatifida: Isolation, structural characteristics, and antitumor activity. *Carbohydr. Res.* **2011**, *346*, 2769–2776. [CrossRef] [PubMed]

169. Badrinathan, S.; Shiju, T.M.; Sharon Christa, A.S.; Arya, R.; Pragasam, V. Purification and structural characterization of sulfated polysaccharide from Sargassum myriocystum and its efficacy in scavenging free radicals. *Indian J. Pharm. Sci.* **2012**, *74*, 549–555. [CrossRef]

170. Tako, M.; Nakada, T.; Hongou, F. Chemical characterization of fucoidan from commercially cultured Nemacystus decipiens (Itomozuku). *Biosci. Biotechnol. Biochem.* **1999**, *63*, 1813–1815. [CrossRef] [PubMed]

171. Bandyopadhyay, S.S.; Navid, M.H.; Ghosh, T.; Schnitzler, P.; Ray, B. Structural features and in vitro antiviral activities of sulfated polysaccharides from Sphacelaria indica. *Phytochemistry* **2011**, *72*, 276–283. [CrossRef]

172. Bilan, M.I.; Grachev, A.A.; Shashkov, A.S.; Kelly, M.; Sanderson, C.J.; Nifantiev, N.E.; Usov, A.I. Further studies on the composition and structure of a fucoidan preparation from the brown alga Saccharina latissima. *Carbohydr. Res.* **2010**, *345*, 2038–2047. [CrossRef]

173. Lim, S.J.; Wan Aida, W.M.; Maskat, M.Y.; Latip, J.; Badri, K.H.; Hassan, O.; Yamin, B.M. Characterisation of fucoidan extracted from Malaysian Sargassum binderi. *Food Chem.* **2016**, *209*, 267–273. [CrossRef]

174. Cai, Y.; Yang, W.; Yin, R.; Zhou, L.; Li, Z.; Wu, M.; Zhao, J. An anticoagulant fucan sulfate with hexasaccharide repeating units from the sea cucumber Holothuria albiventer. *Carbohydr. Res.* **2018**, *464*, 12–18. [CrossRef]
175. Yoshida, K.; Minami, Y.; Nemoto, H.; Numata, K.; Yamanaka, E. Structure of DHG, a depolymerized glycosaminoglycan from sea cucumber, Stichopus japonicus. *Tetrahedron Lett.* **1992**, *33*, 4959–4962. [CrossRef]
176. Shang, F.; Mou, R.; Zhang, Z.; Gao, N.; Lin, L.; Li, Z.; Wu, M.; Zhao, J. Structural analysis and anticoagulant activities of three highly regular fucan sulfates as novel intrinsic factor Xase inhibitors. *Carbohydr. Polym.* **2018**, *195*, 257–266. [CrossRef] [PubMed]
177. Thanh, T.T.; Tran, V.T.; Yuguchi, Y.; Bui, L.M.; Nguyen, T.T. Structure of fucoidan from brown seaweed Turbinaria ornata as studied by electrospray ionization mass spectrometry (ESIMS) and small angle X-ray scattering (SAXS) techniques. *Mar. Drugs* **2013**, *11*, 2431–2443. [CrossRef]
178. Anastyuk, S.D.; Shevchenko, N.M.; Nazarenko, E.L.; Imbs, T.I.; Gorbach, V.I.; Dmitrenok, P.S.; Zvyagintseva, T.N. Structural analysis of a highly sulfated fucan from the brown alga Laminaria cichorioides by tandem MALDI and ESI mass spectrometry. *Carbohydr. Res.* **2010**, *345*, 2206–2212. [CrossRef] [PubMed]
179. Anastyuk, S.D.; Shevchenko, N.M.; Gorbach, V.I. Fucoidan analysis by tandem MALDI-TOF and ESI mass Spectrometry. *Methods Mol. Biol.* **2015**, *1308*, 299–312. [CrossRef] [PubMed]
180. Lang, Y.; Zhao, X.; Liu, L.; Yu, G. Applications of mass spectrometry to structural analysis of marine oligosaccharides. *Mar. Drugs* **2014**, *12*, 4005–4030. [CrossRef]
181. Anastyuk, S.D.; Imbs, T.I.; Dmitrenok, P.S.; Zvyagintseva, T.N. Rapid mass spectrometric analysis of a novel fucoidan, extracted from the brown alga Coccophora langsdorfii. *Sci. World J.* **2014**, *2014*, 972450. [CrossRef]
182. Anastyuk, S.D.; Shevchenko, N.M.; Dmitrenok, P.S.; Zvyagintseva, T.N. Structural similarities of fucoidans from brown algae Silvetia babingtonii and Fucus evanescens, determined by tandem MALDI-TOF mass spectrometry. *Carbohydr. Res.* **2012**, *358*, 78–81. [CrossRef]
183. Domon, B.; Costello, C.E. A systematic nomenclature for carbohydrate fragmentations in FAB-MS/MS spectra of glycoconjugates. *Glycoconj. J.* **1988**, *5*, 397–409. [CrossRef]
184. Tissot, B.; Salpin, J.-Y.; Martinez, M.; Gaigeot, M.-P.; Daniel, R. Differentiation of the fucoidan sulfated l-fucose isomers constituents by CE-ESIMS and molecular modeling. *Carbohydr. Res.* **2006**, *341*, 598–609. [CrossRef]
185. Shevchenko, N.M.; Anastyuk, S.D.; Menshova, R.V.; Vishchuk, O.S.; Isakov, V.I.; Zadorozhny, P.A.; Sikorskaya, T.V.; Zvyagintseva, T.N. Further studies on structure of fucoidan from brown alga Saccharina gurjanovae. *Carbohydr. Polym.* **2015**, *121*, 207–216. [CrossRef] [PubMed]
186. Manivasagan, P.; Oh, J. Production of a novel fucoidanase for the green synthesis of gold nanoparticles by Streptomyces sp. and its cytotoxic effect on HeLa cells. *Mar. Drugs* **2015**, *13*, 6818–6837. [CrossRef]
187. Schultz-Johansen, M.; Cueff, M.; Hardouin, K.; Jam, M.; Larocque, R.; Glaring, M.A.; Hervé, C.; Czjzek, M.; Stougaard, P. Discovery and screening of novel metagenome-derived GH107 enzymes targeting sulfated fucans from brown algae. *FEBS J.* **2018**, *285*, 4281–4295. [CrossRef] [PubMed]
188. Kitamura, K.; Matsuo, M.; Tsuneo, Y. Enzymic degradation of fucoidan by fucoidanase from the Hepatopancreas of Patinopecten yessoensis. *Biosci. Biotechnol. Biochem.* **1992**, *56*, 490–494. [CrossRef] [PubMed]
189. Silchenko, A.S.; Kusaykin, M.I.; Zakharenko, A.M.; Menshova, R.V.; Khanh, H.H.N.; Dmitrenok, P.S.; Isakov, V.V.; Zvyagintseva, T.N. Endo-1,4-fucoidanase from Vietnamese marine mollusk Lambis sp. which producing sulphated fucooligosaccharides. *J. Mol. Catal. B Enzym.* **2014**, *102*, 154–160. [CrossRef]
190. Silchenko, A.S.; Rasin, A.B.; Zueva, A.O.; Kusaykin, M.I.; Zvyagintseva, T.N.; Kalinovsky, A.I.; Kurilenko, V.V.; Ermakova, S.P. Fucoidan Sulfatases from Marine Bacterium Wenyingzhuangia fucanilytica CZ1127(T). *Biomolecules* **2018**, *8*, 98. [CrossRef]
191. Usoltseva, R.V.; Anastyuk, S.D.; Shevchenko, N.M.; Surits, V.V.; Silchenko, A.S.; Isakov, V.V.; Zvyagintseva, T.N.; Thinh, P.D.; Ermakova, S.P. Polysaccharides from brown algae Sargassum duplicatum: The structure and anticancer activity in vitro. *Carbohydr. Polym.* **2017**, *175*, 547–556. [CrossRef] [PubMed]
192. Jo, B.W.; Choi, S.-K. Degradation of fucoidans from Sargassum fulvellum and their biological activities. *Carbohydr. Polym.* **2014**, *111*, 822–829. [CrossRef]
193. Kusaykin, M.; Bakunina, I.; Sova, V.; Ermakova, S.; Kuznetsova, T.; Besednova, N.; Zaporozhets, T.; Zvyagintseva, T. Structure, biological activity, and enzymatic transformation of fucoidans from the brown seaweeds. *Biotechnol. J.* **2008**, *3*, 904–915. [CrossRef]
194. Ohshiro, T.; Ohmoto, Y.; Ono, Y.; Ohkita, R.; Miki, Y.; Kawamoto, H.; Izumi, Y. Isolation and characterization of a novel fucoidan-degrading microorganism. *Biosci. Biotechnol. Biochem.* **2010**, *74*, 1729–1732. [CrossRef]

195. Kusaykin, M.I.; Silchenko, A.S.; Zakharenko, A.M.; Zvyagintseva, T.N. Fucoidanases. *Glycobiology* **2015**, *26*, 3–12. [CrossRef] [PubMed]
196. Silchenko, A.S.; Ustyuzhanina, N.E.; Kusaykin, M.I.; Krylov, V.B.; Shashkov, A.S.; Dmitrenok, A.S.; Usoltseva, R.V.; Zueva, A.O.; Nifantiev, N.E.; Zvyagintseva, T.N. Expression and biochemical characterization and substrate specificity of the fucoidanase from Formosa algae. *Glycobiology* **2017**, *27*, 254–263. [CrossRef] [PubMed]
197. Takayama, M.; Koyama, N.; Sakai, T.; Kato, I. Enzymes Capable of Degrading a Sulfated-Fucose-Containing Polysaccharide and Their Encoding Genes. U.S. Patent 6,489,155,B1, 3 December 2002.
198. Sakai, T.; Ishizuka, K.; Kato, I. Isolation and characterization of a fucoidan-degrading marine bacterium. *Mar. Biotechnol.* **2003**, *5*, 409–416. [CrossRef] [PubMed]
199. Helbert, W. Marine Polysaccharide Sulfatases. *Front. Mar. Sci.* **2017**, *4*, 6. [CrossRef]
200. Colin, S.; Deniaud, E.; Jam, M.; Descamps, V.; Chevolot, Y.; Kervarec, N.; Yvin, J.C.; Barbeyron, T.; Michel, G.; Kloareg, B. Cloning and biochemical characterization of the fucanase FcnA: Definition of a novel glycoside hydrolase family specific for sulfated fucans. *Glycobiology* **2006**, *16*, 1021–1032. [CrossRef] [PubMed]
201. Lombard, V.; Golaconda Ramulu, H.; Drula, E.; Coutinho, P.M.; Henrissat, B. The carbohydrate-active enzymes database (CAZy) in 2013. *Nucleic Acids Res.* **2014**, *42*, D490–D495. [CrossRef] [PubMed]
202. Shen, J.; Chang, Y.; Zhang, Y.; Mei, X.; Xue, C. Discovery and characterization of an endo-1,3-fucanase from marine bacterium Wenyingzhuangia fucanilytica: A novel glycoside hydrolase family. *Front. Microbiol.* **2020**, *11*. [CrossRef]
203. Nagao, T.; Arai, Y.; Yamaoka, M.; Komatsu, F.; Yagi, H.; Suzuki, H.; Ohshiro, T. Identification and characterization of the fucoidanase gene from Luteolibacter algae H18. *J. Biosci. Bioeng.* **2018**, *126*, 567–572. [CrossRef]
204. Ohshiro, T.; Harada, N.; Kobayashi, Y.; Miki, Y.; Kawamoto, H. Microbial fucoidan degradation by Luteolibacter algae H18 with deacetylation. *Biosci. Biotechnol. Biochem.* **2012**, *76*, 620–623. [CrossRef]
205. Sakai, T.; Kawai, T.; Kato, I. Isolation and characterization of a fucoidan-degrading marine bacterial strain and its fucoidanase. *Mar. Biotechnol.* **2004**, *6*, 335–346. [CrossRef]
206. Wu, Q.; Zhang, M.; Wu, K.; Liu, B.; Cai, J.; Pan, R. Purification and characteristics of fucoidanase obtained from Dendryphiella arenaria TM94. *J. Appl. Phycol.* **2011**, *23*, 197–203. [CrossRef]
207. Kusaykin, M.I.; Chizhov, A.O.; Grachev, A.A.; Alekseeva, S.A.; Bakunina, I.Y.; Nedashkovskaya, O.I.; Sova, V.V.; Zvyagintseva, T.N. *A Comparative Study of Specificity of Fucoidanases from Marine Microorganisms and Invertebrates*; Springer: Dordrecht, The Netherlands, 2007; pp. 143–147.
208. Dong, S.; Chang, Y.; Shen, J.; Xue, C.; Chen, F. Purification, expression and characterization of a novel α-l-fucosidase from a marine bacteria Wenyingzhuangia fucanilytica. *Protein Expr. Purif.* **2017**, *129*, 9–17. [CrossRef] [PubMed]
209. Barbeyron, T.; L'Haridon, S.; Michel, G.; Czjzek, M. Mariniflexile fucanivorans sp. nov., a marine member of the Flavobacteriaceae that degrades sulphated fucans from brown algae. *Int. J. Syst. Evol. Microbiol.* **2008**, *58*, 2107–2113. [CrossRef] [PubMed]
210. Sakai, T.; Kimura, H.; Kojima, K.; Shimanaka, K.; Ikai, K.; Kato, I. Marine bacterial sulfated fucoglucuronomannan (SFGM) lyase digests brown algal SFGM into trisaccharides. *Mar. Biotechnol.* **2003**, *5*, 70–78. [CrossRef] [PubMed]
211. Bakunina, I.Y.; Nedashkovskaya, O.I.; Alekseeva, S.A.; Ivanova, E.P.; Romanenko, L.A.; Gorshkova, N.M.; Isakov, V.V.; Zvyagintseva, T.N.; Mikhailov, V.V. Degradation of fucoidan by the marine proteobacterium Pseudoalteromonas citrea. *Microbiology* **2002**, *71*, 41–47. [CrossRef]
212. Bilan, M.I.; Kusaykin, M.I.; Grachev, A.A.; Tsvetkova, E.A.; Zvyagintseva, T.N.; Nifantiev, N.E.; Usov, A.I. Effect of enzyme preparation from the marine mollusk Littorina kurila on fucoidan from the brown alga Fucus distichus. *Biochemistry* **2005**, *70*, 1321. [CrossRef] [PubMed]

Publisher's Note: MDPI stays neutral with regard to jurisdictional claims in published maps and institutional affiliations.

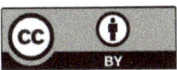

© 2020 by the authors. Licensee MDPI, Basel, Switzerland. This article is an open access article distributed under the terms and conditions of the Creative Commons Attribution (CC BY) license (http://creativecommons.org/licenses/by/4.0/).

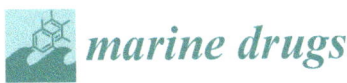

Article

Evaluation of a Brown Seaweed Extract from *Dictyosiphon foeniculaceus* as a Potential Therapeutic Agent for the Treatment of Glioblastoma and Uveal Melanoma

Philipp Dörschmann [1,*], Christina Schmitt [2], Kaya Saskia Bittkau [3], Sandesh Neupane [3], Michael Synowitz [4], Johann Roider [1], Susanne Alban [3], Janka Held-Feindt [4] and Alexa Klettner [1]

1 Department of Ophthalmology, University Medical Center Schleswig-Holstein UKSH, Campus Kiel, D-24105 Kiel, Germany; johann.roider@uksh.de (J.R.); alexakarina.klettner@uksh.de (A.K.)
2 Institute of Anatomy, Kiel University, D-24118 Kiel, Germany
3 Pharmaceutical Institute, Kiel University, D-24118 Kiel, Germany; kbittkau@pharmazie.uni-kiel.de (K.S.B.); sneupane@pharmazie.uni-kiel.de (S.N.); salban@pharmazie.uni-kiel.de (S.A.)
4 Department of Neurosurgery, University Medical Center Schleswig-Holstein UKSH, Campus Kiel, D-24105 Kiel, Germany; michael.synowitz@uksh.de (M.S.); janka.held-feindt@uksh.de (J.H.-F.)
* Correspondence: philipp.doerschmann@uksh.de; Tel.: +49-431-5001-3712

Received: 14 September 2020; Accepted: 3 December 2020; Published: 8 December 2020

Abstract: Ingredients of brown seaweed like fucoidans are often described for their beneficial biological effects, that might be interesting for a medical application. In this study, we tested an extract from *Dictyosiphon foeniculaceus* (DF) to evaluate the effects in glioblastoma and uveal melanoma, looking for a possible anti-cancer treatment. We investigated toxicity, VEGF (vascular endothelial growth factor) secretion and gene expression of tumor and non-tumor cells. SVGA (human fetal astrocytes), the human RPE (retinal pigment epithelium) cell line ARPE-19, the tumor cell line OMM-1 (human uveal melanoma), and two different human primary glioblastoma cultures (116-14 and 118-14) were used. Tests for cell viability were conducted with MTS-Assay (3-(4,5-Dimethylthiazol-2-yl)-5-(3-carboxymethoxyphenyl)-2-(4-sulfophenyl)-2H-tetrazolium), and the proliferation rate was determined with cell counting. VEGF secretion was assessed with ELISA (enzyme-linked immunosorbent assay). The gene expression of VEGF receptor 1 (VEGFR1), VEGF receptor 2 (VEGFR2) and VEGF-A was determined with real-time qPCR (quantitative polymerase chain reaction). DF lowered the cell viability of OMM-1. Proliferation rates of ARPE-19 and OMM-1 were decreased. The VEGF secretion was inhibited in ARPE-19 and OMM-1, whereas it was increased in SVGA and 116-14. The expression of VEGFR1 was absent and not influenced in OMM-1 and ARPE-19. VEGFR2 expression was lowered in 116-14 after 24 h, whereas VEGF-A was increased in 118-14 after 72 h. The extract lowered cell viability slightly and was anti-proliferative depending on the cell type investigated. VEGF was heterogeneously affected. The results in glioblastoma were not promising, but the anti-tumor properties in OMM-1 could make them interesting for further research concerning cancer diseases in the human eye.

Keywords: fucoidan; cancer; VEGF; gene expression; toxicity; *Dictyosiphon foeniculaceus*; retinal pigment epithelium; glioblastoma; astrocytes; uveal melanoma

1. Introduction

Tumor diseases and malignant cancer is a huge challenge and an active research field in medical treatment developments. Cancer is one of the deadliest diseases in industrial nations and a wide variety of cancer types exist. One of these cancer types is glioblastoma multiforme (GBM), one of the most dangerous and most aggressive tumor diseases, which accounts for more than 15% of all intracranial tumors and has a median survival time of 7–15 months from the time of diagnosis [1]. The probability of developing this tumor increases with age. Symptoms of the disease are nausea, vomiting, seizures and severe headaches. The incidence rate is ranges up to 3.69 per 100,000 persons [2]. Standard treatment options include surgery, radiation, and chemotherapy with temozolomide [3]. However, there are still no curative treatment concepts available. Rapid growth and early migration of the tumor cells are responsible for its poor prognosis [4]. The main intraocular cancer type is uveal melanoma (UM) with an incidence of 5.1 per million per year [5]. It generates from melanocytes located in the uvea, most commonly from the choroid. The main problem of this cancer is the potential to metastasize and spreading into the liver which leads often to death [6]. Common harsh therapies like surgery often result in vision loss in the affected eye, while no effective treatment for metastatic tumors are available [7].

The potential of natural marine substances is widely known for the beneficial uses for human health. The regular consummation of algae has been described to be correlated with a longer and healthier life, which is also described for the Okinawa diet [8]. Several marine plants like brown algae, vertebrates like fish and invertebrates contain different agents which are beneficial for the human health [8]. Especially the potential of brown algae extracts, which contain positive ingredients like polyphenols, alginates and sulfated fucans (fucoidans) is often described in the literature [8–11]. Among these positive effects are anti-oxidative, anti-inflammatory, anti-tumor and anti-angiogenic properties [12–15], making it highly interesting for cancer and skin therapies [16,17]. Fucoidans have also been described by our group for their anti-oxidative, VEGF (vascular endothelial growth factor) lowering and binding effects [18–21]. In general they do not lower cell viability as tested in different cell types like ARPE-19 (human retinal pigment epithelium), HL-60 (acute myeloid leukemia), Raji (Burkitt lymphoma), HeLa (cervix carcinoma), A-375 (skin melanoma), HCT-116 (colon carcinoma), Hep G2 (hepatocellular carcinoma) and HaCaT (keratinocytes) after 24 h of treatment [22]. However, in the uveal melanoma cell line OMM-1, certain brown algae extracts above certain concentrations decreased the cell viability [19,22]. Such extracts may be of interest in tumor diseases, such as uveal melanoma or glioblastoma.

Among fucoidan containing extracts from six different brown algae species, that from *Dictyosiphon foeniculaceus* (DF) showed the most pronounced anti-proliferative effects in tumor cell lines OMM-1 after 24 h and in HeLa after 24 and 72 h of treatment [22]. DF, also known as tubular net weed or golden sea hair, belongs to the order of Ectocarpales and is a highly branched brown seaweed species that grows on rocks, other algae, or is free-floating in North Atlantic and Northwest Pacific [23]. Literature on fucose containing sulfated polysaccharides from DF is so far limited to the mentioned DF extract [24,25]. Chemical characterization of the DF extract revealed that the applied fucoidan extraction and purification procedure did not result in fucoidans as known for many other brown algae, but a complex mixture of fucose containing polysaccharides and proteoglycans, respectively, with a relatively low sulfate content [24]. Typical fucoidan activities including antioxidant, elastase inhibiting, anticomplement, and anticoagulant effects turned out to be weaker than those of other fucoidans [24], but contrary to other fucoidans, the DF extract reduced the cell viability of two tumor cell lines [22].

In this work we tested an extract from DF in therapeutically relevant concentration range in terms of cell viability, proliferation, regulation of VEGF secretion and gene expression of VEGF-A, FLT-1/VEGFR1 (fms related receptor tyrosine kinase 1/VEGF receptor 1) and KDR/VEGFR2 (kinase insert domain receptor/VEGF receptor 2) after short- and mid-term time period stimulation of the tumor cell line OMM-1 and the human primary glioblastoma cultures 116-14 and 118-14. As a comparison, we used the healthy cells of ARPE-19 and human astrocytes SVGA. This study is well-equipped for investigation of the currently unknown effects of DF extract on tumor relevant properties like angiogenesis, cell viability and proliferation and to make a comparison between two non-tumor and three tumor cell lines as well as between two ocular and three brain cell cultures.

2. Results

2.1. Chemical Characterization of the Extract

The extraction and purification of DF was performed by a procedure usually resulting in relatively pure fucoidans. The chemical analysis of the DF extract (Table 1) conducted by Bittkau et al., 2020 and Neupane et al., 2020 [24,25] revealed that the DF extract strongly differs from the fucoidans obtained from five other brown algae species and cannot be considered as typical fucoidan. Compared to other five extracts, its sulfate content (8.8% vs. 12.3–28.8%), which resulted in a calculated apparent degree of sulfation of only 0.1, and its fucose content (38.7% vs. 40.6–96.1%) were the lowest, whereas its protein content (24.1% vs. 1.9–15.3%) was the highest (Table 1). Also the contents of other monosaccharides were considerably higher than those of the other five fucoidans, namely 32.0% xylose, 16.2% galactose and 5.6% mannose. The average molecular weight of the DF extract was 194 kDa (vs. 188–1340 kDa) with a quite high polydispersity of 3.9, its contents of glucose (5.0%) and uronic acids amounted to 98% and its content of phenolic compounds was 2.2–4.5 times lower than that of the three *Fucus* fucoidans. According to analysis by size exclusion chromatography with multiple detection, the main fraction of the DF extract had a compact spherical conformation, whereas typical fucoidans exist as random coil with expanded structure. This conformation is in line with the high protein content and suggests polysaccharides tightly associated with protein (glycoproteins, proteoglycans) [25]. Especially due these pronounced structural differences of the DF extract, it was of interest to investigate its effects on VEGF secretion, gene expression as well as cell viability and proliferation of tumor cells.

Table 1. Chemical characterization of extract from *Dictyosiphon feoniculaceus* [1].

Characteristics	Value
Molecular mass	193 ± 0.8 kDa
Sulfate content [2]	8.8%
Fucose content	38.7%
Uronic acid	9.8 ± 0.6%
Total phenolic content	11.0 ± 3.2 µg GAE/mg [3]
Protein content	24.1%

[1] data from Bittkau et al., 2020 and Neupane et al., 2020 [24,25]; [2] apparent degree of sulfation amounts to only 0.1; [3] µg GAE/mg = gallic acid equivalents/mg.

2.2. Cell Viability Assay

Cell viability of the five different cell types was assessed with the commercially available MTS (3-(4,5-Dimethylthiazol-2-yl)-5-(3-carboxymethoxyphenyl)-2-(4-sulfophenyl)-2H- tetrazolium) assay by Promega Corporation. Cells were treated for 24 and 72 h. Cell viability of SVGA, 116-14 and 118-14 was unaffected (Figure 1) except for 118-14; here 100 µg/mL DF slightly lowered the viability to 93% ± 4% after 24 h of treatment ($p < 0.05$). ARPE-19 viability was decreased after the application of 100 µg/mL of the DF extract for 24 h to 94% ± 3% ($p < 0.001$). The DF extract showed slight anti-proliferative effects in the OMM-1 cell line. In detail, 10 µg/mL DF lowered the viability of OMM-1 cells to 91% ± 6% ($p < 0.05$), and 100 µg/mL DF lowered it to 73% ± 9% ($p < 0.001$) after 24 h. Contrary, 10 µg/mL DF reduced OMM-1 cell viability to 91% ± 6% ($p < 0.01$), and 100 µg/mL DF reduced it to 93% ± 5% ($p < 0.05$) after 72 h.

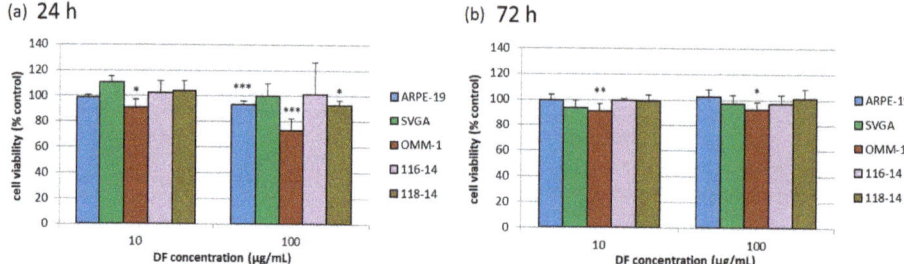

Figure 1. Cell viability of five different cell cultures was investigated, namely the human RPE (retinal pigment epithelium) cell line (ARPE-19), human, uveal melanoma cell line OMM-1, human fetal astrocytes SVGA and human glioblastoma cells 116-14 and 118-14. MTS-Assay (3-(4,5-Dimethylthiazol-2-yl)-5-(3-carboxymethoxyphenyl)-2-(4-sulfophenyl)-2H-tetrazolium) was performed after treatment with 10 or 100 µg/mL DF (*Dictyosiphon foeniculaceus*) extract for 24 (**a**) or 72 h (**b**). The mean values and standard deviation were calculated in relation to the untreated control (set to 100%, not shown). Significance tests were performed with One-Way ANOVA with multiple comparison test; * $p < 0.05$, ** $p < 0.01$, *** $p < 0.001$ compared to control group ($n \geq 4$; number of independent experiments).

2.3. Cell Proliferation Test

The influence of the DF extract on cell proliferation was determined with cell counting after trypan blue staining. The diagrams represent the relative cell number in percent to the untreated control (Figure 2). The cell numbers of ARPE-19, SVGA and 116-14 were not significantly influenced. After 24 h of treatment, the cell number of 118-14 was reduced to 77 ± 10% (10 µg/mL DF) ($p < 0.05$). An application of 100 µg/mL DF lowered the cell number of OMM-1 to 21 ± 10% ($p < 0.05$) after 24 h and to 9 ± 7% ($p < 0.05$) after 72 h of stimulation. These lowered proliferation rates of OMM-1 correspond to the lowered cell viabilities as described in Section 2.2.

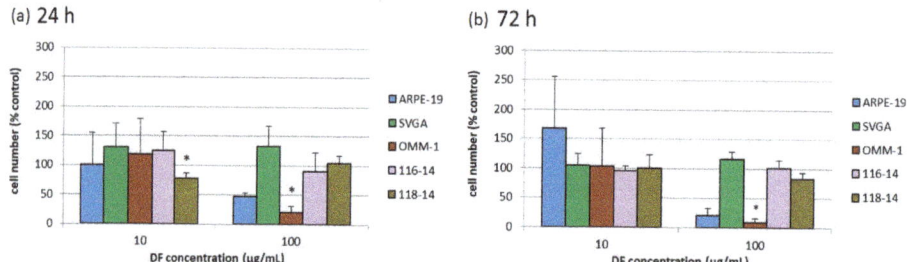

Figure 2. Cell proliferation of ARPE-19, SVGA, OMM-1, 116-14 and 118-14 was investigated by cell counting with trypan blue staining after treatment with 10 or 100 µg/mL DF extract for 24 (**a**) and 72 h (**b**), respectively. The mean values and standard deviation represent the mean of the cell number in relation to an untreated control in percent (set to 100%, not shown). Significance tests were performed with One-Way ANOVA with multiple comparison test; * $p < 0.05$, compared to untreated control group ($n \geq 4$).

2.4. VEGF Secretion

The secreted VEGF amounts of ARPE-19, SVGA, OMM-1, 116-14 and 118-14 were determined with ELISA (enzyme-linked immunosorbent assay). The individual VEGF amount in pg/mL was set in relation to the corresponding cell viability in % (cell viability assay performed, data not shown), compared to controls, to exclude the dependency of the measured VEGF secretion on the cell viability and number. The normalized, relative VEGF amounts compared to untreated controls are depicted in

Figure 3. After 10 µg/mL DF application, SVGA cells responded with a high increase of VEGF secretion up to 3.7 [a.u.] ± 1.8 [a.u.] (arbitrary units) ($p < 0.05$). Additional effects could be determined after 100 µg/mL DF treatment: The secreted VEGF amount of 116-14 was increased to 2.2 [a.u.] ± 0.3 [a.u.] ($p < 0.05$), whereas VEGF of ARPE-19 and OMM-1 was decreased to 0.7 [a.u.] ± 0.3 [a.u.] ($p < 0.05$) and 0.8 [a.u.] ± 0.0 [a.u.] ($p < 0.05$), respectively. Thus, it seems that DF extracts can promote pro-angiogenic effects in brain cells and small anti-angiogenic effects in ocular cells.

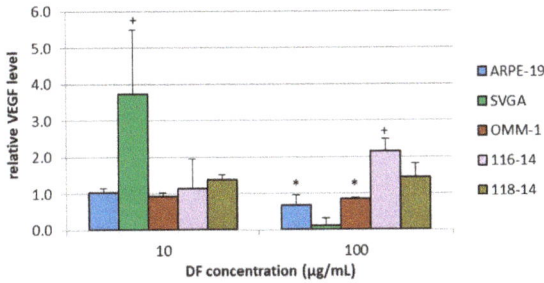

Figure 3. VEGF (vascular endothelial growth factor) secretion of ARPE-19, SVGA, OMM-1, 116-14 and 118-14 was assessed with ELISA (enzyme-linked immunosorbent assay) after treatment with 10 or 100 µg/mL DF extract for three days. The secreted individual VEGF amount in pg/mL was set in relation to the corresponding cell viability, which was determined in parallel. The mean values and standard deviation represent the mean of this calculated relative VEGF amount. Significance tests were performed with One-Way ANOVA with multiple comparison test; */+ $p < 0.05$, compared to untreated control group ($n \geq 4$).

2.5. Gene Expression

The effects of 10 and 100 µg/mL DF extract on the gene expression of VEGFR1, VEGFR2 and VEGF-A were determined with qPCR (quantitative polymerase chain reaction) after 24 and 72 h. The diagrams in Figures 4–6 depict the potentiated ΔΔCT values, which are determined in relation to the corresponding untreated controls, respectively (control = 1). Expression of VEGFR1 could not be determined in ARPE-19 or OMM-1. In addition, the DF extract had no significant influence on the VEGFR1 expression of SVGA, 116-14 and 118-14.

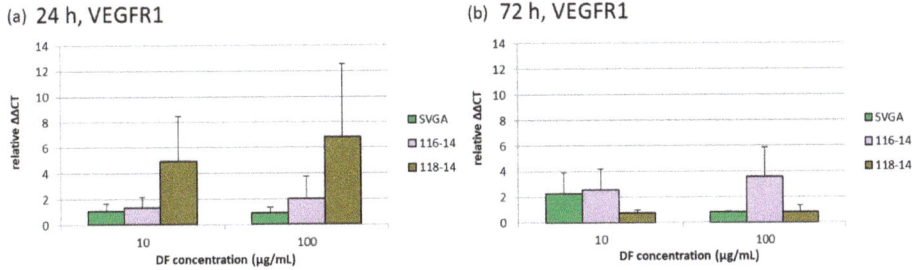

Figure 4. Relative gene expression of VEGFR1 (VEGF receptor 1) was determined with qPCR (quantitative polymerase chain reaction) after 24 (a) and 72 h (b) of treatment with 10 or 100 µg/mL DF extract. The potentiated ΔΔCT values are determined in relation to the corresponding untreated controls, respectively (control = 1). Significance tests were performed with One-Way ANOVA with multiple comparison test, compared to the untreated control group ($n \geq 4$).

VEGFR2 was expressed in all five cell cultures. There were no significant effects of the DF extract on the gene expression of VEGFR2 after 24 and 72 h of treatment, respectively, with one exception: the application of 100 µg/mL of the DF extract lowered the relative VEGFR2 expression in 116-14 to

0.66 [a.u.] ± 0.07 [a.u.] after 24 h. Although a statistical significance of this effect was determined, the biological relevance of this very small reduction of VEGFR2 in 116-14 must be considered critically.

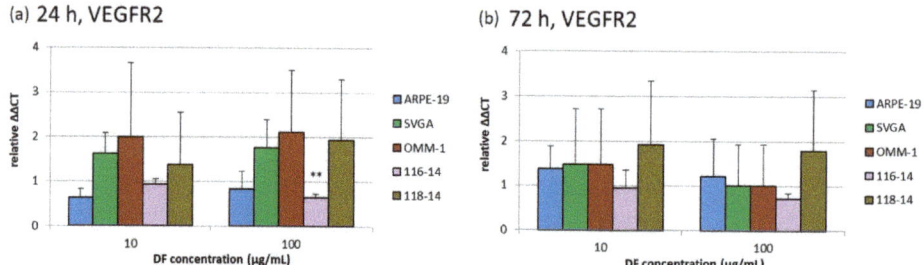

Figure 5. Relative gene expression of VEGFR2 (VEGF receptor 2) was determined with qPCR after 24 (**a**) and 72 h (**b**) of treatment with 10 and 100 µg/mL of the DF extract. The potentiated ΔΔCT values are determined in relation to the individual untreated controls, respectively (control = 1). Significance tests were performed with One-Way ANOVA with multiple comparison test; ** $p < 0.01$, compared to untreated control group ($n \geq 4$).

VEGF-A was expressed in all five cell types. Only 100 µg/mL DF increased the relative VEGF-A expression in 118-14 to 1.66 [a.u.] ± 0.13 [a.u.]. Despite the statistical significance of this effect, the very small increase of VEGF-A expression in 118-14 has to be considered to be of little biological relevance.

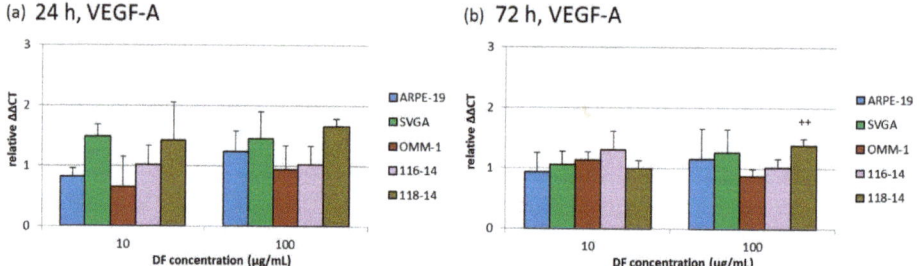

Figure 6. Relative gene expression of VEGF-A was determined with qPCR after 24 (**a**) and 72 h (**b**) of treatment with 10 or 100 µg/mL DF extract. The potentiated ΔΔCT values are determined in relation to the individual untreated controls, respectively (control = 1). Significance tests were performed with One-Way ANOVA with multiple comparison test; ++ $p < 0.01$, compared to untreated control group ($n \geq 4$).

3. Discussion

The DF extract investigated in this study strongly differs from other brown algae extracts usually consisting of fucose-rich sulfated polysaccharides. The main aim of this study was to evaluate potential anti-tumor effects of the DF extract on uveal melanoma and glioblastoma cell lines. For this purpose, we tested the effects of 10 and 100 µg/mL DF extract on the non-tumor cell lines ARPE-19 and SVGA as well as on the tumor cell line OMM-1, and the primary tumor cells 116-14 and 118-14. A first indication of anti-tumor effects of DF was described by Bittkau, Dörschmann et al., 2019. Here, 100 µg/mL DF extract reduced the cell viability of OMM-1 to nearly 75% after 24 h of treatment [22]. Futhermore, the cell viability of the cervical cancer cell line HeLa was reduced to 61–69% after 24 h, and to 70% after 72 h [22]. This corresponds to the data of this work where the OMM-1 viability was also reduced to 73% after 24 h, whereas the viability regenerated after 72 h to over 90%. Although DF lowered the viability of 118-14, this effect was quite small. The data of the viability assay also corresponds partially to the proliferation rate in case of OMM-1. In contrast to viability, ARPE-19 proliferation was not significantly inhibited and the cell number of 118-14 was reduced with a different concentration than in the cell viability assay. However, the small effects on the viability of 118-14 seem to be of little biological relevance. Regarding the effects on the gene expression of VEGF-A and its receptors, VEGFR1 and VEGFR2, only slightly increased or reduced expression levels could be detected. In detail, for VEGFR1 no significant effect was seen in the brain cells and for ARPE-19 and OMM-1 no expression of VEGFR1 was determined, which is in contrast to the literature for ARPE-19 [26] and could depend on the passage number or mutation level of these cells. An only very slight decrease of VEGFR2 expression was detected for 116-14 and a very small increase for VEGF-A was determined for 118-14. Since VEGF-A is well known to promote tumor progression [27], even a small effect is not desirable as an anticancer effect. However, an influence of fucoidans on the gene expression level is shown for commercially available fucoidan from *Undaria pinnatifida* (Marinova), which is able to change the gene expression of cancer-related and cell surface signaling-related pathways [28]. But this alga is from another brown algae order and was used in a clinical study with human blood serum, which could explain the differences. Nevertheless, the DF extract used in our study did not influence the expression of VEGF-A, VEGFR1 and VEGFR2 in our experimental setting.

So far, there are no further data or studies about cellular effects of extracts from the brown algae DF. However, a few other species of the order of Ectocarpales are described to contain fucoidans. Among these, fucoidans from *Cladosiphon okamuranus* were shown to exhibit anti-tumor effects after oral administration in a colon cancer mouse model by slowing down tumor growth and increasing the survival time depending on the molecular weight of the fucoidan [29]. This effect is suspected to correlate with an activation of the colon-associated immune cells [29].

In contrast, there are numerous reports on various anti-tumor effects of fucoidans from brown algae belonging to the orders of Laminariales and Fucales. For example, fucoidans from Fucus vesiculosus and Laminaria japonica, which are also commercially available, are often described to exhibit anti-tumor activities [30–37]. We previously found that any potential anti-tumor effects depended on the fucoidan source and the specific extract, respectively [18,19]. Middle- and low-molecular weight fucoidans from Laminaria hyperborea lowered the cell viability of OMM-1 cells [19], whereas enzymatically treated extracts from Laminaria digitata, Fucus distichus subsp. evanescens as well as various extracts from Saccharina latissima with different fucose content and degree of sulfation did not exhibit any anti-tumor effects on OMM-1 [20]. Dithmer et al., 2017 tested the effects of Fucus vesiculosus fucoidan from Sigma Aldrich on five different uveal melanoma cell types and on the one hand, this fucoidan had an anti-proliferative effect on the primary uveal melanoma cells Mel270, but not on the OMM-1 cells [38]. On the other hand, it decreased only the VEGF secretion by OMM-1 cells after three-day stimulation with the fucoidan [38]. The latter effect is consistent with the present results showing that DF extract reduced the VEGF secretion also by about 20%. However, in contrast to the Fucus vesiculosus fucoidan, the DF extract additionally had an antiproliferative effect on the OMM-1 cells. Thus, the two test compounds differed in their activities, which is probably due to their considerably different structural composition. Compared to the fucoidan, the DF extract has a more than two-fold lower sulfate and fucose content, but is characterized by 24.1% proteins [24,39]. These proteins were shown to be tightly associated with the glycans [25] as previously found for certain fractions of other fucoidans [40,41]. Since the DF extract displayed much weaker effects than other fucoidans in various activity assays (i.e., elastase inhibiting, anticomplement, and anticoagulant activities) [24], it can be assumed that its similar result in the VEGF secretion assay is mediated by molecules structurally different from those in the Fucus vesiculosus fucoidan and possibly also by a different mechanism. Regarding the antiproliferative activity of DF extract on OMM-1, it is known that the total phenolic content of fucoidans correlates with both their cell viability reducing effect and antioxidant capacity [18,39,42,43]. However, the DF extract has only a low content of phenols compared to other fucoidans [25], which is in line with its low antioxidant capacity [24]. Consequently, also its antiproliferative effect seems to be caused by other components. Comprehensive and challenging further analyses are needed to get more information on the structure of the glycan-protein-associates of the DF extract.

Regarding the effects of algae-derived substances on glioblastoma cells, knowledge is still limited. Nevertheless, studies with pheophorbide (chlorophyll breakdown product) from the red seaweed Grateloupia elliptica showed anticancer effects in U87MG cells (a human glioma cell line) by inducing G0/G1 cell cycle arrest, apoptosis and DNA degradation [44]. Further, nano-micro particles loaded with microalgae from Chlorella protothecoides and Nannochloropsis oculata had cytotoxic effects on human A-172 glioblastoma cells and HCT-116 (human colon colorectal carcinoma), whereas HUVEC (human umbilical vein endothelial cells) were not influenced [45]. It was speculated that microalgae contain anti-proliferative and apoptotic compounds and therefore, represent a source for the development of potential therapeutics [45]. Liao et al., 2019 showed that oligo-fucoidan from brown seaweed markedly suppressed the proliferation of U87MG cells and also regulated the gene expression of several differentiation markers [46]. Interestingly, Lv et al., 2012 stated that conditioned media taken from fucoidan-pretreated T98G glioblastoma cells inhibited endothelial cell tube formation leading to the assumption that at least *Fucus vesiculosus* (Sigma Aldrich) significantly inhibits angiogenesis induced by glioma cells. An up-regulation of sFlt-1 played an important role in this process [47]. In the presented study, however, relevant anti-proliferative effects on glioblastoma cells were absent, and DF extract even increased the VEGF secretion by 116-18 cells. These results might be due to the used experimental set-up, glioblastoma cell types and/or the test compound.

In general, this study again confirms the exact effects of fucoidans and brown algae extracts, respectively, on the reactions of tumor cell lines are highly dependent on the used cell line as well as on the structural composition and characteristics of the tested compound [22]. Thus, each fucoidan or brown algae extract has to be examined for each individual purpose.

Furthermore, the question of pharmaceutical applications for a possible tumor treatment is of high relevance. The bioavailability after oral administration of fucoidan is still under investigation [48–51]. However, different studies described that fucoidans can be taken up depending on the kind of application and the chemical characteristics. A *Fucus vesiculosus* fucoidan of 735 kDa in ointments can be applied topically and penetrate the skin reaching the blood plasma [50]. The same fucoidan was also detected in kidney, spleen and liver after oral administration of rats with long absorption and blood circulation times [49]. Furthermore, Japanese researches detected a high molecular weight fucoidan (3200 kDa) from *Okinawa mozuku* in urine after oral administration in human and rats [51]. Nevertheless, reaching clinical concentration in the desired tissue is a challenge and carrier/delivery systems for fucoidans would be of high interest.

In this study, we examined an extract from the brown alga DF with a composition different from that of typical fucoidans, for its potential anti-tumor effects in uveal melanoma and glioblastoma cells. However, it had no influence on glioblastoma cells, it showed some activities in the experiments with the uvea melanoma cell line OMM-1 by lowering the cell viability and exhibiting anti-proliferative and anti-angiogenic effects. The absence of negative effects on healthy cells like ARPE-19 and SVGA can be considered as beneficial, too.

Currently, there is no medicinal product approved for the treatment of uveal melanoma, the most important tumor disease of the eye, and thus a medical need for new therapies. Although the basic experiments with the DF extract look promising, this extract as well as fucoidans are associated with some obstacles regarding medical applications. This includes their complex composition and the strong requirements on the pharmaceutical quality of drug substances as well as the biopharmaceutical properties of these negatively charged macromolecules. For the treatment of uveal melanoma intravitreal application would also be of interest.

4. Material and Methods

4.1. Extraction and Chemical Characterization

The DF alga was harvested in May 2017 in the Baltic Sea (Kiel Fjord) and provided by Coastal Research and Management GmbH (Kiel, Germany). Extraction and purification was performed as described before [40]. In short: The pulverized algal material was defatted with Soxhlet extraction (99% *v/v* ethanol). The main extraction was performed with aqueous 2% $CaCl_2$ at 85 °C for 2 h (reflux condition). The supernatant was evaporated and precipitated with ethanol (final concentration 60% *v/v*) at 4 °C. Further steps involved centrifugation, dissolving in demineralized water, dialysis and lyophilisation. The following chemical parameters of the DF extract were analyzed as previously described [24,25]: Sulfate content and degree of sulfation, weight average molecular weight, monosaccharide composition, contents of protein, uronic acid content, and phenolic compounds as well as size distribution and chain conformation.

The dried extract was solved in Ampuwa bidest. (Fresenius, Schweinfurt, Germany) to a stock concentration of 1 mg/mL. Before use in experiments, the stock solution was diluted to 100 µg/mL in appropriate medium, sterile filtered with 0.2 µm Sarstedt filters (Nümbrecht, Germany) and further diluted with medium to 10 µg/mL. Final medium concentrations were 10 and 100 µg/mL in each case. The final medium volume was 1 mL per well in 12 well plates (Sections 2.3–2.5 assays) and 100 µL per well in 96 well plates (Section 2.2), respectively.

4.2. Cell Culture and Reagents

Used cell lines were the uveal melanoma cell line OMM-1 [52], the human RPE cell line ARPE-19 [53], the human fetal astrocyte cell line SVGA and the human glioblastoma (GBM) primary cells 116-14 and 118-14. ARPE-19 was purchased from ATCC (ATCC, Manassas, VA, USA). OMM-1 was kindly provided by Dr. Sarah Coupland, University of Liverpool. The human fetal astrocyte cell line SVGA was kindly provided by the group of Christine Hanssen Rinaldo, University Hospital of North Norway [54] with the permission of W. J. Altwood [55]. RPMI 1640 (Merck, Darmstadt, Germany), which was supplemented with 10% fetal calf serum (Linaris GmbH, Wertheim-Bettingen, Germany) and 1% penicillin/streptomycin (Merck), was used for OMM-1. Cultivation medium for ARPE-19 was HyClone Dulbecco's modified Eagle's medium (DMEM; GE Healthcare, München, Germany), with 10% fetal calf serum, 1% penicillin/streptomycin, 2.5% HEPES (4-(2-hydroxyethyl)-1-piperazineethanesulfonic acid, Merck) and 1% non-essential amino acids (Merck). Cultured human primary GBM cells were generated by dissociation of surgically dissected tumor materials and cultured in DMEM (Life Technologies, Carlsbad, CA, USA) supplemented with 10% fetal bovine serum (FBS; Invitrogen, Carlsbad, CA, USA or PAN-Biotech GmbH, Aidenbach, Germany), 1% Penicillin–Streptomycin (10,000 U/mL; Thermo Fisher Scientific, Waltham, MA, USA), and 2 mM additional L-glutamine (Thermo Fisher Scientific). Materials were obtained in accordance with the Helsinki Declaration of 1964 and its later amendments and with approval of the ethics committee of the University of Kiel, Germany after written informed consent of donors (file references: D571/15 and D524/17). Tumors were diagnosed and classified according to WHO criteria by a pathologist. All cell lines were stored at 37 °C and 5% CO_2 in a humidified incubator, seeded at 100,000 cells/mL and treated at 80% subconfluence. For the experiments adequate medium without phenol red was used.

4.3. Cell Viability Assay

To measure cell viability after treatment with DF extract for 24 and 72 h, the MTS assay was performed after seeding the cells in a 96 well plate. The commercially available CellTiter 96® AQueous One Solution Cell Proliferation Assay from Promega Corporation (Mannheim, Germany) was used. The assay was conducted according to the supplier's instructions. In brief, 20 µL MTS solution was put into each well and the plates were incubated for 1 h in the 37 °C incubator. Measurements were taken at 490 nm with the Elx800 (BioTek Instruments Inc., Bad Friedrichshall, Germany).

4.4. Cell Proliferation Assay

Cells were seeded at 100,000 cells/mL in a 24-well plate. The cell number was counted before seeding and after 24 h as well as 72 h of incubation. For the counting trypan blue solution was used (Merck). Cells were counted with an inverted light microscope Axiovert 100 (Carl Zeiss AG, Oberkochen, Germany).

4.5. VEGF ELISA

Cells were seeded into 24 well plates and treated with DF for three days, followed by the collection of the supernatant. A media exchange was conducted 24 h before supernatant collection. To determine the secreted VEGF amount the human VEGF DuoSet ELISA from R&D Systems (Wiesbaden, Germany) was used. The assay was performed according to the producer's instructions. In parallel, the cell viability of the cells was determined to set it in relation to the secreted VEGF.

4.6. Real-Time PCR

RNA was isolated with the TRIZOL reagent (Invitrogen, Carlsbad, CA, USA), digested by DNase (Promega, Madison, WI, USA), and cDNA was synthesized using RevertAidTM H minus reverse transcriptase, (Thermo Scientific, Schwerte, Germany). Quantitative reverse transcription real time PCR (qRT-PCR) was performed using TaqMan primer probes (Applied Biosystems, Foster City, CA, USA) as described before [56]: glycerinaldehyde-3-phosphate-dehydrogenase (GAPDH) (Hs99999905_m1), VEGF-A (Hs_00173626_m1), FLT-1/VEGFR1 (Hs00176573_m1), KDR/VEGFR2 (Hs_00176676_m1). Fluorescent data were converted into cycle threshold (CT) measurements. ΔCT values of each sample were calculated as $CT_{gene\ of\ interest} - CT_{GAPDH}$. A ΔCT value of 3.33 corresponds to one magnitude lower gene expression compared to GAPDH. Relative gene expression ($\Delta\Delta$CT values) was calculated with $2^{(normalized\ CT\ non-stimulated\ -\ normalized\ CT\ stimulated)}$ = n-fold of control.

4.7. Statistics

Four independent experiments per test were conducted at least. Diagrams, data tables and statistics were created with Microsoft Excel (Excel 2010, Microsoft, Redmond, WA, USA). The mean and standard deviation were calculated and pictured in the diagrams. Significances were calculated via One-Way ANOVA and multiple comparison tests with GraphPad PRISM 7 (GraphPad Software, Inc., San Diego, CA, USA, 2017). p-values under 0.05 were considered significant.

5. Conclusions

In contrast to other fucoidans, an extract from the brown alga *Dictyosiphon foeniculaceus* (DF extract) showed anti-proliferative effects on two tumor cell lines in a previous study. The aim of this work was, therefore, to evaluate potential antitumor effects of the DF extract on uveal melanoma (OMM-1) and glioblastoma cells (116-14, 118-14). For comparison, two healthy human cell lines (ARPE-19, SVGA) were included in the study. Tests for cell viability, VEGF secretion, proliferation and gene expression of VEGF-A, VEGFR1 and VEGFR2 were conducted after treatment with the DF extract. The extract decreased the cell viability and the proliferation of the OMM-1 cell line after 72 h, whereas neither the glioblastoma nor the healthy cells were affected. The gene expression of VEGFR1 was not influenced. The VEGFR2 mRNA expression was slightly decreased after 24 h in 116-14 cells, whereas the VEGF-A mRNA expression was increased in 118-14 cells after 72 h of stimulation. VEGF secretion by SVGA and 116-14 cells was increased after three days, but, conversely, that by ARPE-19 and OMM-1 was decreased, which indicates a potential anti-angiogenic effect. Thus, these initial experiments suggest that DF extract does not influence glioblastoma cells, but could exhibit anti-tumor effects on uveal melanoma.

Finally, the study with an DF extract demonstrated that not each brown alga contains considerable amounts of typical fucoidans, but these cell wall components may be "replaced" by other protein-associated glycans. Extracts from such algae do not exhibit activities as expected for typical fucoidans, but may have other activities as observed in this study.

Author Contributions: Conceptualization, A.K., J.H.-F., M.S. and S.A.; Methodology, C.S., K.S.B., S.N. and P.D.; Validation, C.S. and P.D.; Formal Analysis, A.K., J.H.-F. and P.D.; Investigation, P.D.; Resources, A.K., M.S. and J.R.; Data Curation, C.S. and P.D.; Writing—Original Draft Preparation, P.D.; Writing—Review and Editing, A.K., C.S., K.S.B., J.H.-F., J.R., M.S., P.D., S.A. and S.N.; Visualization, P.D.; Supervision, A.K., J.H.-F., J.R. and M.S. All authors have read and agreed to the published version of the manuscript.

Funding: This study is part of the FucoSan-Health from the Sea Project, is supported by EU InterReg-Deutschland-Denmark and the European Fund of Regional Development, and was funded by the German Research Foundation (DFG) as part of the Research Training Group "Materials4Brain" (RTG2154).

Acknowledgments: We thank the Coastal Research & Management for the provision of the algae, and Fereshteh Ebrahim and Brigitte Rehmke for expert technical assistance.

Conflicts of Interest: The authors declare no conflict of interest.

References

1. Ohgaki, H.; Kleihues, P. Epidemiology and etiology of gliomas. *Acta Neuropathol.* **2005**, *109*, 93–108. [CrossRef]
2. Gousias, K.; Markou, M.; Voulgaris, S.; Goussia, A.; Voulgari, P.; Bai, M.; Polyzoidis, K.; Kyritsis, A.; Alamanos, Y. Descriptive Epidemiology of Cerebral Gliomas in Northwest Greece and Study of Potential Predisposing Factors, 2005–2007. *Neuroepidemiology* **2009**, *33*, 89–95. [CrossRef] [PubMed]
3. Braun, K.; Ahluwalia, M.S. Treatment of Glioblastoma in Older Adults. *Curr. Oncol. Rep.* **2017**, *19*, 81. [CrossRef]
4. Thakkar, J.P.; Dolecek, T.A.; Horbinski, C.; Ostrom, Q.T.; Lightner, D.D.; Barnholtz-Sloan, J.S.; Villano, J.L. Epidemiologic and Molecular Prognostic Review of Glioblastoma. *Cancer Epidemiol. Biomark. Prev.* **2014**, *23*, 1985–1996. [CrossRef] [PubMed]
5. Kaliki, S.; Shields, C.L. Uveal melanoma: Relatively rare but deadly cancer. *Eye* **2017**, *31*, 241–257. [CrossRef] [PubMed]
6. Voelter, V.; Schalenbourg, A.; Pampallona, S.; Peters, S.; Halkic, N.; Denys, A.; Goitein, G.; Zografos, L.; Leyvraz, S. Adjuvant intra-arterial hepatic fotemustine for high-risk uveal melanoma patients. *Melanoma Res.* **2008**, *18*, 220–224. [CrossRef] [PubMed]
7. Chattopadhyay, C.; Kim, D.W.; Gombos, D.S.; Oba, J.; Qin, Y.; Williams, M.D.; Esmaeli, B.; Grimm, E.A.; Wargo, J.A.; Woodman, S.E.; et al. Uveal melanoma: From diagnosis to treatment and the science in between. *Cancer* **2016**, *122*, 2299–2312. [CrossRef]
8. Willcox, D.C.; Scapagnini, G.; Willcox, B.J. Healthy aging diets other than the Mediterranean: A focus on the Okinawan diet. *Mech. Ageing Dev.* **2014**, *136–137*, 148–162. [CrossRef]
9. Ford, L.; Stratakos, A.C.; Theodoridou, K.; Dick, J.T.A.; Sheldrake, G.N.; Linton, M.; Corcionivoschi, N.; Walsh, P.J. Polyphenols from Brown Seaweeds as a Potential Antimicrobial Agent in Animal Feeds. *ACS Omega* **2020**, *5*, 9093–9103. [CrossRef]
10. Dobrinčić, A.; Balbino, S.; Zorić, Z.; Pedisić, S.; Bursać Kovačević, D.; Elez Garofulić, I.; Dragović-Uzelac, V. Advanced Technologies for the Extraction of Marine Brown Algal Polysaccharides. *Mar. Drugs* **2020**, *18*, 168. [CrossRef]
11. Klettner, A. Fucoidan as a Potential Therapeutic for Major Blinding Diseases—A Hypothesis. *Mar. Drugs* **2016**, *14*, 31. [CrossRef] [PubMed]
12. Freitas, R.; Martins, A.; Silva, J.; Alves, C.; Pinteus, S.; Alves, J.; Teodoro, F.; Ribeiro, H.M.; Gonçalves, L.M.D.; Petrovski, Ž.; et al. Highlighting the Biological Potential of the Brown Seaweed *Fucus spiralis* for Skin Applications. *Antioxidants* **2020**, *9*, 611. [CrossRef] [PubMed]
13. Hsu, H.-Y.; Hwang, P. Clinical applications of fucoidan in translational medicine for adjuvant cancer therapy. *Clin. Transl. Med.* **2019**, *8*, 15. [CrossRef] [PubMed]
14. Pozharitskaya, O.; Obluchinskaya, E.; Shikov, A. Mechanisms of Bioactivities of Fucoidan from the Brown Seaweed Fucus vesiculosus L. of the Barents Sea. *Mar. Drugs* **2020**, *18*, 275. [CrossRef] [PubMed]
15. Wang, L.; Oh, J.Y.; Kim, Y.-S.; Jeon, Y.-J.; Lee, J.-S.; Jeon, Y.-J. Anti-Photoaging and Anti-Melanogenesis Effects of Fucoidan Isolated from *Hizikia fusiforme* and Its Underlying Mechanisms. *Mar. Drugs* **2020**, *18*, 427. [CrossRef]
16. Fitton, J.H.; Dell'Acqua, G.; Gardiner, V.-A.; Karpiniec, S.; Stringer, D.N.; Davis, E. Topical Benefits of Two Fucoidan-Rich Extracts from Marine Macroalgae. *Cosmetics* **2015**, *2*, 66–81. [CrossRef]

17. Fitton, J.H.; Stringer, D.N.; Karpiniec, S. Therapies from Fucoidan: An Update. *Mar. Drugs* **2015**, *13*, 5920–5946. [CrossRef]
18. Dörschmann, P.; Bittkau, K.S.; Neupane, S.; Roider, J.; Alban, S.; Klettner, A. Effects of Fucoidans from Five Different Brown Algae on Oxidative Stress and VEGF Interference in Ocular Cells. *Mar. Drugs* **2019**, *17*, 258. [CrossRef]
19. Dörschmann, P.; Kopplin, G.; Roider, J.; Klettner, A. Effects of Sulfated Fucans from Laminaria hyperborea Regarding VEGF Secretion, Cell Viability, and Oxidative Stress and Correlation with Molecular Weight. *Mar. Drugs* **2019**, *17*, 548. [CrossRef]
20. Dörschmann, P.; Mikkelsen, M.D.; Nguyen, T.T.; Roider, J.; Meyer, A.S.; Klettner, A. Effects of a Newly Developed Enzyme-Assisted Extraction Method on the Biological Activities of Fucoidans in Ocular Cells. *Mar. Drugs* **2020**, *18*, 282. [CrossRef]
21. Rohwer, K.; Neupane, S.; Bittkau, K.S.; Galarza Pérez, M.; Dörschmann, P.; Roider, J.; Alban, S.; Klettner, A. Effects of Crude Fucus distichus Subspecies evanescens Fucoidan Extract on Retinal Pigment Epithelium Cells-Implications for Use in Age-Related Macular Degeneration. *Mar. Drugs* **2019**, *17*, 538. [CrossRef] [PubMed]
22. Bittkau, K.S.; Dörschmann, P.; Blümel, M.; Tasdemir, D.; Roider, J.; Klettner, A.; Alban, S. Comparison of the Effects of Fucoidans on the Cell Viability of Tumor and Non-Tumor Cell Lines. *Mar. Drugs* **2019**, *17*, 441. [CrossRef] [PubMed]
23. Greville, R.K. *Algae Britannicae, or Descriptions of the Marine and Other Inarticulated Plants of the British Islands, Belonging to the Order Algae; with Plates Illustrative of the Genera*; McLachlan & Stewart: Edinburgh, Scotland; Baldwin & Cradock: London, UK, 1830; pp. 1–218.
24. Bittkau, K.S.; Neupane, S.; Alban, S. Initial evaluation of six different brown algae species as source for crude bioactive fucoidans. *Algal Res.* **2020**, *45*, 101759. [CrossRef]
25. Neupane, S.; Bittkau, K.S.; Alban, S. Size distribution and chain conformation of six different fucoidans using size-exclusion chromatography with multiple detection. *J. Chromatogr. A* **2020**, *1612*, 460658. [CrossRef]
26. Miyamoto, N.; De Kozak, Y.; Jeanny, J.C.; Glotin, A.; Mascarelli, F.; Massin, P.; Benezra, D.; Behar-Cohen, F.F. Placental growth factor-1 and epithelial haemato–retinal barrier breakdown: Potential implication in the pathogenesis of diabetic retinopathy. *Diabetologia* **2006**, *50*, 461–470. [CrossRef] [PubMed]
27. Ameratunga, M.; Pavlakis, N.; Wheeler, H.; Grant, R.; Simes, J.; Khasraw, M. Anti-angiogenic therapy for high-grade glioma. *Cochrane Database Syst. Rev.* **2018**, *11*, 008218. [CrossRef] [PubMed]
28. Gueven, N.; Spring, K.J.; Holmes, S.; Ahuja, K.D.K.; Eri, R.; Park, A.Y.; Fitton, J.H. Micro RNA Expression after Ingestion of Fucoidan; A Clinical Study. *Mar. Drugs* **2020**, *18*, 143. [CrossRef]
29. Azuma, K.; Ishihara, T.; Nakamoto, H.; Amaha, T.; Osaki, T.; Tsuka, T.; Imagawa, T.; Minami, S.; Takashima, O.; Ifuku, S.; et al. Effects of Oral Administration of Fucoidan Extracted from Cladosiphon okamuranus on Tumor Growth and Survival Time in a Tumor-Bearing Mouse Model. *Mar. Drugs* **2012**, *10*, 2337–2348. [CrossRef]
30. Venkatesan, J.; Singh, S.K.; Anil, S.; Kim, S.-K.; Shim, M.S. Preparation, Characterization and Biological Applications of Biosynthesized Silver Nanoparticles with Chitosan-Fucoidan Coating. *Molecules* **2018**, *23*, 1429. [CrossRef]
31. Huang, Y.-C.; Lam, U.-I. Chitosan/Fucoidan pH Sensitive Nanoparticles for Oral Delivery System. *J. Chin. Chem. Soc.* **2011**, *58*, 779–785. [CrossRef]
32. Jang, B.; Moorthy, M.S.; Manivasagan, P.; Xu, L.; Song, K.; Lee, K.D.; Kwak, M.; Oh, J.; Jin, J.-O. Fucoidan-coated CuS nanoparticles for chemo-and photothermal therapy against cancer. *Oncotarget* **2018**, *9*, 12649–12661. [CrossRef] [PubMed]
33. Kim, H.; Nguyen, V.P.; Manivasagan, P.; Jung, M.J.; Kim, S.W.; Oh, J.; Kang, H.W. Doxorubicin-fucoidan-gold nanoparticles composite for dual-chemo-photothermal treatment on eye tumors. *Oncotarget* **2017**, *8*, 113719–113733. [CrossRef] [PubMed]
34. Lee, K.W.; Jeong, D.; Na, K. Doxorubicin loading fucoidan acetate nanoparticles for immune and chemotherapy in cancer treatment. *Carbohydr. Polym.* **2013**, *94*, 850–856. [CrossRef] [PubMed]
35. Lu, K.-Y.; Li, R.; Hsu, C.-H.; Lin, C.; Chou, S.-C.; Tsai, M.-L.; Mi, F.-L. Development of a new type of multifunctional fucoidan-based nanoparticles for anticancer drug delivery. *Carbohydr. Polym.* **2017**, *165*, 410–420. [CrossRef] [PubMed]

36. Pawar, V.K.; Singh, Y.; Sharma, K.; Shrivastav, A.; Sharma, A.; Singh, A.; Meher, J.G.; Singh, P.; Raval, K.; Kumar, A.; et al. Improved chemotherapy against breast cancer through immunotherapeutic activity of fucoidan decorated electrostatically assembled nanoparticles bearing doxorubicin. *Int. J. Biol. Macromol.* **2019**, *122*, 1100–1114. [CrossRef]
37. Wang, P.; Kankala, R.K.; Chen, B.; Long, R.; Cai, D.; Liu, Y.; Wang, S. Poly-allylamine hydrochloride and fucoidan-based self-assembled polyelectrolyte complex nanoparticles for cancer therapeutics. *J. Biomed. Mater. Res. Part A* **2018**, *107*, 339–347. [CrossRef]
38. Dithmer, M.; Kirsch, A.-M.; Richert, E.; Fuchs, S.; Wang, F.; Schmidt, H.; Coupland, S.E.; Roider, J.; Klettner, A. Fucoidan Does Not Exert Anti-Tumorigenic Effects on Uveal Melanoma Cell Lines. *Mar. Drugs* **2017**, *15*, 193. [CrossRef]
39. Lahrsen, E.; Liewert, I.; Alban, S. Gradual degradation of fucoidan from Fucus vesiculosus and its effect on structure, antioxidant and antiproliferative activities. *Carbohydr. Polym.* **2018**, *192*, 208–216. [CrossRef]
40. Ehrig, K.; Alban, S. Sulfated Galactofucan from the Brown Alga Saccharina latissima—Variability of Yield, Structural Composition and Bioactivity. *Mar. Drugs* **2014**, *13*, 76–101. [CrossRef]
41. Deniaud-Bouët, E.; Kervarec, N.; Michel, G.; Tonon, T.; Kloareg, B.; Hervé, C. Chemical and enzymatic fractionation of cell walls from Fucales: Insights into the structure of the extracellular matrix of brown algae. *Ann. Bot.* **2014**, *114*, 1203–1216. [CrossRef]
42. Schneider, T.; Ehrig, K.; Liewert, I.; Alban, S. Interference with the CXCL12/CXCR4 axis as potential antitumor strategy: Superiority of a sulfated galactofucan from the brown algaSaccharina latissimaand Fucoidan over heparins. *Glycobiology* **2015**, *25*, 812–824. [CrossRef] [PubMed]
43. Yuan, Y.V.; Walsh, N.A. Antioxidant and antiproliferative activities of extracts from a variety of edible seaweeds. *Food Chem. Toxicol.* **2006**, *44*, 1144–1150. [CrossRef] [PubMed]
44. Cho, M.; Park, G.-M.; Kim, S.-N.; Amna, T.; Lee, S.; Shin, W.-S. Glioblastoma-Specific Anticancer Activity of Pheophorbide a from the Edible Red Seaweed Grateloupia elliptica. *J. Microbiol. Biotechnol.* **2014**, *24*, 346–353. [CrossRef] [PubMed]
45. Karakaş, C.Y.; Şahin, H.T.; Inan, B.; Özçimen, D.; Erginer, Y.Ö. In vitro cytotoxic activity of microalgal extracts loaded nano–micro particles produced via electrospraying and microemulsion methods. *Biotechnol. Prog.* **2019**, *35*, e2876. [CrossRef]
46. Liao, C.-H.; Lai, I.-C.; Kuo, H.-C.; Chuang, S.-E.; Lee, H.-L.; Whang-Peng, J.; Lai, G.-M.; Lai, G.-M. Epigenetic Modification and Differentiation Induction of Malignant Glioma Cells by Oligo-Fucoidan. *Mar. Drugs* **2019**, *17*, 525. [CrossRef] [PubMed]
47. Lv, Y.; Song, Q.; Shao, Q.; Gao, W.; Mao, H.; Lou, H.; Qu, X.; Li, X. Comparison of the effects of marchantin C and fucoidan on sFlt-1 and angiogenesis in glioma microenvironment. *J. Pharm. Pharmacol.* **2012**, *64*, 604–609. [CrossRef] [PubMed]
48. Zhao, X.; Guo, F.; Hu, J.; Zhang, L.; Xue, C.; Zhang, Z.; Li, B. Antithrombotic activity of oral administered low molecular weight fucoidan from Laminaria Japonica. *Thromb. Res.* **2016**, *144*, 46–52. [CrossRef]
49. Pozharitskaya, O.N.; Shikov, A.N.; Faustova, N.M.; Obluchinskaya, E.; Kosman, V.M.; Vuorela, H.; Makarov, V.G. Pharmacokinetic and Tissue Distribution of Fucoidan from Fucus vesiculosus after Oral Administration to Rats. *Mar. Drugs* **2018**, *16*, 132. [CrossRef]
50. Pozharitskaya, O.; Shikov, A.; Obluchinskaya, E.; Vuorela, H. The Pharmacokinetics of Fucoidan after Topical Application to Rats. *Mar. Drugs* **2019**, *17*, 687. [CrossRef]
51. Tokita, Y.; Hirayama, M.; Nakajima, K.; Tamaki, K.; Iha, M.; Nagamine, T. Detection of Fucoidan in Urine after Oral Intake of Traditional Japanese Seaweed, Okinawa mozuku (Cladosiphon okamuranus Tokida). *J. Nutr. Sci. Vitaminol.* **2017**, *63*, 419–421. [CrossRef]
52. Luyten, G.P.M.; Naus, N.C.; Mooy, C.M.; Hagemeijer, A.; Kan-Mitchell, J.; Van Drunen, E.; Vuzevski, V.; De Jong, P.T.V.M.; Luider, T.M. Establishment and characterization of primary and metastatic uveal melanoma cell lines. *Int. J. Cancer* **1996**, *66*, 380–387. [CrossRef]
53. Dunn, K.; Aotaki-Keen, A.; Putkey, F.; Hjelmeland, L. ARPE-19, A Human Retinal Pigment Epithelial Cell Line with Differentiated Properties. *Exp. Eye Res.* **1996**, *62*, 155–170. [CrossRef] [PubMed]
54. Henriksen, S.; Tylden, G.D.; Dumoulin, A.; Sharma, B.N.; Hirsch, H.H.; Rinaldo, C.H. The Human Fetal Glial Cell Line SVG p12 Contains Infectious BK Polyomavirus. *J. Virol.* **2014**, *88*, 7556–7568. [CrossRef] [PubMed]
55. Schweighardt, J.T.S.B.; Shieh, J.T.C.; Atwood, W.J. CD4/CXCR4-independent infection of human astrocytes by a T-tropic strain of HIV-1. *J. NeuroVirol.* **2001**, *7*, 155–162. [CrossRef] [PubMed]

56. Adamski, V.; Hempelmann, A.; Flüh, C.; Lucius, R.; Synowitz, M.; Hattermann, K.; Held-Feindt, J. Dormant glioblastoma cells acquire stem cell characteristics and are differentially affected by Temozolomide and AT101 treatment. *Oncotarget* **2017**, *8*, 108064–108078. [CrossRef]

Publisher's Note: MDPI stays neutral with regard to jurisdictional claims in published maps and institutional affiliations.

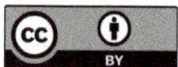 © 2020 by the authors. Licensee MDPI, Basel, Switzerland. This article is an open access article distributed under the terms and conditions of the Creative Commons Attribution (CC BY) license (http://creativecommons.org/licenses/by/4.0/).

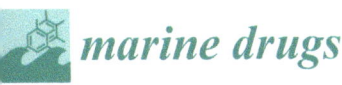

Article

The Inhibition Effect of the Seaweed Polyphenol, 7-Phloro-Eckol from *Ecklonia cava* on Alcohol-Induced Oxidative Stress in HepG2/CYP2E1 Cells

Liyuan Lin [1,2,†], Shengtao Yang [1,2,†], Zhenbang Xiao [1,2], Pengzhi Hong [1,2], Shengli Sun [1], Chunxia Zhou [1,2] and Zhong-Ji Qian [1,2,*]

[1] School of Chemistry and Environment, Shenzhen Institute of Guangdong Ocean University, College of Food Science and Technology, Guangdong Ocean University, Zhanjiang 524-088, China; liyuanlin1024@163.com (L.L.); 15766385620@163.com (S.Y.); xzhenbang@163.com (Z.X.); hongpengzhigdou@163.com (P.H.); xinglsun@126.com (S.S.); chunxia.zhou@163.com (C.Z.)
[2] Southern Marine Science and Engineering Guangdong Laboratory, Zhanjiang 524-088, China
* Correspondence: zjqian@gdou.edu.cn; Tel.: +86-1860-759-6590
† These authors contribute equally in this work.

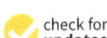

Citation: Lin, L.; Yang, S.; Xiao, Z.; Hong, P.; Sun, S.; Zhou, C.; Qian, Z.-J. The Inhibition Effect of the Seaweed Polyphenol, 7-Phloro-Eckol from *Ecklonia cava* on Alcohol-Induced Oxidative Stress in HepG2/CYP2E1 Cells. *Mar. Drugs* 2021, 19, 158. https://doi.org/10.3390/md19030158

Academic Editor: Roland Ulber

Received: 12 February 2021
Accepted: 16 March 2021
Published: 17 March 2021

Publisher's Note: MDPI stays neutral with regard to jurisdictional claims in published maps and institutional affiliations.

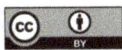

Copyright: © 2021 by the authors. Licensee MDPI, Basel, Switzerland. This article is an open access article distributed under the terms and conditions of the Creative Commons Attribution (CC BY) license (https:// creativecommons.org/licenses/by/ 4.0/).

Abstract: The liver is vulnerable to oxidative stress-induced damage, which leads to many diseases, including alcoholic liver disease (ALD). Liver disease endanger people's health, and the incidence of ALD is increasing; therefore, prevention is very important. 7-phloro-eckol (7PE) is a seaweed polyphenol, which was isolated from *Ecklonia cava* in a previous study. In this study, the antioxidative stress effect of 7PE on HepG2/CYP2E1 cells was evaluated by alcohol-induced cytotoxicity, DNA damage, and expression of related inflammation and apoptosis proteins. The results showed that 7PE caused alcohol-induced cytotoxicity to abate, reduced the amount of reactive oxygen species (ROS) and nitric oxide (NO), and effectively inhibited DNA damage in HepG2/CYP2E1 cells. Additionally, the expression levels of glutathione (GSH), superoxide dismutase (SOD), B cell lymphoma 2 (Bcl-2), and Akt increased, while γ-glutamyltransferase (GGT), Bcl-2 related x (Bax), cleaved caspase-3, cleaved caspase-9, nuclear factor-κB (NF-κB), and JNK decreased. Finally, molecular docking proved that 7PE could bind to BCL-2 and GSH protein. These results indicate that 7PE can alleviate the alcohol-induced oxidative stress injury of HepG2 cells and that 7PE may have a potential application prospect in the future development of antioxidants.

Keywords: 7-phloro-eckol; HepG2/CYP2E1 cells; oxidative stress; apoptosis

1. Introduction

The liver is the main organ of alcohol metabolism, and the adverse reaction of alcohol metabolism will damage the liver [1]. The main cause of alcoholic liver disease (ALD) is long-term excessive drinking. ALD symptoms, including alcohol fatty liver disease and alcohol hepatitis, can further lead to steatohepatitis, liver fibrosis, cirrhosis, and the most severe form of liver cancer [2]. In China, liver disease affects about 300 million people, and the number of cases of ALD is increasing, with a major impact on the global burden of liver disease [3]. Fat accumulation in the liver occurs in the early stages of ALD, and only this stage can be reversed without any medical intervention; therefore, early diagnosis and proper treatment of ALD are essential before irreversible liver damage occurs [4].

Due to the production of reactive oxygen species (ROS) during alcohol metabolism, the liver is vulnerable to oxidative stress-induced injury [5]. Oxidative stress induced by free radicals has been reported to play a key role in the degeneration, inflammation, apoptosis, and necrosis of hepatocytes [6]. ROS molecules are highly active and play an important role in cell functions but are also closely related to pathology. High levels of ROS can cause cell death by damaging the cell structure by oxidation of nucleic acids, proteins, and lipids [7]. Nitric Oxide (NO) is also involved in a wide range of toxic oxidative reactions with ROS [8].

Therefore, inhibiting the level of reactive oxygen species may be a way to prevent ALD. Among them, ROS can be eliminated by antioxidant metalloenzymes, such as superoxide dismutase (SOD) [9]. Glutathione (GSH), as an important antioxidant, can scavenge free radicals in the body [10]. The activity of γ -glutamyltransferases (GGT) also can be used as a marker for ALD evaluation [11,12]. Moreover, when free radicals damage the kidney, the inflammatory reaction, which is usually the mechanism of protection and repair, will appear and may stimulate the formation of other free radicals [13]. In addition, ROS can act as the second messengers of intracellular signal transduction cascades and regulate the expression of apoptotic genes through MAPK activation, thus increasing apoptosis. It is reported that Bcl-2 related x (Bax) proteins related to caspase-3 and B cell lymphoma 2 (BCL-2) play a key role in apoptosis [14]. Apoptosis can also be activated by other signal molecules [8], such as Akt [15], nuclear factor-κB (NF-κB) [16], and JNK [17], a member of mitogen-activated protein kinase.

In recent decades, a large number of highly effective and low-toxicity marine active substances have been discovered in the vast ocean [18]. Among them, seaweed, as one of the important plants in the marine, has a variety of active components and has been widely studied [19,20]. The active ingredients of seaweed include Sulfated seaweed polysaccharides [21], polyphenols [22], proteins [23], terpenes [24], alkaloids [25], phenolic compounds [26], and halogenated compounds [27]. Among these ingredients, seaweed polyphenols are considered a good source of antioxidants [28]. 7-phloro-eckol (7PE), a seaweed polyphenol, was extracted from edible brown algae, *Ecklonia cava* [29], and its structure was similar to eckol and dieckol. It is noteworthy that eckol and dieckol have been reported to have anticancer [30,31] and antioxidant [31–35] properties and modulate anti-monoamine oxidases [36], but the role of 7PE has received little attention. Therefore, 7PE, with a structure similar to eckol and dieckol, has high research value.

In order to prove that 7PE can be used as a potential preventive substance against oxidative stress, ethanol-induced oxidative stress in HepG2/CYP2E1 cells was used as a mature model [37,38]. Our data suggest that 7PE inhibits ethanol-induced oxidative stress, which indicates that 7PE has antioxidant potential and is expected to be the source of antioxidant development in the future.

2. Results

2.1. Effects of 7PE on Cell Viability of HepG2/CYP2E1 Cells

The results showed no significant change in the viability of HepG2/CYP2E1 cells (Figure 1b), which indicated that there was no toxic effect of 7PE treatment of up to 100 μM. Thus, the employed concentrations (0, 10, 20, 50, and 100 μM) of 7PE were used in all the subsequent experiments. Figure 1c shows that ethanol decreased cell viability in a dose-dependent manner. Cell viability was approximately 50% when cells were exposed to 0.5 M ethanol. As depicted in Figure 1d, treatment with 7PE significantly increased the viability of HepG2/CYP2E1 cells following exposure to 0.5 M ethanol. The results showed that 7PE (20, 50, and 100 μM) could effectively prevent damage to HepG2/CYP2E1 cells from ethanol.

2.2. Determination of Intracellular ROS and NO

The cells were treated as shown in Figure 2, then treated with 2,7-dichlorodi-hydrofluorescein diacetate (DCFH-DA) and 3-amino,4-aminomethyl-2′,7′-difluorescein diacetate (DAF-FM-DA), respectively, for 30 min, and an inverted fluoroscope was used to obtain Figure 2a,c. In the blank group, there was no significant fluorescence. On the other hand, in the control group, high ROS levels were observed. Treatment with different concentrations of 7PE for 2 h downregulated ROS levels in a dose-dependent manner. The result of NO is similar (Figure 2c,d). These results show that 7PE had a protective effect against alcohol-induced cytotoxicity in HepG2/CYP2E1 cells by inhibiting ROS and NO.

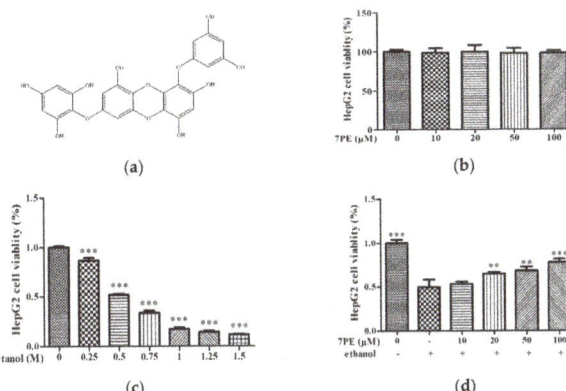

Figure 1. Effect of 7-phloro-eckol (7PE) on cell viability of HepG2/CYP2E1 cells. (**a**) Chemical structure of 7PE from marine brown alga, *Ecklonia cava*. Effect of 7PE (0, 10, 20, 50, and 100 μM) on the viability of HepG2/CYP2E1 cells; (**b**) HepG2/CYP2E1 cells were evaluated by MTT assay, respectively; (**c**) the viability of various doses of ethanol (0, 0.25, 0.5, 0.75, 1.0, 1.25, and 1.5 M) on HepG2/CYP2E1 cells; (**d**) protective effects of 7PE (0, 10, 20, 50, and 100 μM) on ethanol-induced (0.5 M) HepG2/CYP2E1 cell injury. Data are shown as mean ± SD (n = 3). * Compared with the control group (ethanol-induced group). ** $p < 0.01$; *** $p < 0.001$.

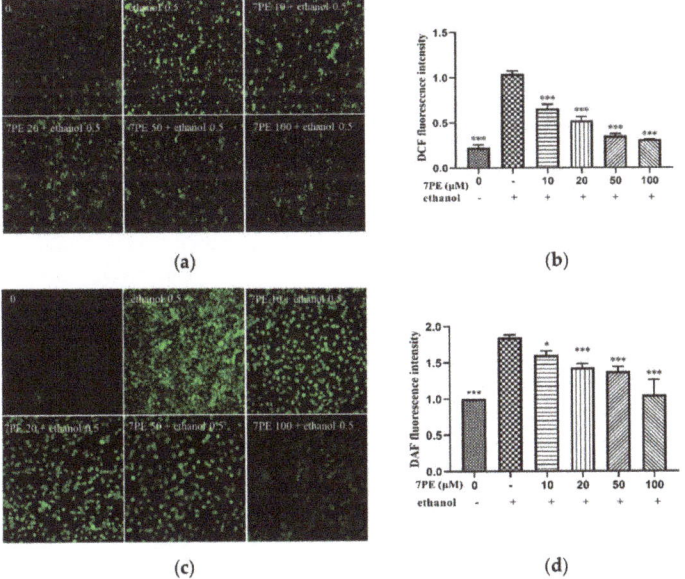

Figure 2. Effect of 7PE on intercellular reactive oxygen species (ROS) and (NO) generation in HepG2/CYP2E1 cells damaged by ethanol. (**a**) Then, the cells were exposed to 2,7-dichlorodihydrofluorescein diacetate (DCFH-DA) for 30 min. DCF fluorescence of the treated cells was measured using an inverted fluorescence microscope; (**b**) the relative DCF fluorescence intensity analysis of image; (**c**) the cells were exposed to 3-amino,4-aminomethyl-2′,7′-difluorescein diacetate (DAF-FM-DA) for 30 min. DAF fluorescence of the treated cells was measured using an inverted fluorescence microscope; (**d**) the relative DAF fluorescence intensity analysis of the images. Data are shown as mean ± SD (n = 3). * Compared with the control group (ethanol-induced group). * $p < 0.05$; ** $p < 0.01$; *** $p < 0.001$.

2.3. Determination of Intracellular DNA Damage

Cells were obtained by comet assay with DAPI and then imaged using an inverted fluorescence microscope to obtain Figure 3. In the blank group, there was no obvious tailing fluorescence. In the control group, HepG2/CYP2E1 cells showed obvious tailing fluorescence in 0.5 M ethanol. However, with the increase in 7PE concentration, the length of the comet tail decreased, which proves that 7PE could prevent alcohol-induced oxidative damage at the cellular level.

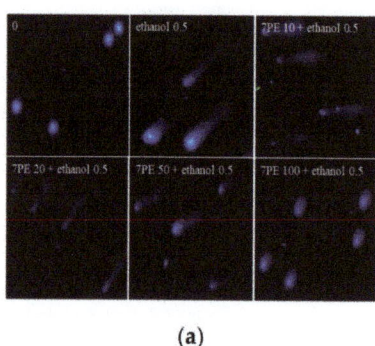
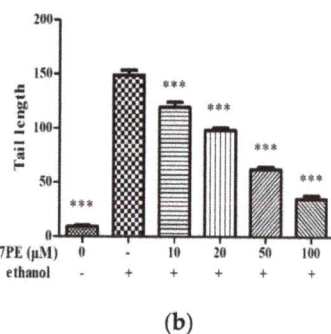

(a) (b)

Figure 3. (a) The cells were stained with DAPI. Images were obtained using an inverted fluorescence microscope; (b) tail lengths of the comets were analyzed by CASP. HepG2/CYP2E1 cells without treatment formed the blank group. Data are shown as mean ± SD (n = 3). * Compared with the control group (ethanol-induced group). ** $p < 0.01$; *** $p < 0.001$.

2.4. Effect of 7PE on the Level of Oxidative Stress-Related Proteins

As shown in Figure 4a–d, the protein levels of GSH and SOD in the control group decreased significantly, and the protein levels of the GGT increased significantly in the control group. In addition, compared with the control group, after treatment with 7PE, the protein levels of GSH and SOD increased significantly and were dose-dependent, while the protein level of GGT decreased.

The results of ELISA showed that the levels of interleukin-1 (IL-1), IL-6, and tumor necrosis factor-α (TNF-α) in the control group were higher than those in the blank group (Figure 4e–g). Then, compared with the control group, the inflammatory factors IL-1 and TNF-α decreased after 7PE treatment, but IL-6 did not change significantly.

2.5. Detection of Related Apoptosis Proteins

In order to determine whether 7PE has an anti-apoptotic effect on alcohol-induced cytotoxicity in HepG2/CYP2E1 cells, the expressions of Bcl-2 and Bax were determined (Figure 5). In comparison with the blank group, the expression of the bcl-2 protein decreased, and the expression of bax protein increased in the control group. Compared with the control group, after 7PE treatment, the expression of bcl-2 increased while the expression of bax decreased in a dose-dependent manner. Additionally, compared with the blank group, the p-pi3k protein, cleaved caspase-9 (c-c-9) protein, and cleaved caspase-3 (c-c-3) protein in the control group increased, while p-akt decreased (Figure 5c–f). These results indicate that 7PE could alleviate the oxidative stress induced by ethanol by regulating the production of apoptosis-related proteins.

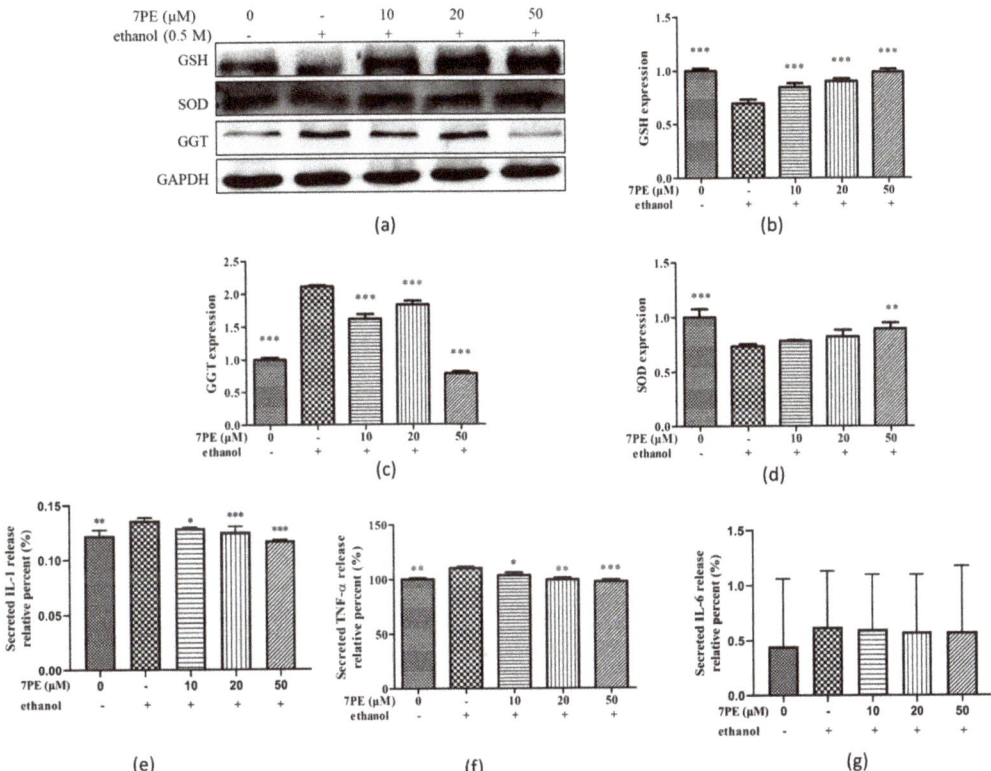

Figure 4. Effect of 7PE on superoxide dismutase (SOD), glutathione (GSH), and γ-glutamyl transferase (GGT) protein levels by Western blot and detection of related inflammatory factors by ELISA in HepG2 cells. Cells were treated with 7PE (10, 20, and 50 μM) for 2 h and then treated with 0.5 M ethanol for 24 h. GAPDH was used as an internal control. (a) Protein expression (relative to GAPDH) was evaluated; (b) GSH protein expression was evaluated; (c) GGT protein expression was evaluated; (d) SOD protein expression was evaluated; (e) interleukin-1 (IL-1) expression was evaluated; (f) tumor necrosis factor-α (TNF-α) expression was evaluated; (g) IL-6 expression was evaluated. Data are shown as mean ± SD ($n = 3$). * Compared with the control group (ethanol-induced group). * $p < 0.05$; ** $p < 0.01$; *** $p < 0.001$.

2.6. Effect of 7PE on the NF-κB Signal Pathway

The effect of 7PE on the NF-κB signal pathway was studied. As shown in Figure 6, compared with the blank group, the phosphorylation levels of p65 and IκBα in the control group were significantly increased. After 7PE treatment, the values of p-p65/p65 and p-IκBα/IκBα showed a dose-dependent decrease (Figure 6b,c). This indicated that 7PE inhibited the phosphorylation of NF-κB at the protein level to inhibit apoptosis.

2.7. JNK and p53 Protein Levels

Apoptosis depends on the activation of receptors for the mitochondrial-dependent death pathway, and the process is also affected by many other signaling pathways, such as p53 and c-Jun N-terminal kinase (JNK). Therefore, the effects of 7PE on p53 and JNK were studied (Figure 7). The results showed the phosphorylation level of JNK in the control group was significantly increased, and after 7PE treatment, the value of p-JNK/JNK showed a dose-dependent decrease. However, p53 did not change significantly. This indicated that 7PE only inhibited the phosphorylation of JNK at the protein level but had little effect on p53.

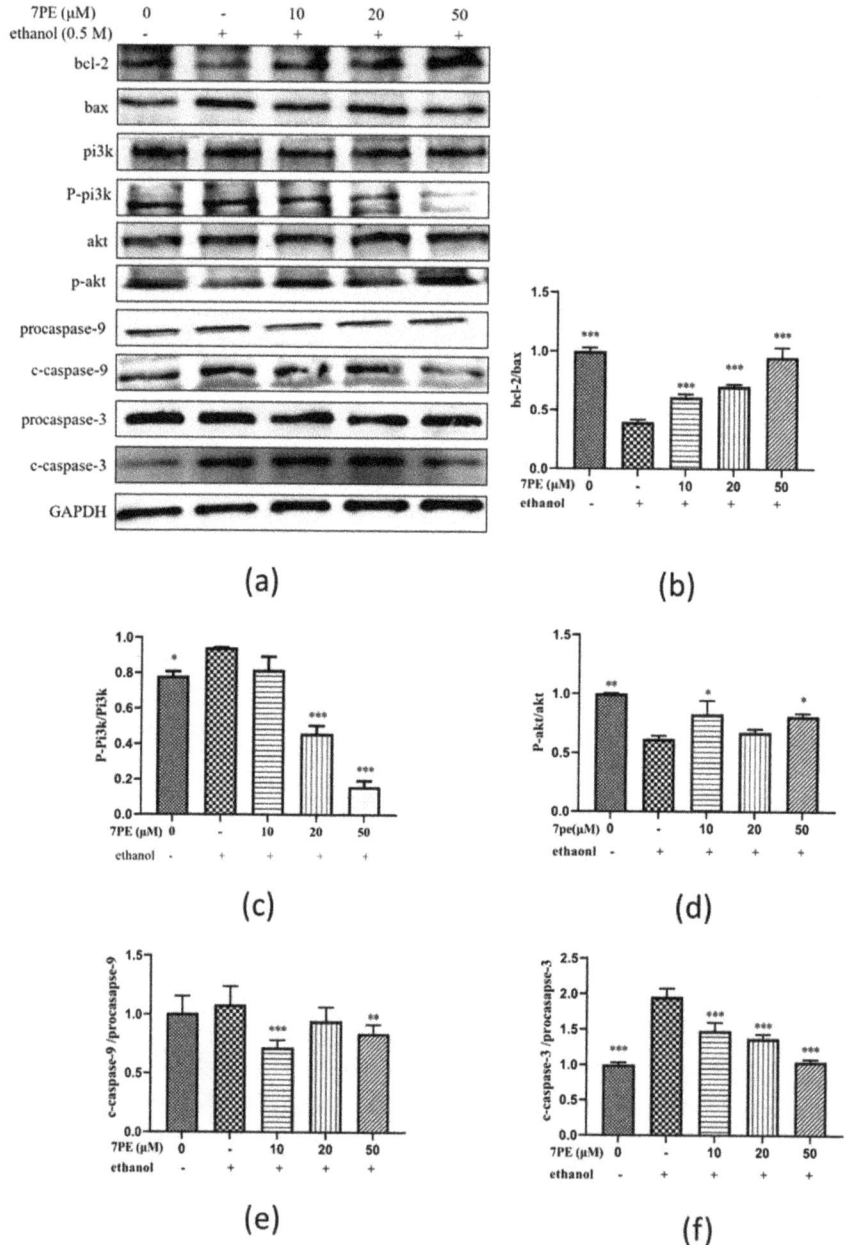

Figure 5. The effect of 7PE on the levels of related apoptosis proteins in HepG2/CYP2E1 cells treated with ethanol (0.5 M) by Western blot. GAPDH was used as an internal control. (**a**) Western blot analysis of bcl-2, bax, pi3k, p-pi3k, akt, p-akt, caspase-9, cleaved caspase-9, caspase-3 (c-3), and cleaved caspase-3 (c-c-3) protein levels; (**b**) the ratios of bcl-2 and bax proteins were calculated; (**c**) the ratios of p-pi3k and pi3k were calculated; (**d**) the ratios of p-akt and akt were calculated; (**e**) the ratios of cleaved caspase-9 and procaspase-9 were calculated; (**f**) the rations of cleaved caspase-3 and procaspase-3 were calculated. Data are shown as mean ± SD (n = 3). * Compared with the control group (ethanol-induced group). * $p < 0.05$; ** $p < 0.01$; *** $p < 0.001$.

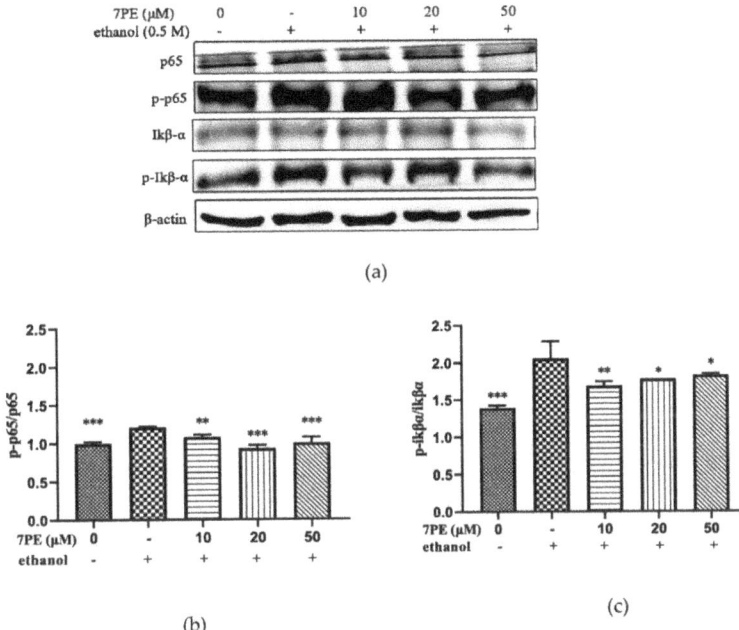

Figure 6. (a) The phosphorylation levels of p65, p-p65, IκBα, and p-IκBα proteins in HepG2/CYP2E1 cells. Cells were treated with 7PE (10, 20, and 50 μM) for 2 h, then treated with 0.5 M ethanol for 24 h; (b) the ratios of p-p65/p65 were calculated; (c) the ratios of p-IκBα/IκBα were calculated. Data are shown as mean ± SD ($n = 3$). * Compared with the control group (ethanol-induced group). * $p < 0.05$; ** $p < 0.01$; *** $p < 0.001$.

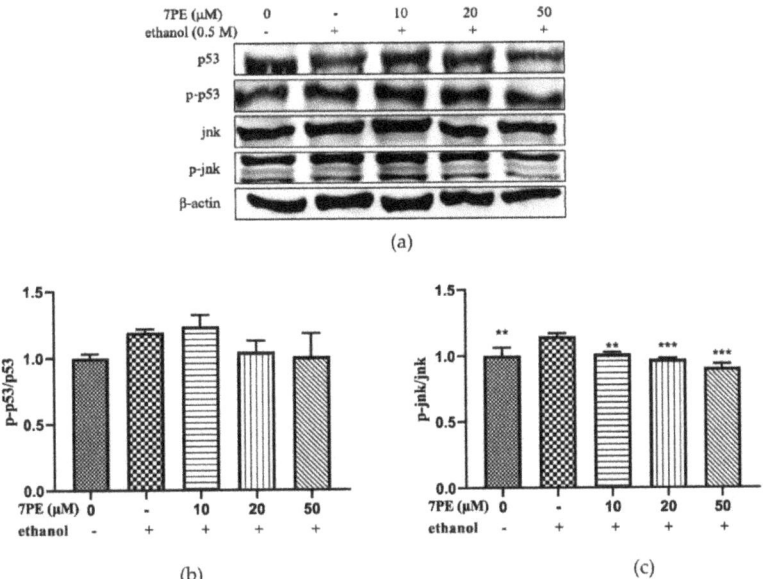

Figure 7. (a) The phosphorylation levels of p53, p-p53, JNK, and p-JNK proteins in HepG2/CYP2E1 cells. Cells were treated with 7PE (10, 20, and 50μM) for 2 h and then treated with 0.5 M ethanol for 24 h; (b) the ratios of p-p53/p53 were calculated; (c) the ratios of p-JNK/JNK were calculated. Data are shown as mean ± SD ($n = 3$). * Compared with the control group (ethanol-induced group). ** $p < 0.01$, *** $p < 0.001$.

2.8. GSH and bcl-2 Molecular Docking Analysis

In order to elucidate the structure-activity relationship of 7PE, the molecular interaction modes of GSH, bcl-2 protein, and 7PE were studied by molecular docking analysis. 7PE was docked with the active pockets of GSH and bcl-2 proteins to obtain the optimal docking structure (Figure 8a,c). The affinity of GSH and bcl-2 proteins to 7PE was −8.7 kcal/mol and −8.0 kcal/mol, respectively. As shown in Figure 8b, 7PE exhibits a tight binding pattern in the active pocket of GSH protein. 7PE was enclosed in a cavity bag composed of amino acids PHE31, CYS32, PRO33, PHE34, LEU56, ASN67, LEU71, VAL72, PRO73, and GLU85. Through a detailed analysis, it could be concluded that the four hydroxyl groups of 7PE could form six hydrogen bonds with amino acids PHE31, ASN67, LEU71, VAL72, PRO73, and GLU85, which were the main forces between 7PE and GSH. As shown in Figure 8d, 7PE was located in the active pocket composed of amino acids TYR18, SER19, ARG21, ARG46, ARG50, GLU98, ARG99, and LEU102. It is important that the five hydroxyl groups of 7PE could form six hydrogen bonds with amino acids SER19, ARG46, ARG50, GLU98, and ARG99, respectively. These hydrogen bonds were the main force between 7PE and bcl-2. All these interactions allowed 7PE to form stable complexes with GSH and bcl-2.

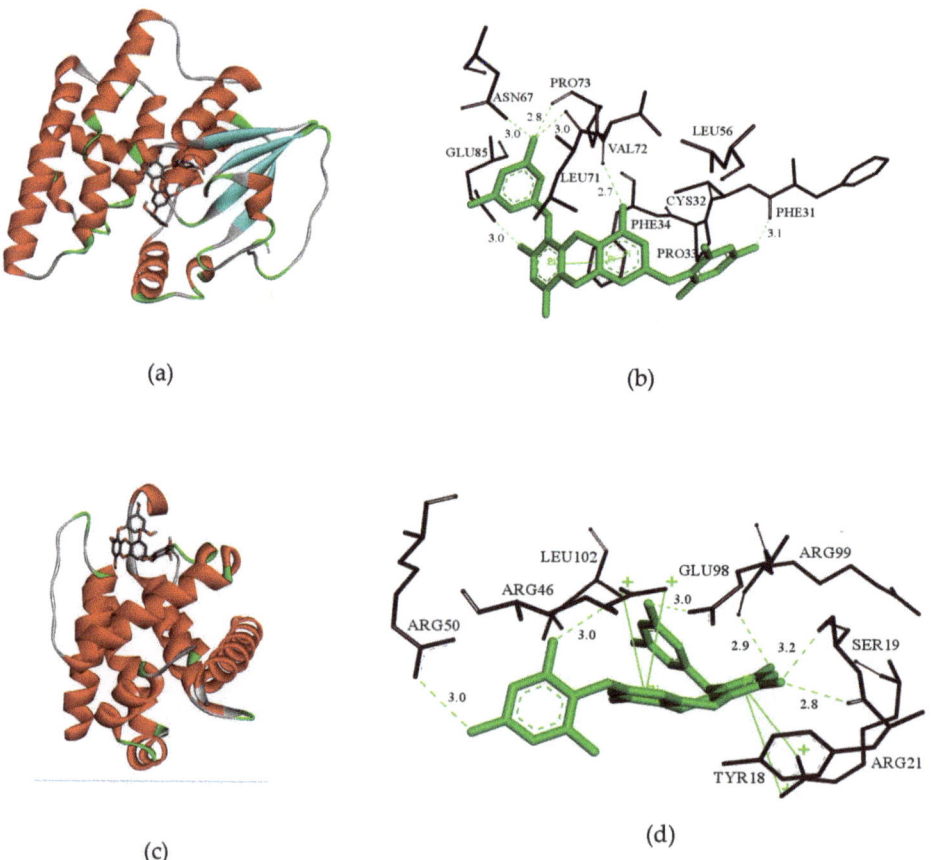

Figure 8. (a,c) 3D model of the interaction between 7PE and GSH and between 7PE and bcl-2, respectively. (b,d) 3D model of the optimal docking structure interaction between 7PE and the active sites of GSH and bcl-2, respectively.

The aforementioned molecular docking studies provide a reasonable explanation for the interaction of 7PE with GSH and bcl-2 and lay the foundation for further research on 7PE.

3. Discussion

The structure of the 7PE compound was first isolated and identified by Yoshihito Okada [39] in the brown algae *Eisenia bicyclis*, and proved it had antidiabetic biological activity. However, Li [29] first isolated this structural compound in *Ecklonia cava*, and proved it had an antioxidant action. *Ecklonia cava* is an edible marine brown algae that was abundant in the subtidal areas of South Korea, Japan, and China. In addition, a variety of active substances have been extracted from the brown algae, including polysaccharides [40], carotenoids, fucoidans, and polyphenols [38]. These active substances show different biological activities in pharmaceuticals, nutraceuticals, cosmeceuticals, and functional foods, including antioxidant, anticoagulant, antibacterial, anti-human immunodeficiency virus, anti-inflammatory, and anti-tumor actions [41]. Among them, the polyphenol compounds were the main research objects of brown algae, *Ecklonia cava*.

The antioxidant activity of polyphenols is in direct relation with their chemical structures, such as the number as well as the position of the hydroxyl groups [42]. The greater the number of hydroxyl groups, the stronger the antioxidant activity of polyphenols, but as the number of hydroxyl groups increases, the stability of polyphenols will decrease [29,42]. In addition, from the perspective of molecular docking, the interaction between the polyphenols and the target protein mainly depends on the hydrogen bonding force, and the hydroxyl structure happens to be the best site for hydrogen bonding with the protein [34]. Therefore, the number of hydroxyl groups is one of the important indicators for the binding of polyphenol molecules to target proteins, and it was also one of the foundations for studying the stability and antioxidant activity of polyphenols. And among the polyphenolic compounds of *Ecklonia cava*, research on the two structures of eckol and dieckol is relatively mature, and both compounds have antioxidant activity [33,43]. According to research, eckol and dieckol have six and eleven hydroxyl groups, respectively, while 7PE has eight hydroxyl groups. Therefore, it is possible that 7PE with hydroxyl group number between eckol and dieckol will have better performance in both antioxidant activity and structural stability. This study proved that 7PE had excellent antioxidant activity and inhibited ROS-induced apoptosis.

The MTT assay (Figure 1d) showed that 7PE with a concentration of 10–100 μM had no cytotoxicity. When the concentration of ethanol stimulation is 0.5 M, the cell viability decreased by half, but when 7PE (20–100 μM) was added, the cell viability increased significantly, which showed that 7PE had an obvious relative repair effect on alcohol-induced injury. The experimental results also showed that the expression of reactive oxygen species and nitric oxide increased after ethanol treatment. However, 7PE treatment can reduce the production of reactive oxygen species (ROS) and nitric oxide (NO), increase the levels of superoxide dismutase (SOD) and glutathione protein (GSH), and reduce the level of GGT protein. Finally, the comet assay (Figure 3) showed that 7PE could reduce DNA damage caused by alcohol. Severe ALD can lead to hepatitis and liver cancer. In the process of ALD developing into a liver tumor, the growth and metastasis of liver cells need the support of a large number of cytokines and nutrients [44]. Oxidative stress can induce liver cells to secrete TNF-α, which leads to inflammation. Long-term sustained oxidative stress can lead to inflammatory responses [45] and further increase the expression of inflammatory factors. TNF-α is associated with a number of inflammatory diseases. According to ELISA results, alcohol induction will lead to the overexpression of TNF-α and inflammatory factors, but 7PE can regulate TNF-α and IL-1 and inhibit inflammation (Figure 4e,f). However, studies have shown that IL-6 is a hepatoprotective factor, which can predict alcoholic liver injury [46,47]. The experimental results also showed that the expression of IL-6 did not decrease significantly after 7PE treatment, indicating that 7PE did not decrease the content of liver-protective factors. At the same time, the amount of

IL-6 did not increase, possibly due to other reasons, such as insufficient stimulation. In summary, 7PE could reduce the production of inflammatory factors, but whether it can increase the role of liver-protective factors remains to be further studied.

Studies have shown that alcohol can lead to oxidative stress and ROS overexpression [10,48], coupled with the synergistic reaction of NO. ROS and NO can act as second messengers and activate the expression of apoptotic genes, thus increasing apoptosis [43]. Apoptosis can be controlled by various apoptosis-related proteins, including bcl-2 family proteins, death receptors, and caspase [49]. Caspase-3 is considered to be the key protein in the farthest effect pathway of apoptosis [50]. In this study, Western blot detected that the cleaved caspase-3/procaspase-3 and bcl-2/bax values decreased. Many factors can activate the PI3K pathway, which leads to the activation of Akt. Akt plays an important role in cell survival signal transduction [51]. Akt can phosphorylate and inhibit the pro-apoptotic Bcl-2 family members Bad, Bax, and caspase-9. Western blot showed that the ratio of p-akt/akt increased (as observed in Figure 5d), while the ratio of cleaved caspase-9/procaspase-9 decreased (Figure 5f), which proved that 7PE could resist apoptosis by activating Akt.

Nuclear factor-κB (NF-κB), composed of proteins p50, p65, and IκB, is related to the control of apoptosis and autophagy [52]. Without being stimulated, NF-κB is located in the cytoplasm. Extracellular stimulation causes rapid phosphorylation and subsequent degradation of IκB, thus exposing the nuclear localization sequence on p50–p65 heterodimer [53]. Then, p65 protein is phosphorylated, resulting in nuclear translocation. The results of the Western blot showed that ethanol treatment increased the phosphorylation of IκB-α and p65 in HepG2 cells. 7PE inhibits apoptosis by inhibiting phosphorylation of p65 and IκB-α (Figure 6).

Although the initiation and execution of apoptosis depending on the activation of receptors for the mitochondrial-dependent death pathway, the process is also affected by many other signaling pathways, such as p53 and c-JunN-terminal kinase (JNK) from the MAPK family [54]. After DNA damage, p53 can be activated to induce Bax transcription [55], but experiments show that p53 phosphorylation has no significant change after 7PE treatment. JNK is one of the important mitogen-activated protein kinases and is involved in stress response and apoptosis [56]. The results also showed that 7PE could significantly reduce the phosphorylation of JNK in the process of apoptosis induced by alcohol (Figure 7c), which indicates that alcohol may activate MAPKs pathways, although more proof is required. Finally, the interaction of 7PE with GSH and bcl-2 was studied by molecular docking. The results showed that the hydroxyl group of 7PE could form stable hydrogen bonds with GSH and bcl-2 (Figure 8b,d). This is the main function of molecular compounds and proteins. The results provide a theoretical basis for further verifying the role of 7PE in antioxidation at the molecular level.

Combined with the experimental results of this study, it can be concluded that 7PE could repair liver injury caused by alcohol, but the specific mechanism of action should be further studied.

4. Materials and Methods

4.1. Chemicals and Materials

7-phloro-eckol (7PE, Figure 1a) was isolated from *Ecklonia cava* in a previous study [26–29]. Dulbecco's modified Eagle's medium (DMEM), fetal bovine serum (FBS), trypsin-EDTA (0.25%), and penicillin/streptomycin were purchased from Gibco (New York, USA). Dimethyl sulfoxide (DMSO), DCFH-DA, 4′,6-diamidino-2-phenylindole (DAPI), and 3-(4,5-Dimethylthiazol-2-yl)-2,5-diphenyltetrazolium bromide (MTT) were purchased from Sigma-Aldrich (St. Louis, MO, USA). TNF-α (EHC103a), IL-1, and IL-6 kits were purchased from Neobio Science Technology Co., Ltd. (Shenzhen, Guangdong, China). p-pi3k (17366), AKT (4691), p-AKT (4060), c-c-9 (2075s), and c9 (9508) were provided by Cell Signaling Technology (CST, MA, USA). Pi3k (SC-376112), SOD (sc-271014), GGT (sc-100746), GSH (sc-71155), p65 (sc-8008), p-p65 (sc-136548), JNK (sc-7345), p-JNK (sc-6254), GAPDH (sc-47724), β-acting (47778), and secondary antibodies (goat anti-rabbit IgG-HRP, sc-2004; goat anti-mouse IgG-HRP, sc-

2005) were purchased from Santa Cruz Biotechnology Inc. (Santa Cruz, CA, USA). All other chemicals and solvents were of analytical grade.

4.2. Cell Culture

HepG2/CYP2E1 cells (HepG2 cells transfected with human CYP2E1 cDNA) were provided by the Cell Bank of the Chinese Academy of Sciences (Shanghai, China). HepG2/CYP2E1 cells were cultured respectively in DMEM, 10% FBS, 100 mg/mL streptomycin, and 100 U/mL penicillin in a humidified incubator of 5% CO_2 at 37 °C.

4.3. Cell Viability Assay

Cells were cultured in 96-well plates (4×10^3 cells/mL) for 24 h. This was changed to a fresh serum-free medium containing different concentrations of 7PE (0, 10, 20, 50, and 100 µM) for 24 h. An amount of 100 µL MTT (1 mg/mL) was added to each well, and cells were incubated for 4 h at 37 °C. Subsequently, 100 µL DMSO was added to dissolve the formazan crystals. The absorbance was measured using a microplate reader (BioTek, Winooski, VT, USA) at 570 nm.

4.4. Cell ROS Analysis

ROS content was directly proportional to the fluorescence intensity of DCFH-DA. Cells were cultured in 24-well plates, and 7PE (0, 1, 10, 20, 50, and 100 µM) was added for 2 h. Cells were treated with 0.5 M ethanol for 24 h in a CO_2 incubator. Subsequently, DCFH-DA (10 µM) was added for 30 min at 37 °C in the dark. Finally, the fluorescence intensity was examined under an inverted fluorescence microscope (Olympus, Tokyo, Japan).

4.5. Cell NO Analysis

No content was directly proportional to the fluorescence intensity of DAF-FM-DA. Cells were cultured in 24-well plates, and 7PE (0, 1, 10, 20, 50, and 100 µM) was added for 2 h. Cells were treated with 0.5 M ethanol for 24 h in a CO_2 incubator. Subsequently, DAF-DA (10 µM) was added for 30 min at 37 °C in the dark. Finally, the fluorescence intensity was examined under an inverted fluorescence microscope (Olympus, Tokyo, Japan).

4.6. Comet Assay

HepG2/CYP2E1 cells were treated with 7PE (0, 10, 20, 50, and 100 µM) and 0.5 M ethanol for 24 h in a CO_2 incubator. Subsequently, the cells were treated with EDTA-trypsin to form a cell suspension (1×10^5 cells/mL). The cell suspension (20 µL) and 1% low-melting-point agarose (LMA, 80 µL) were mixed and dropped onto 0.8% normal-melting-point agarose (NMA, 100 µL). After the gel was cured, the slides were immersed in a precooled lysate solution (2.5 M NaCl, 200 mM NaOH, 100 mM Na2EDTA, 10 mM Tris, 1%Triton X-100, and 1% sodium lauroyl sarcosinate; pH 10) at 4 °C for 90 min. The slides were then gently immersed in an alkaline electrophoresis solution (200 mM NaOH and 1 mM Na_2EDTA; pH > 13) at 4 °C for 30 min. Next, electrophoresis (25 V; 20 min) was performed, and the slides were stained with DAPI (20 µg/mL; 20 µL) in the dark for 10 min. Finally, the fluorescence intensity was observed under an inverted fluorescence microscope (Olympus, Tokyo, Japan), and the CASP software was applied to analyzed comet images.

4.7. Western Blot

Total protein from the treated HepG2/CYP2E1 cells was isolated using radio immunoprecipitation assay (RIPA) lysis buffer containing 1% phenylmethylsulfonyl fluoride (PMSF) RIPA buffer. The BCA protein assay kit was used to quantify the sample. An equal amount of protein was used for electrophoresis. The target protein was transferred to a nitrocellulose (NC) membrane (Boston, MA, USA) using SDS-PAGE. The membrane was visualized by blocking for 2 h, incubating the primary antibodies, and secondary antibody incubation was performed with enhanced chemiluminescence (ECL) detection system (Syngene, Cambridge, UK).

4.8. Enzyme-Linked Immunosorbent Assay (ELISA)

Cells were treated with various concentrations of 7PE (0, 10, 20, and 50 µM) for 24 h. Conditional media or cell lysates were harvested in sterile tubes and centrifuged (12,000 rpm; 4 °C) for 10 min to get the supernatants. The concentration of protein was analyzed according to the manufacturer's protocol.

4.9. Molecular Docking

The chemical structure of 7PE was drawn using ChemDraw (PerkinElmer, Waltham, MA, USA) (Figure 1A), then converted into a 3D structure by Chem3D (PerkinElmer, Waltham, MA, USA), and optimized using the MMFF94 force field. The 3D structure of GSH (PDB ID: 6PNN), BCL-2 (PDB ID: 4B4S) can be downloaded from the RCSB Protein Data Bank (www.rcsb.org, accessed on 25 January 2021). GSH, BCL -2, and compound 7PE were converted to a PDBQT grid using Autodock Tools (Scr ipps Research Institute, La Jolla, CA, USA). Autodock vina (Scripps Research Institute, La Jolla, CA, USA) was used for molecular docking research. In order to increase the accuracy of the calculation, the parameter exhaustiveness was set to 100, and other parameters used the default values. Finally, the constellation with the highest score was selected for analysis using PyMoL (DeLano Scientific LLC, San Carlos, CA, USA) and Discovery Studio (Biovia, Waltham, MA, USA).

4.10. Statistical Analysis

Image J (Version 1.46r, NIH), GraphPad Prism 5 (Graphpad Software, San Diego, CA, USA), and the CAPS (Version 1.2.3 beta1 Krzysztof Konca, urlCaspLab.com, accessed on 1 February 2021) were used for data analyses. All data were analyzed by one-way ANOVA accompanied by Dunnett's multiple comparison test for group comparison. Data are expressed as the mean ± SD (n = 3).

5. Conclusions

In summary, the current research results show that 7PE could increase the expression of SOD, GSH, and IL-1, downregulate the levels of GGT, ROS, NO, TNF-α, and IL-6, and reduce DNA damage. Therefore, 7PE could alleviate the oxidative stress induced by ethanol. In addition, 7PE can prevent ethanol-induced apoptosis by upregulating the expression of bcl-2 and AKT, downregulating the expression of bax, caspase-9, and caspase-3, and inhibiting the activation of NF-κB and JNK pathways.

The results show that 7PE could protect the liver by preventing oxidative stress and apoptosis of hepatocytes induced by alcohol. Therefore, this study lays the foundation for 7PE to be used as functional liver-protecting food and preventive substance of ALD.

Author Contributions: L.L. and S.Y. performed the experiment and wrote the manuscript; Z.-J.Q. and C.Z. conceived the research and revised the manuscripts; Z.X. analyzed the data; P.H. and S.S. contributed materials and analysis tools. All authors have read and agreed to the published version of the manuscript.

Funding: The research was funded by the 2020 Shenzhen International Scientific and Technological Cooperation R&D Project and the Natural Science Foundation of Guangdong Province (2020A1515011075). The supported by the Development Project about Marine Economy Demonstration of Zhanjiang City (XM-202008-01B1) and Southern Marine Science and Engineering Guangdong Laboratory (Zhanjiang, ZJW-2019-07).

Institutional Review Board Statement: Not applicable.

Informed Consent Statement: Not applicable.

Conflicts of Interest: The authors declare no conflict of interest.

References

1. Samir, Z. Overview: How is alcohol metabolized by the body? *Alcohol Res. Health* **2006**, *29*, 245–254.
2. Lieber, C.S. Alcohol and the liver: 1994 update. *Gastroenterology* **1994**, *106*, 1085–1105. [CrossRef]
3. Wang, F.S.; Fan, J.G.; Zhang, Z.; Gao, B.; Wang, H.Y. The global burden of liver disease: The major impact of China. *Hepatology* **2014**, *60*, 2099–2108. [CrossRef]
4. Orman, E.S.; Odena, G.; Bataller, R. Alcoholic liver disease: Pathogenesis, management, and novel targets for therapy. *J. Gastroenterol. Hepatol.* **2013**, *28*, 77–84. [CrossRef]
5. Yang, S.T.; Chen, M.F.; Ryu, B.; Chen, J.; Xiao, Z.; Hong, P.Z.; Sun, S.L.; Wang, D.; Qian, Z.J.; Zhou, C.X. The Protective Effect of the Polysaccharide Precursor, D-Isofloridoside, from Laurencia undulata on Alcohol-Induced Hepatotoxicity in HepG2 Cells. *Molecules* **2020**, *25*, 1024. [CrossRef] [PubMed]
6. Castán, A.; Navarro, Y.; Sarría, L.; Larrosa, R.; Serradilla, M.; Serrablo, A. Radiological diagnosis of hepatocellular carcinoma in non-cirrhotic patients. *Hepatoma Res.* **2017**, *3*, 1–17. [CrossRef]
7. Ron, M. Oxidative stress, antioxidants and stress tolerance. *Trends Plant. Sci.* **2002**, *7*, 405–410.
8. Liu, Y.; Wang, J.; Li, L.; Hu, W.; Qu, Y.; Ding, Y.; Meng, L.; Teng, L.; Wang, D. Hepatoprotective Effects of Antrodia cinnamomea: The Modulation of Oxidative Stress Signaling in a Mouse Model of Alcohol-Induced Acute Liver Injury. *Oxid. Med. Cell Longev.* **2017**, *2017*, 7841823. [CrossRef] [PubMed]
9. Chen, M.F.; Gong, F.; Zhang, Y.Y.; Li, C.Y.; Zhou, C.X.; Hong, P.Z.; Sun, S.L.; Qian, Z.J. Preventive Effect of YGDEY from Tilapia Fish Skin Gelatin Hydrolysates against Alcohol-Induced Damage in HepG2 Cells through ROS-Mediated Signaling Pathways. *Nutrients* **2019**, *11*, 392. [CrossRef] [PubMed]
10. Chen, M.F.; Zhang, Y.Y.; Di He, M.; Li, C.Y.; Zhou, C.X.; Hong, P.Z.; Qian, Z.J. Antioxidant Peptide Purified from Enzymatic Hydrolysates of Isochrysis Zhanjiangensis and Its Protective Effect against Ethanol Induced Oxidative Stress of HepG2 Cells. *Biotechnol. Bioprocess Eng.* **2019**, *24*, 308–317. [CrossRef]
11. Singh, M.; Gupta, S.; Singhal, U.; Pandey, R.; Aggarwal, S.K. Evaluation of the oxidative stress in chronic alcoholics. *J. Clin. Diagn. Res.* **2013**, *7*, 1568–1571.
12. Praetorius Bjork, M.; Johansson, B. Gamma-Glutamyltransferase (GGT) as a biomarker of cognitive decline at the end of life: Contrasting age and time to death trajectories. *Int. Psychogeriatr.* **2018**, *30*, 981–990. [CrossRef]
13. Closa, D.; Folch Puy, E. Oxygen free radicals and the systemic inflammatory response. *IUBMB Life* **2004**, *56*, 185–191. [CrossRef] [PubMed]
14. Tatsuya, K.; Junya, M.; Tsuyoshi, T.; Tetsuo, N.; Kazuhiro, H.; Jun, N. Prognostic significance of the immunohistochemical staining of cleaved caspase-3, an activated form of caspase-3, in gliomas. *Clin. Cancer Res.* **2007**, *13*, 3868–3874.
15. Yi, G.; Li, H.; Li, Y.; Zhao, F.; Ying, Z.; Liu, M.; Zhang, J.; Liu, X. The protective effect of soybean protein-derived peptides on apoptosis via the activation of PI3K-AKT and inhibition on apoptosis pathway. *Food Sci. Nutr.* **2020**, *8*, 4591–4600. [CrossRef]
16. Jiang, T.; Tian, F.; Zheng, H.T.; Whitman Samantha, A.; Lin, Y.F.; Zhang, Z.G.; Zhang, N.; Zhang, D.N. Nrf2 suppresses lupus nephritis through inhibition of oxidative injury and the NF-κB mediated inflammatory response. *Kidney Int.* **2014**, *85*, 333–343. [CrossRef] [PubMed]
17. Kluwe, J.; Pradere, J.P.; Gwak, G.Y.; Mencin, A.; De Minicis, S.; Osterreicher, C.H.; Colmenero, J.; Bataller, R.; Schwabe, R.F. Modulation of hepatic fibrosis by c-Jun-N-terminal kinase inhibition. *Gastroenterology* **2010**, *138*, 347–359. [CrossRef] [PubMed]
18. Wali, A.F.; Majid, S.; Rasool, S.; Shehada, S.B.; Abdulkareem, S.K.; Firdous, A.; Beigh, S.; Shakeel, S.; Mushtaq, S.; Akbar, I.; et al. Natural products against cancer: Review on phytochemicals from marine sources in preventing cancer. *Saudi Pharm. J.* **2019**, *27*, 767–777. [CrossRef] [PubMed]
19. Li, S.; Ji, L.; Shi, Q.; Wu, H.; Fan, J. Advances in the production of bioactive substances from marine unicellular microalgae Porphyridium spp. *Bioresour. Technol.* **2019**, *292*, 122048. [CrossRef]
20. Scieszka, S.; Klewicka, E. Algae in food: A general review. *Crit. Rev. Food Sci. Nutr.* **2019**, *59*, 3538–3547. [CrossRef] [PubMed]
21. Zargarzadeh, M.; Amaral, A.J.R.; Custodio, C.A.; Mano, J.F. Biomedical applications of laminarin. *Carbohydr. Polym.* **2020**, *232*, 115774. [CrossRef]
22. Zenthoefer, M.; Geisen, U.; Hofmann Peiker, K.; Fuhrmann, M.; Kerber, J.; Kirchhöfer, R.; Hennig, S.; Peipp, M.; Geyer, R.; Piker, L.; et al. Isolation of polyphenols with anticancer activity from the Baltic Sea brown seaweed Fucus vesiculosus using bioassay-guided fractionation. *J. Appl. Phycol.* **2017**, *29*, 1007. [CrossRef]
23. Cao, J.; Wang, J.; Wang, S.; Xu, X. Porphyra Species: A Mini-Review of Its Pharmacological and Nutritional Properties. *J. Med. Food* **2016**, *19*, 111–119. [CrossRef]
24. Peres, J.C.F.; de Carvalho, L.R.; Goncalez, E.; Berian, L.O.S.; Felicio, J.D. Evaluation of antifungal activity of seaweed extracts. *Ciência Agrotecnologia* **2012**, *36*, 294–299. [CrossRef]
25. Bhadury, P.; Wright, P.C. Exploitation of marine algae: Biogenic compounds for potential antifouling applications. *Planta* **2004**, *219*, 561–578. [CrossRef] [PubMed]
26. Mhadhebi, L.; Mhadhebi, A.; Robert, J.; Bouraoui, A. Antioxidant, Anti-inflammatory and Antiproliferative Effects of Aqueous Extracts of Three Mediterranean Brown Seaweeds of the Genus Cystoseira. *Iran J. Pharm. Res.* **2014**, *13*, 207–220. [PubMed]
27. Smyrniotopoulos, V.; de Andrade Tomaz, A.C.; Vanderlei de Souza, M.F.; Leitao da Cunha, E.V.; Kiss, R.; Mathieu, V.; Ioannou, E.; Roussis, V. Halogenated Diterpenes with In Vitro Antitumor Activity from the Red Alga Sphaerococcus corono-pifolius. *Mar. Drugs* **2019**, *18*, 29. [CrossRef]

28. Montero, L.; Del Pilar Sanchez Camargo, A.; Ibanez, E.; Gilbert Lopez, B. Phenolic Compounds from Edible Algae: Bioactivity and Health Benefits. *Curr. Med. Chem.* **2018**, *25*, 4808–4826. [CrossRef] [PubMed]
29. Li, Y.; Qian, Z.J.; Ryu, B.; Lee, S.H.; Kim, M.M.; Kim, S.K. Chemical components and its antioxidant properties in vitro: An edible marine brown alga, Ecklonia cava. *Bioorg. Med. Chem.* **2009**, *17*, 1963–1973. [CrossRef] [PubMed]
30. Zhang, M.; Zhou, W.; Zhao, S.; Li, S.; Yan, D.; Wang, J. Eckol inhibits Reg3A-induced proliferation of human SW1990 pan-creatic cancer cells. *Exp. Ther. Med.* **2019**, *18*, 2825–2832. [PubMed]
31. Zhang, M.Y.; Guo, J.; Hu, X.M.; Zhao, S.Q.; Li, S.L.; Wang, J. An in vivo anti-tumor effect of eckol from marine brown algae by improving the immune response. *Food Funct.* **2019**, *10*, 4361–4371. [CrossRef]
32. Li, S.; Liu, J.; Zhang, M.; Chen, Y.; Zhu, T.; Wang, J. Protective Effect of Eckol against Acute Hepatic Injury Induced by Carbon Tetrachloride in Mice. *Mar. Drugs* **2018**, *16*, 300. [CrossRef] [PubMed]
33. Kang, M.C.; Kim, K.N.; Kang, S.M.; Yang, X.; Kim, E.A.; Song, C.B.; Nah, J.W.; Jang, M.K.; Lee, J.S.; Jung, W.K.; et al. Protective effect of dieckol isolated from Ecklonia cava against ethanol caused damage in vitro and in zebrafish model. *Environ. Toxicol. Pharmacol.* **2013**, *36*, 1217–1226. [CrossRef]
34. Kang, S.M.; Cha, S.H.; Ko, J.Y.; Kang, M.C.; Kim, D.; Heo, S.J.; Kim, J.S.; Heu, M.S.; Kim, Y.T.; Jung, W.K.; et al. Neuroprotective effects of phlorotannins isolated from a brown alga, Ecklonia cava, against H2O2-induced oxidative stress in murine hippocampal HT22 cells. *Environ. Toxicol. Pharmacol.* **2012**, *34*, 96–105. [CrossRef]
35. Kim, A.D.; Kang, K.A.; Piao, M.J.; Kim, K.C.; Zheng, J.; Yao, C.W.; Cha, J.W.; Hyun, C.L.; Kang, H.K.; Lee, N.H.; et al. Cytoprotective effect of eckol against oxidative stress-induced mitochondrial dysfunction: Involvement of the FoxO3a/AMPK pathway. *J. Cell Biochem.* **2014**, *115*, 1403–1411. [CrossRef] [PubMed]
36. Ah Jung, H.; Roy, A.; Jung, J.H.; Choi, J.S. Evaluation of the inhibitory effects of eckol and dieckol isolated from edible brown alga Eisenia bicyclis on human monoamine oxidases A and B. *Arch. Pharmacal Res.* **2017**, *40*, 480–491. [CrossRef] [PubMed]
37. Kang, K.H.; Qian, Z.J.; Ryu, B.; Karadeniz, F.; Kim, D.; Kim, S.K. Antioxidant peptides from protein hydrolysate of microalgae Navicula incerta and their protective effects in HepG2/CYP2E1 cells induced by ethanol. *Phytother. Res.* **2012**, *26*, 1555–1563. [CrossRef] [PubMed]
38. Kang, K.H.; Qian, Z.-J.; Ryu, B.; Kim, D.; Kim, S.K. Protective effects of protein hydrolysate from marine microalgae Navicula incerta on ethanol-induced toxicity in HepG2/CYP2E1 cells. *Food Chem.* **2012**, *132*, 677–685. [CrossRef]
39. Yoshihito, O.; Akiko, I.; Ryuichiro, S.; Toru, O. A new phloroglucinol derivative from the brown alga Eisenia bicyclis: Potential for the effective treatment of diabetic complications. *J. Nat. Prod.* **2004**, *67*, 1318–1323.
40. Athukorala, Y.; Jung, W.K.; Vasanthan, T.; Jeon, Y.J. An anticoagulative polysaccharide from an enzymatic hydrolysate of Ecklonia cava. *Carbohydr. Polym.* **2006**, *66*, 184–191. [CrossRef]
41. Wijesinghe, W.A.; Jeon, Y.J. Exploiting biological activities of brown seaweed Ecklonia cava for potential industrial applications: A review. *Int. J. Food Sci. Nutr.* **2012**, *63*, 225–235. [CrossRef]
42. Singh, B.; Singh, J.P.; Kaur, A.; Singh, N. Phenolic composition and antioxidant potential of grain legume seeds: A review. *Food Res. Int.* **2017**, *101*, 1–16. [CrossRef] [PubMed]
43. Kim, E.K.; Tang, Y.; Kim, Y.S.; Hwang, J.W.; Choi, E.J.; Lee, J.H.; Lee, S.H.; Jeon, Y.J.; Park, P.J. First evidence that Ecklonia cava-derived dieckol attenuates MCF-7 human breast carcinoma cell migration. *Mar. Drugs* **2015**, *13*, 1785–1797. [CrossRef] [PubMed]
44. Strathearn, L.S.; Stepanov, A.I.; Font-Burgada, J. Inflammation in Primary and Metastatic Liver Tumorigenesis–Under the Influence of Alcohol and High-Fat Diets. *Nutrients* **2020**, *12*, 933. [CrossRef] [PubMed]
45. Cannon, A.R.; Morris, N.L.; Hammer, A.M.; Curtis, B.; Remick, D.G.; Yeligar, S.M.; Poole, L.; Burnham, E.L.; Wyatt, T.A.; Molina, P.E.; et al. Alcohol and inflammatory responses: Highlights of the 2015 Alcohol and Immunology Research Interest Group (AIRIG) meeting. *Alcohol* **2016**, *54*, 73–77. [CrossRef]
46. Congcong, Z.; Yulin, L.; Yina, W.; Luya, W.; Xiaonan, W.; Jie, D. Interleukin-6/signal transducer and activator of transcription 3 (STAT3) pathway is essential for macrophage infiltration and myoblast proliferation during muscle regeneration. *J. Biol. Chem.* **2013**, *288*, 1489–1499.
47. Horiguchi, N.; Wang, L.; Mukhopadhyay, P.; Park, O.; Jeong, W.I.; Lafdil, F.; Osei Hyiaman, D.; Moh, A.; Fu, X.Y.; Pacher, P.; et al. Cell type-dependent pro- and anti-inflammatory role of signal transducer and activator of transcription 3 in alcoholic liver injury. *Gastroenterology* **2008**, *134*, 1148–1158. [CrossRef] [PubMed]
48. You, Y.; Min, S.; Lee, Y.H.; Hwang, K.; Jun, W. Hepatoprotective effect of 10% ethanolic extract from Curdrania tricuspidata leaves against ethanol-induced oxidative stress through suppression of CYP2E1. *Food Chem. Toxicol.* **2017**, *108*, 298–304. [CrossRef] [PubMed]
49. Hidayat, A.F.A.; Chan, C.K.; Mohamad, J.; Kadir, H.A. Dioscorea bulbifera induced apoptosis through inhibition of ERK 1/2 and activation of JNK signaling pathways in HCT116 human colorectal carcinoma cells. *Biomed. Pharmacother.* **2018**, *104*, 806–816. [CrossRef]
50. Zou, H.; Henzel, W.J.; Liu, X.; Lutschg, A.; Wang, X. Apaf-1, a Human Protein Homologous to C. elegans CED-4, Participates in Cytochrome c–Dependent Activation of Caspase-3. *Cell* **1997**, *90*, 405–413. [CrossRef]
51. Zhang, X.; Tang, N.; Hadden, T.J.; Rishi, A.K. Akt, FoxO and regulation of apoptosis. *Biochim. Biophys. Acta* **2011**, *1813*, 1978–1986. [CrossRef] [PubMed]

2. Sun, X.; Li, L.; Ma, H.G.; Sun, P.; Wang, Q.L.; Zhang, T.T.; Shen, Y.M.; Zhu, W.M.; Li, X. Bisindolylmaleimide alkaloid BMA-155Cl induces autophagy and apoptosis in human hepatocarcinoma HepG-2 cells through the NF-κB p65 pathway. *Acta Pharmacol. Sin.* **2017**, *38*, 524–538. [CrossRef] [PubMed]
3. Li, N.; Xin, W.Y.; Yao, B.R.; Cong, W.; Wang, C.H.; Hou, G.G. N-phenylsulfonyl-3,5-bis(arylidene)-4-piperidone derivatives as activation NF-κB inhibitors in hepatic carcinoma cell lines. *Eur. J. Med. Chem.* **2018**, *155*, 531–544. [CrossRef] [PubMed]
4. Anning, L. Activation of the JNK signaling pathway: Breaking the brake on apoptosis. *Bioessays* **2003**, *25*, 17–24.
5. Speidel, D. Transcription-independent p53 apoptosis: An alternative route to death. *Trends Cell Biol.* **2010**, *20*, 14–24. [CrossRef] [PubMed]
6. Feng, W.; Li, J.; Liao, S.; Ma, S.; Li, F.; Zhong, C.; Li, G.; Wei, Y.; Huang, H.; Wei, Q.; et al. Go6983 attenuates titanium particle-induced osteolysis and RANKL mediated osteoclastogenesis through the suppression of NFkappaB/JNK/p38 pathways. *Biochem. Biophys. Res. Commun.* **2018**, *503*, 62–70. [CrossRef] [PubMed]

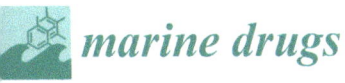

Article

Effect of Oversulfation on the Composition, Structure, and In Vitro Anti-Lung Cancer Activity of Fucoidans Extracted from *Sargassum aquifolium*

Hui-Hua Hsiao [1,2,3,4,5], Tien-Chiu Wu [4,5], Yung-Hsiang Tsai [6], Chia-Hung Kuo [6], Ren-Han Huang [7], Yong-Han Hong [8,*] and Chun-Yung Huang [6,*]

1. Faculty of Medicine, Kaohsiung Medical University, Kaohsiung 80708, Taiwan; huhuhs@kmu.edu.tw
2. Center for Cancer Research, Kaohsiung Medical University, Kaohsiung 80708, Taiwan
3. Center for Liquid Biopsy and Cohort Research, Kaohsiung Medical University, Kaohsiung 80708, Taiwan
4. Division of Hematology and Oncology, Department of Internal Medicine, Kaohsiung Medical University Hospital, Kaohsiung Medical University, Kaohsiung 80756, Taiwan; 960552@ms.kmuh.org.tw
5. Cancer Center, Kaohsiung Medical University Hospital, Kaohsiung Medical University, Kaohsiung 80756, Taiwan
6. Department of Seafood Science, National Kaohsiung University of Science and Technology, No. 142, Haijhuan Rd., Nanzih District, Kaohsiung City 81157, Taiwan; yht@nkust.edu.tw (Y.-H.T.); kuoch@nkust.edu.tw (C.-H.K.)
7. Mackay Memorial Hospital Emergency Department, No. 92, Sec. 2, Zhongshan North Rd., Taipei City 10449, Taiwan; lisa68850@gmail.com
8. Department of Nutrition, Yanchao Campus, I-Shou University, No. 8, Yida Rd., Jiaosu Village, Yanchao District, Kaohsiung City 82445, Taiwan
* Correspondence: yonghan@isu.edu.tw (Y.-H.H.); cyhuang@nkust.edu.tw (C.-Y.H.); Tel.: +886-7-6151100 (ext. 7914) (Y.-H.H.); +886-7-3617141 (ext. 23606) (C.-Y.H.)

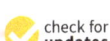

Citation: Hsiao, H.-H.; Wu, T.-C.; Tsai, Y.-H.; Kuo, C.-H.; Huang, R.-H.; Hong, Y.-H.; Huang, C.-Y. Effect of Oversulfation on the Composition, Structure, and In Vitro Anti-Lung Cancer Activity of Fucoidans Extracted from *Sargassum aquifolium*. *Mar. Drugs* 2021, 19, 215. https://doi.org/10.3390/md19040215

Academic Editor: Roland Ulber

Received: 14 March 2021
Accepted: 8 April 2021
Published: 12 April 2021

Publisher's Note: MDPI stays neutral with regard to jurisdictional claims in published maps and institutional affiliations.

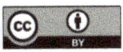

Copyright: © 2021 by the authors. Licensee MDPI, Basel, Switzerland. This article is an open access article distributed under the terms and conditions of the Creative Commons Attribution (CC BY) license (https://creativecommons.org/licenses/by/4.0/).

Abstract: Intensive efforts have been undertaken in the fields of prevention, diagnosis, and therapy of lung cancer. Fucoidans exhibit a wide range of biological activities, which are dependent on the degree of sulfation, sulfation pattern, glycosidic branches, and molecular weight of fucoidan. The determination of oversulfation of fucoidan and its effect on anti-lung cancer activity and related signaling cascades is challenging. In this investigation, we used a previously developed fucoidan (SCA), which served as a native fucoidan, to generate two oversulfated fucoidan derivatives (SCA-S1 and SCA-S2). SCA, SCA-S1, and SCA-S2 showed differences in compositions and had the characteristic structural features of fucoidan by Fourier transform infrared (FTIR) and nuclear magnetic resonance (NMR) analyses. The anticancer properties of SCA, SCA-S1, and SCA-S2 against human lung carcinoma A-549 cells were analyzed in terms of cytotoxicity, cell cycle, Bcl-2 expression, mitochondrial membrane potential (MMP), expression of caspase-3, cytochrome *c* release, Annexin V/propidium iodide (PI) staining, DNA fragmentation, and the underlying signaling cascades. Our findings indicate that the oversulfation of fucoidan promotes apoptosis of lung cancer cells and the mechanism may involve the Akt/mTOR/S6 pathway. Further in vivo research is needed to establish the precise mechanism whereby oversulfated fucoidan mitigates the progression of lung cancer.

Keywords: anti-lung cancer; apoptosis; brown algae; fucoidan; human lung carcinoma A-549 cells; oversulfation; *Sargassum aquifolium*

1. Introduction

Lung cancer is the most common cancer worldwide and has high morbidity and mortality rates. Thus, considerable research efforts have been undertaken aimed at improving the prevention, diagnosis, and treatment of this disease [1]. The biggest risk factors for lung cancer are habitual smoking of tobacco, air pollution (indoor and outdoor), radiation, and occupational exposure to hazardous chemicals [2]. Lung cancer is the most prevalent form of cancer in Taiwan and is the most common cause of cancer-related mortality [3].

While therapeutic approaches for lung cancer have seen significant advances in recent years, the treatment of this disease remains a considerable clinical challenge. Hence, in order to improve patient outcomes, there is a crucial need for novel agents and targets for the treatment of lung cancer.

Fucoidan has been shown to exhibit impressive biological activities, such as antioxidant, immunoregulatory, anti-inflammatory, antitumor, and antithrombotic effects [4]. The degree of sulfation, sulfation pattern, molecular weight (MW), and glycosidic branches of various fucoidans influence the aforementioned biological activities [4]. Sulfate content appears to be the most critical variable [5]. According to a study conducted by Soeda et al. [5], fucoidan derivatives with varying sulfate contents were capable of promoting tissue plasminogen activator (t-PA)-induced plasma clot lysis and preventing the formation of fibrin polymers. These activities were enhanced in direct proportion to the degree of sulfation. In another study by Koyanagi et al. [6], it was shown that oversulfated fucoidans demonstrated greater anti-angiogenic activity compared with native fucoidans, and therefore they were able to inhibit the growth of tumor cells more effectively by suppressing angiogenesis. Moreover, in comparison with native fucoidans, oversulfated fucoidans appeared to show more potent anticancer activity against AGS, a human stomach cancer cell line [7]. The above-mentioned studies indicate that the sulfate content of fucoidans has a significant influence on their biological properties and that the modification of sulfate content could thus potentially enhance said properties. A number of studies have explored the biological activities of oversulfated fucoidans, but relatively little is known about the effects that varying levels of sulfation of fucoidan have on anti-lung cancer activity, and the mechanism involved remains poorly understood.

This investigation is an extension of our previous study, in which a native fucoidan (SC) was created from single-screw extrusion pretreated *Sargassum aquifolium*. Three degraded fucoidan products were developed: SCA (degradation of SC by ascorbic acid), SCH (degradation of SC by hydrogen peroxide), and SCAH (degradation of SC by ascorbic acid + hydrogen peroxide). The results of the study showed that SCA had high cytotoxicity to lung cancer cells as well as a strong ability to suppress Bcl-2 expression in lung cancer cells. Moreover, SCA showed high efficacy with respect to induction of cytochrome c release, promotion of late apoptosis of lung cancer cells, and activation of caspase-9 and -3 [8]. In the present study, SCA served as a native fucoidan from which two fucoidan derivatives with different levels of sulfation were generated: SCA-S1 and SCA-S2. Then we analyzed the anticancer activities of SCA, SCA-S1, and SCA-S2 against human lung carcinoma A-549 cells in terms of cell cycle, cytotoxicity, expression of caspase-3, mitochondrial membrane potential (MMP), cytochrome c release, Bcl-2 expression, Annexin V/ propidium iodide (PI) staining, and DNA fragmentation, as well as the underlying signaling transduction cascades. To the best of the authors' knowledge, this is the first study to investigate a potential mechanism of anti-lung cancer activity involving oversulfated fucoidans obtained from single-screw extrusion pretreated *S. aquifolium*. In future research, we intend to explore the clinical applications of oversulfated fucoidans in the treatment and prevention of lung cancer and possibly other cancers.

2. Results

2.1. Preparation of Oversulfated Fucoidans (SCA-S1 and SCA-S2) and Compositional Analysis

SCA is a degraded fucoidan product, which was previously produced by our laboratory. The results of our in vitro analyses demonstrated that SCA possesses anti-lung cancer properties [8]. We used SCA in the present study as a native fucoidan and created two oversulfated fucoidans termed SCA-S1 and SCA-S2. Table 1 displays the chemical and monosaccharide compositions of SCA, SCA-S1, and SCA-S2. The percentages of sulfate content for SCA, SCA-S1, and SCA-S2 were $13.67 \pm 2.19\%$, $34.67 \pm 3.73\%$, and $60.63 \pm 3.69\%$, respectively. The greater sulfate content in SCA-S1 and SCA-S2 indicates that the addition of sulfate in SCA was successful. The total sugar contents of SCA, SCA-S1, and SCA-S2 ranged from $28.95 \pm 0.24\%$ to $41.70 \pm 0.91\%$ (w/w, dry basis). The addition of sulfate to fucoidan generally resulted in a reduction in total sugar content. The fucose contents of SCA, SCA-S1, and SCA-S2 were 35.22 ± 2.79%, 20.36 ± 1.52%, and 12.58 ± 0.46%, respectively. Similarly, the fucose content of fucoidan was found to be lower following oversulfation. These results suggest that the addition of sulfate to fucoidan lowers its total sugar and fucose contents. Table 1 shows the monosaccharide compositions of these fucoidans. The major neutral sugar constituents in SCA were galactose, fucose, and galacturonic acid, while the minor sugar units consisted of xylose, mannose, and glucuronic acid. The monosaccharide composition of fucoidan did not appear to change significantly following oversulfation, although SCA-S1 and SCA-S2 showed a reduction in galacturonic acid. Taken together, the aforementioned results indicate that oversulfated fucoidans had higher sulfate content, lower total sugar and fucose contents, and monosaccharide compositions were altered, albeit only slightly. Our results demonstrated differences in compositions among SCA, SCA-S1, and SCA-S2, and thus further analyses of the biological functions of these fucoidans are warranted.

Table 1. Compositional analysis of SCA, SCA-S1, and SCA-S2.

Chemical Composition	SCA [2]	SCA-S1 [2]	SCA-S2 [2]
Sulfate (%) [1]	13.67 ± 2.19 [a]	34.67 ± 3.73 [b]	60.63 ± 3.69 [c]
Total sugar (%) [1]	41.70 ± 0.91 [c]	28.95 ± 0.24 [a]	35.08 ± 0.21 [b]
Fucose (%) [1]	35.22 ± 2.79 [c]	20.36 ± 1.52 [b]	12.58 ± 0.46 [a]
Monosaccharide Composition (Molar Ratio)	SCA	SCA-S1	SCA-S2
Fucose	1	1	1
Galactose	0.30	0.28	0.27
Glucuronic acid	0.01	ND [3]	ND
Galacturonic acid	0.11	ND	ND
Mannose	0.05	0.05	0.05
Xylose	0.05	ND	0.04

[1] Total sugars (%), fucose (%), and sulfate (%) = (g/g, dry basis) × 100; [2] Experiments were performed in triplicate; values in the same row with varying letters differ ($p < 0.05$); [3] ND: not detected.

2.2. Structural Analysis of SCA, SCA-S1, and SCA-S2

Fourier transform infrared (FTIR) and nuclear magnetic resonance (NMR) techniques were employed to conduct structural analyses of SCA, SCA-S1, and SCA-S2. Figure 1 depicts IR bands at 3401 and 2940 cm^{-1} which correspond to the presence of OH and H$_2$O stretching vibration and C–H stretching of the pyranoid ring or the C-6 group of fucose and galactose units [9,10]. Absorption bands were detected at 1621 and 1421 cm^{-1} which can be attributed to the scissoring vibration of H$_2$O and in-plane ring CCH, COH, and OCH vibrations, characteristic of the absorption pattern of polysaccharide [9–11]. The peaks at 1243 and 1055 cm^{-1} can be ascribed to the presence of the asymmetric stretching of S=O and the C–O–C stretching vibrations in ring or C–O–H in the glucosidal bond [9,10]. The absorption bands at 900 and 840 cm^{-1} were due to the presence of C1–H bending in the β-anomeric link of galactose and equatorial C–O–S bending vibration of sulfate substituents at the axial C-4 position [12]. The bands at 620 and 580 cm^{-1} may correspond to symmetric and anti-symmetric O=S=O deformations [13]. Figure 2A shows the ^{1}H-NMR spectra for SCA, SCA-S1, and SCA-S2. The signals from 5.5 to 5.0 ppm can be attributed to L-fucopyranosyl units [14]. The signal at 4.46 ppm, which was most apparent in SCA, denotes the presence of H-2 in a 2-sulfated fucopyranose residue [14], and the signal at 4.13 ppm (4[H]) indicates the presence of 3-linked α-L-fucose [14]. Signals with a ppm of 4.07/3.95 (6[H]/6′[H]), which were pronounced in SCA, can be explained by the presence of a (1-6)-β-D-linked galacton [15]. Moreover, the signals from 3.9 to 3.6 ppm could be characteristic signals of mannitol [16,17], which is frequently extracted along with fucoidan. The signal obtained at 3.72 ppm may denote the presence of (4[H]) 2,3-linkedα-β-mannose [11], and the signal at 2.14 ppm may indicate methyl protons in

O-acetyls [11,18], which are frequently detected in algal polysaccharides [18]. The signals at 1.92 (1[H]) and 1.23 ppm (6[H]) demonstrate the existence of alkyl at a sulfonyl-attached proton and an alkane proton in two methyl groups, respectively [19]. Other signals, including 7.91, 2.87, and 2.71 ppm, were detected in SCA-S1 and SCA-S2 and these may correspond to N, N-dimethylformamide (DMF), which is a sulfation reagent utilized in the oversulfate treatment of fucoidan. The ^{13}C-NMR spectra (Figure 2B) for SCA, SCA-S1, and SCA-S2 revealed that the prominent signal at 101.6 ppm and peaks between 65–80 ppm correspond to (1-6)-β-D-linked galacton [15]. The signal at 100.3 ppm can be assigned to a (1,3)-linked α-L-fucopyranose residue [17]. The signals at 62.0 and 66.7 ppm signified β-D-galactopyranose residues [20]. Peaks at 19–20 ppm revealed the presence of O-acetyl groups [21], which is often visible in algal polysaccharides. Additional signals can be found in SCA-S1 and SCA-S2 including 164.9, 36.8, and 31.3 ppm, which can be assigned to DMF, a sulfation reagent used for oversulfation of fucoidan [22]. In summary, the data pertaining to FTIR, ^{1}H NMR, and ^{13}C-NMR indicate that SCA, SCA-S1, and SCA-S2 have the characteristic structural features of fucoidan, and that DMF signals could only be detected in SCA-S1 and SCA-S2 using NMR spectra.

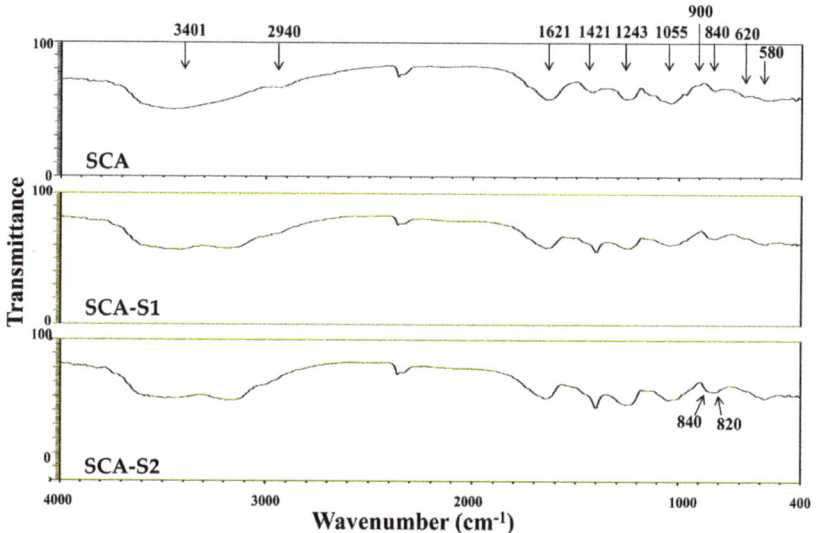

Figure 1. FTIR spectra for SCA, SCA-S1, and SCA-S2. The characteristic peaks at 3401, 2940, 1621, 1421, 1243, 1055, 900, 840, 820, 620, and 580 cm^{-1} are labeled.

2.3. SCA, SCA-S1, and SCA-S2 Exhibited Cytotoxic Effects on A-549 Cells

The human lung carcinoma A-549 cell line is considered a useful in vitro model for investigations of the anti-lung cancer effects of fucoidans [8]. Figure 3A shows the cytotoxic effects of SCA, SCA-S1, and SCA-S2 on A-549 cells. All fucoidans, namely SCA, SCA-S1, and SCA-S2, had reduced ratios of live A-549 cells in a dose-dependent manner, and SCA-S1 exhibited more potent cytotoxic effects on A-549 cells compared with those of SCA and SCA-S2. BEAS-2B, a non-cancerous bronchial epithelial cell line, can be used to represent normal human lung cells [23]. Hence, we conducted a similar experiment using BEAS-2B cells to determine whether these fucoidans exert cytotoxic effects on normal cells. As shown in Figure 3B, the results suggest that SCA-S1 conferred the largest cytotoxicities on BEAS-2B cells, followed by SCA-S2 and SCA. This response was similar to that seen in A-549 cells. In addition, SCA, SCA-S1, and SCA-S2 showed lower cytotoxicities to BEAS-2B in comparison with A-549 cells (Figure 3A,B). Moreover, SCA, SCA-S1, and SCA-S2 had survival rates of A-549 cells ranging from 25.9% to 53.8% at a concentration of 200 µg/mL, and of BEAS-2B cells, survival rates ranged from 64.4% to 94.1%, suggesting these fucoidans were less cytotoxic to normal cells. In our preliminary experiment, a treatment time of 48 h was found to be optimal for the induction of cytotoxicity in A-549 cells. As the survival rates of A-549 cells were reduced to less than 50% (approx.) following treatment of these fucoidans, a concentration of 200 µg/mL and a treatment duration of 48 h were adopted for further in vitro anti-lung cancer experiments.

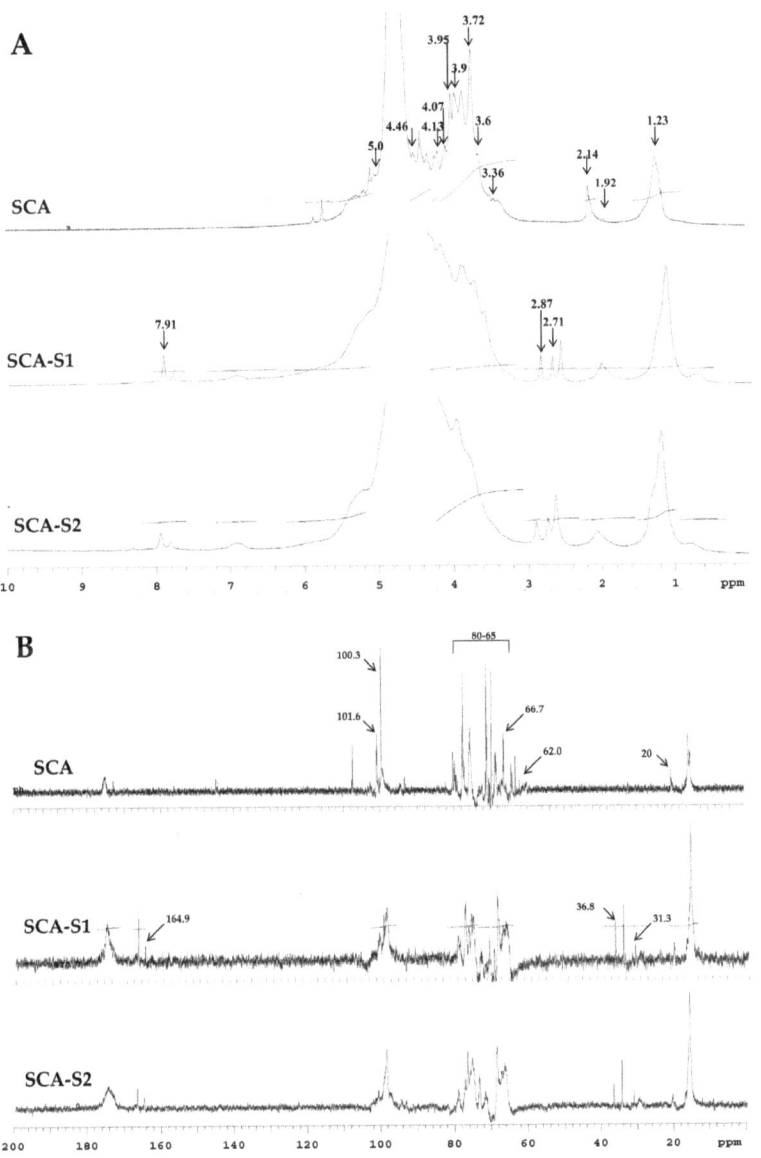

Figure 2. NMR analyses of SCA, SCA-S1, and SCA-S2. (**A**) ^{1}H-NMR spectra for SCA, SCA-S1, and SCA-S2. The characteristic peaks at 7.91, 5.0, 4.46, 4.13, 4.07, 3.95, 3.9, 3.72, 3.6, 3.36, 2.87, 2.71, 2.14, 1.92, and 1.23 ppm are indicated. (**B**) ^{13}C-NMR spectra for SCA, SCA-S1, and SCA-S2. The characteristic peaks at 164.9, 101.6, 100.3, 80–65, 66.7, 62.0, 36.8, 31.3, and 20 ppm are indicated.

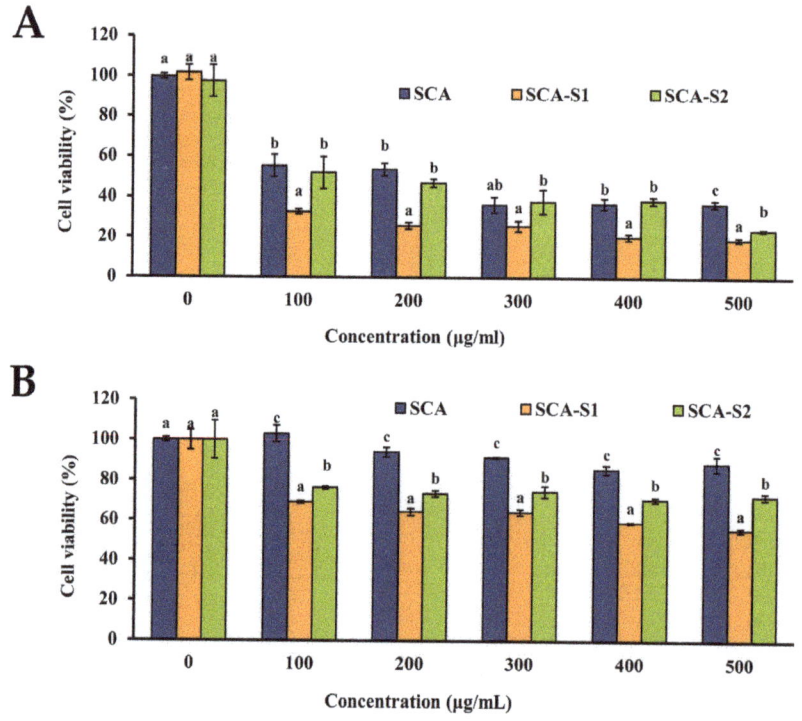

Figure 3. Effects of SCA, SCA-S1, and SCA-S2 on cell viabilities of A-549 and BEAS-2B cells: (**A**) A-549 cells were cotreated with 0–500 μg/mL of SCA, SCA-S1, and SCA-S2 for 48 h, and the cell viability was measured by MTT assays; (**B**) BEAS-2B cells were coincubated with 0–500 μg/mL of SCA, SCA-S1, and SCA-S2 for 48 h, and the cell viability was determined by MTT assays. Experiments were performed in triplicate. Bars with different letters significantly differ at the level of 0.05.

2.4. Effects of SCA, SCA-S1, and SCA-S2 on Cell Cycle Profile of A-549 Cells

Figure 4 shows that when A-549 cells were treated with 200 μg/mL SCA, SCA-S1, and SCA-S2 for 48 h, SCA-S2 had the highest percentage of cells in the sub-G_1 phase (25.0 ± 0.6%), followed by SCA-S1 (13.9 ± 0.4%), SCA (5.33 ± 0.12%), and untreated cells (2.50 ± 0.14%). The cell population in the sub-G_1 phase rose in direct proportion to the induction of DNA fragmentation [24]. As such, SCA-S2 showed the greatest DNA fragmentation (also termed sub-G_1 cell cycle arrest), followed by SCA-S1, SCA, and untreated cells. In summary, all of the tested fucoidans were capable of inducing sub-G_1 cell cycle arrest. SCA-S2 displayed the greatest ability to induce DNA fragmentation of A-549 cells.

2.5. Effects of SCA, SCA-S1, and SCA-S2 on Mitochondrial Membrane Potential, Bcl-2 Expression, and Cytochrome c Release of A-549 Cells

It is thought that TMRE binds to active mitochondria owing to its ability to permeate cells in addition to its positive charge. Loss of MMP is directly related to reduced TMRE binding [25]. In Figure 5, the percentage of cells with low TMRE intensity in the control was 16.7 ± 0.4%. Following treatment of A-549 cells with 200 μg/mL SCA, SCA-S1, and SCA-S2 for 48 h, the percentage of cells with low TMRE intensity increased significantly to 27.3 ± 0.4%, 58.2 ± 2.0%, and 65.9 ± 0.2%, respectively ($p < 0.05$), indicating the occurrence of fucoidan-induced mitochondrial dysfunction. Bcl-2 is a member of the anti-apoptotic class of B cell leukemia-2 gene product (Bcl-2) family proteins and it has been postulated that it blocks MMP depolarization [26]. In contrast, suppressed Bcl-2 expression results in cellular apoptosis. In Figure 6 it can be seen that the percentage of cells with high Bcl-2 intensity in the control was 64.5 ± 0.3%. Treatment of A-549 cells with 200 μg/mL SCA, SCA-S1, and SCA-S2 for 48 h resulted in a reduction of the percentage of cells with high Bcl-2 intensity to 48.4 ± 0.2%, 50.7 ± 0.2%, and 54.5 ± 0.4%, respectively, suggesting the occurrence of fucoidan-mediated suppression of Bcl-2. The release of cytochrome c from mitochondria is a nearly apoptotic event and is an upstream signal of the mitochondria-dependent apoptotic pathway [27,28]. Figure 7 shows that in the control, the percentage of cells with low cytochrome c intensity was 5.07 ± 0.26%. The percentage of cells with low cytochrome c intensity significantly increased to 9.57 ± 0.21%, 13.2 ± 0.1%, and 16.4 ± 0.2%, respectively ($p < 0.05$), when A-549 cells were treated with 200 μg/mL SCA, SCA-S1, and SCA-S2 for 48 h, suggesting the involvement of fucoidan-mediated release of cytochrome c from mitochondria. In summary, these findings indicate that SCA, SCA-S1, and SCA-S2 induced mitochondria-dependent apoptotic effects, as evidenced by the loss of MMP, release of cytochrome c, and suppression of Bcl-2.

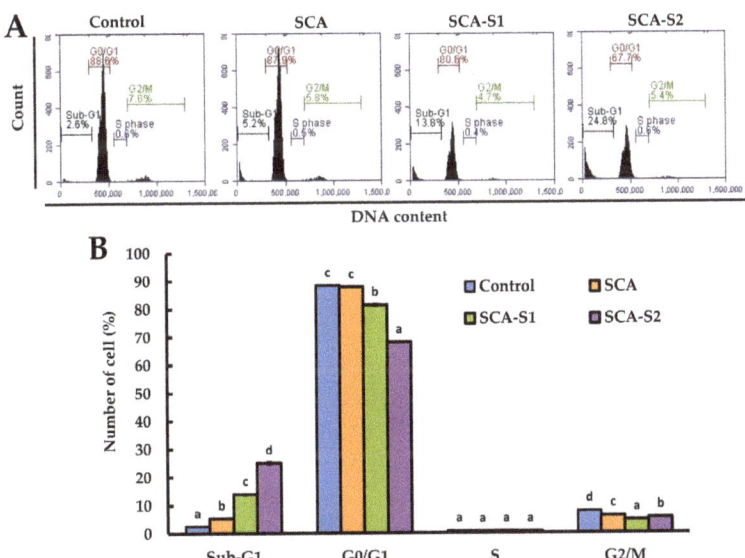

Figure 4. Effects of SCA, SCA-S1, and SCA-S2 treatments on cell cycle profiles of A-549 cells: (**A**) A-549 cells were treated with SCA, SCA-S1, and SCA-S2 at a concentration of 200 μg/mL for 48 h, and cell cycle profiles were measured; (**B**) summary bar graph of three cell cytometric analyses showing the percentages of cells in the sub-G_1, G_0/G_1, S, and G_2/M phases of the cell cycle according to treatments. Results are shown as mean ± SD of three separate experiments. Differences exist between columns labeled with different letters at the level of 0.05.

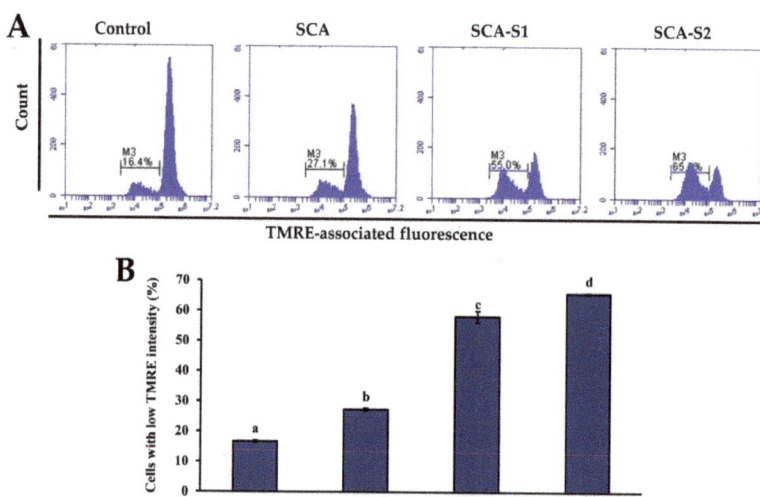

Figure 5. Effects of SCA, SCA-S1, and SCA-S2 treatments on MMP of A-549 cells. A-549 cells were treated with and without 200 µg/mL SCA, SCA-S1, and SCA-S2 for 48 h, and MMP was determined by TMRE staining and flow cytometry. (**A**) Histograms; (**B**) summary bar graph of three cell cytometric analyses showing the percentages of cells with low TMRE intensity according to treatments. Results are shown as mean ± SD of three separate experiments. Differences exist between columns labeled with different letters at the level of 0.05.

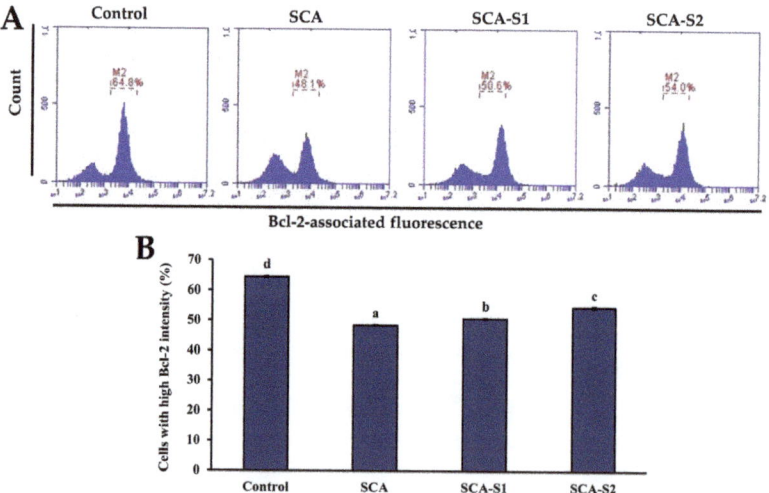

Figure 6. Effects of SCA, SCA-S1, and SCA-S2 treatments on the Bcl-2 expression in A-549 cells. A-549 cells were treated with and without 200 µg/mL SCA, SCA-S1, and SCA-S2 for 48 h, and the level of immunolabeled Bcl-2 was determined by flow cytometry. (**A**) Histograms; (**B**) summary bar graph of three cell cytometric analyses showing the percentages of cells with high Bcl-2 intensity according to treatments. Results are shown as mean ± SD of three separate experiments. Differences exist between columns labeled with different letters at the level of 0.05.

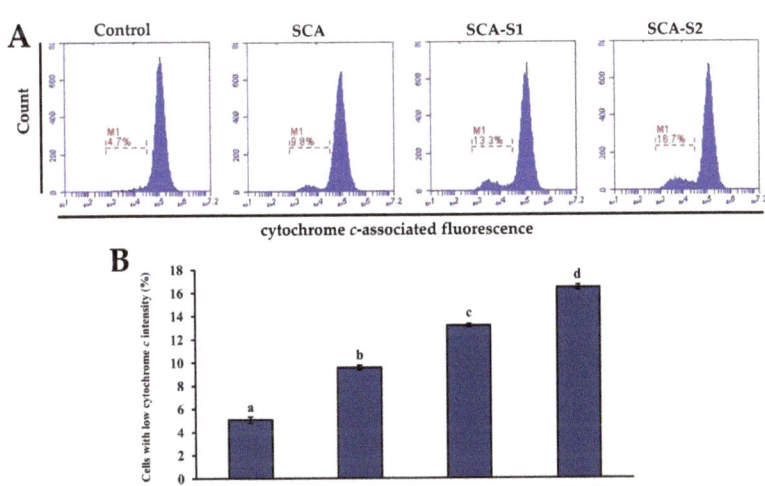

Figure 7. Effects of SCA, SCA-S1, and SCA-S2 treatments on the amount of cytochrome *c* release in A-549 cells. A-549 cells were treated with and without 200 µg/mL SCA, SCA-S1, and SCA-S2 for 48 h, and the level of immunolabeled cytochrome *c* was determined by flow cytometry. (**A**) Histograms; (**B**) summary bar graph of three cell cytometric analyses showing the percentages of cells with low cytochrome *c* intensity according to treatments. Results are shown as mean ± SD of three separate experiments. Differences exist between columns labeled with different letters at the level of 0.05.

2.6. Effects of SCA, SCA-S1, and SCA-S2 on Activation of Caspase-3 and DNA Fragmentation of A-549 Cells

When cytochrome *c* is released from the mitochondrial intermembrane space, apoptosome formation is triggered, leading to the induction of caspase-9 and caspase-3 activation [29]. In Figure 8, it can be seen that the percentage of cells in the control with high caspase-3 intensity was 39.6 ± 0.3%. Treatment of A-549 cells with 200 µg/mL SCA, SCA-S1, and SCA-S2 for 48 h led to an increase in the percentage of cells with high caspase-3 intensity to 63.1 ± 0.5%, 48.8 ± 0.9%, and 59.5 ± 0.4%, respectively, thus providing evidence that activation of caspase-3 was mediated by fucoidan. Activation of caspase-3 was shown to be a vital component of apoptotic cascades and triggers fragmentation of DNA, resulting in late phase apoptosis [30,31]. Figure 9 demonstrates that the percentage of cells in the control with a high DNA break-associated fluorescent intensity was 10.3 ± 1.8%. Treatment of A-549 cells with 200 µg/mL SCA, SCA-S1, and SCA-S2 for 48 h significantly enhanced the percentage of cells with high DNA break-associated fluorescent intensity by 15.6 ± 1.2%, 25.0 ± 1.7%, and 20.1 ± 1.1% ($p < 0.05$), respectively, suggesting the occurrence of fucoidan-mediated DNA fragmentation.

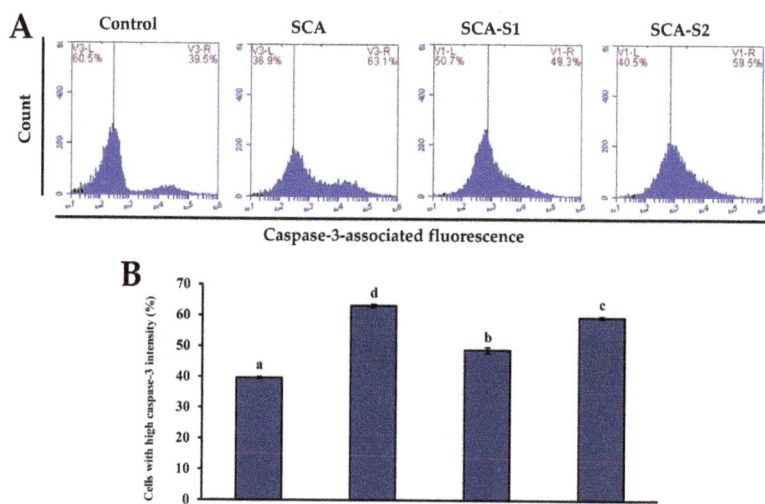

Figure 8. Effects of SCA, SCA-S1, and SCA-S2 treatments on the activation of caspase-3 in A-549 cells. A-549 cells were treated with and without 200 µg/mL SCA, SCA-S1, and SCA-S2 for 48 h, and the level of immunolabeled caspase-3 was determined by flow cytometry. (**A**) Histograms; (**B**) summary bar graph of three cell cytometric analyses showing the percentages of cells with high caspase-3 intensity according to treatments. Results are shown as mean ± SD of three separate experiments. Differences exist between columns labeled with different letters at the level of 0.05.

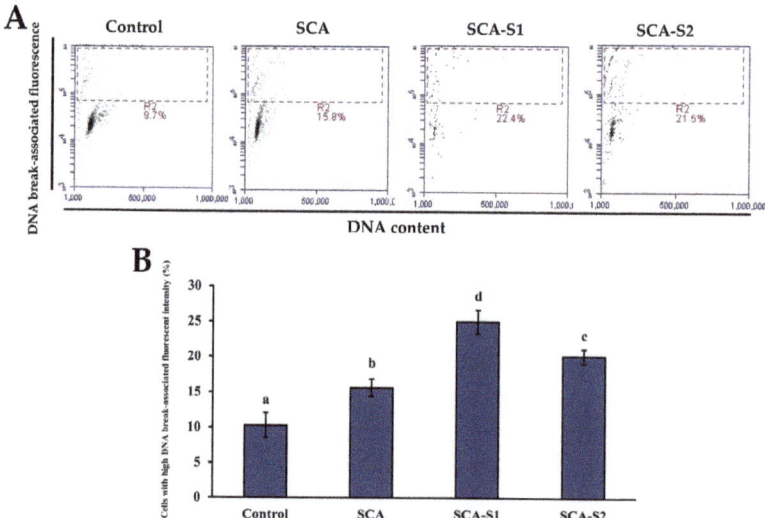

Figure 9. Effects of SCA, SCA-S1, and SCA-S2 treatments on the extent of DNA fragmentation in A-549 cells. A-549 cells were treated with and without 200 µg/mL SCA, SCA-S1, and SCA-S2 for 48 h, and the level of immunolabeled BrdU was determined by flow cytometry. (**A**) Histograms; (**B**) summary bar graph of three cell cytometric analyses showing the percentages of cells with high DNA break-associated fluorescent intensity according to treatments. Results are shown as mean ± SD of three separate experiments. Differences exist between columns labeled with different letters at the level of 0.05.

2.7. Effects of SCA, SCA-S1, and SCA-S2 on the Induction of Apoptosis in A-549 Cells

Loss of plasma membrane asymmetry occurs early in apoptosis, leading to exposure of phosphatidylserine (PS) residues at the outer plasma membrane [32]. The specific binding of Annexin V to PS means that loss of plasma membrane integrity can be used in the detection of apoptosis [32]. The Annexin V-FITC and PI double-staining method is also capable of providing information related to necrotic cells as well as early- and late-stage apoptosis. Figure 10 shows that, in the control, the percentage of live cells was 68.0 ± 0.8%. Furthermore, treatment of A-549 cells with 200 µg/mL SCA, SCA-S1, and SCA-S2 for 48 h led to a decrease in the percentage of live cells to 27.2 ± 1.3%, 2.38 ± 0.83%, and 2.93 ± 0.40%, respectively. Meanwhile, the percentage of late apoptotic cells in the control was 13.2 ± 0.6%. When A-549 cells were subjected to 200 µg/mL SCA, SCA-S1, and SCA-S2 for 48 h, the percentage of late apoptotic cells rose to 45.2 ± 1.0%, 75.9 ± 0.7%, and 80.5 ± 1.1%, respectively. The aforementioned findings clearly demonstrate that A-549 cellular death (primary late apoptosis) was induced by SCA, SCA-S1, and SCA-S2.

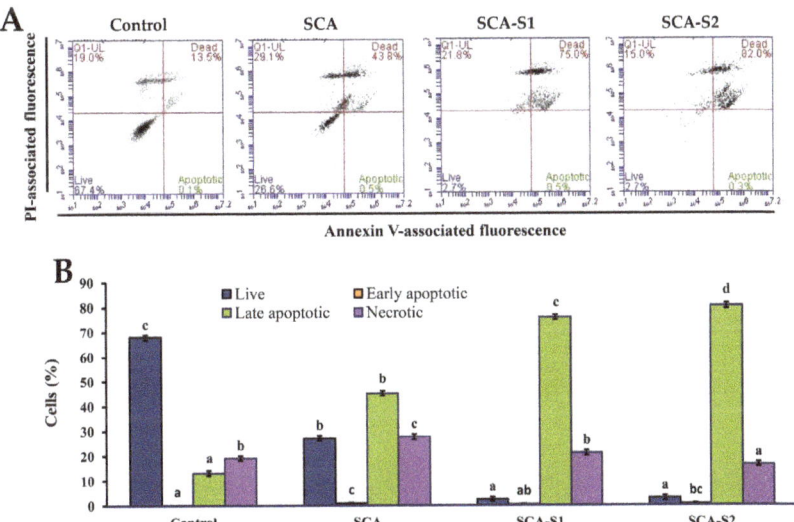

Figure 10. Effects of SCA, SCA-S1, and SCA-S2 treatments on the induction of apoptosis in A-549 cells. A-549 cells were treated with and without 200 µg/mL SCA, SCA-S1, and SCA-S2 for 48 h, and the Annexin V-FITC/PI-stained cells were determined by flow cytometry. (**A**) Histograms; (**B**) summary bar graph of three cell cytometric analyses showing the percentages of Annexin V-FITC/PI-stained cells according to treatments. Results are shown as mean ± SD of three separate experiments. Differences exist between columns labeled with different letters at the level of 0.05.

2.8. SCA, SCA-S1, and SCA-S2 Induced Dephosphorylation of Akt, mTOR, and S6 in A-549 Cells

Figure 11 depicts the percentage of cells in the control with high p-Akt intensity: 91.0 ± 0.2%. When A-549 cells were exposed to 200 µg/mL SCA, SCA-S1, and SCA-S2 for 48 h, the percentage of cells with high p-Akt intensity fell to 88.6 ± 1.9%, 65.3 ± 3.0%, and 67.6 ± 3.5%, respectively. Moreover, the percentage of cells with high Akt1 intensity in the control was 95.2 ± 0.3%. When A-549 cells were subjected to 200 µg/mL SCA, SCA-S1, and SCA-S2 for 48 h, the percentage of cells with high Akt1 intensity was 94.1 ± 1.0%, 85.4 ± 1.2%, and 86.7 ± 0.1%, respectively. The percentage of cells with high p-mTOR intensity in the control was 81.0 ± 0.4%. Following the treatment of A-549 cells with 200 µg/mL SCA, SCA-S1, and SCA-S2 for 48 h, the percentage of cells with high p-mTOR intensity was reduced to 79.3 ± 0.4%, 66.0 ± 0.8%, and 66.1 ± 0.8%, respectively. In the control, the percentage of cells with high p-S6 intensity was 88.2 ± 0.7%. The percentage of cells with high p-S6 intensity dropped to 69.2 ± 0.9%, 50.3 ± 2.3%, and 64.1 ± 1.2%, respectively, when A-549 cells had been treated with 200 µg/mL SCA, SCA-S1, and SCA-S2 for 48 h. The data above provide clear evidence of fucoidan-mediated dephosphorylation of Akt, mTOR, and S6 in A-549 cells.

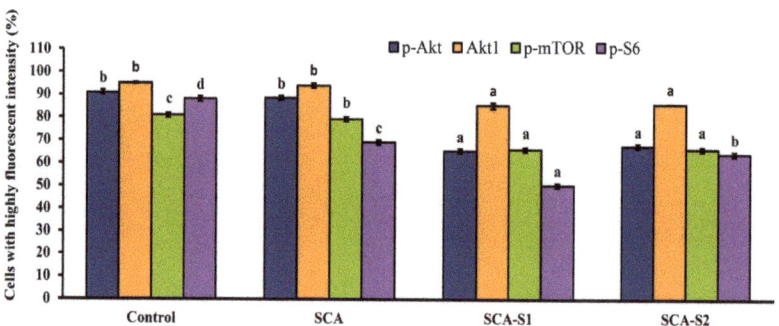

Figure 11. Effects of SCA, SCA-S1, and SCA-S2 treatments on the levels of p-Akt, Akt1, p-mTOR, and p-S6 in A-549 cells. A-549 cells were treated with and without 200 µg/mL SCA, SCA-S1, and SCA-S2 for 48 h, and the cells with highly fluorescent intensity were determined by flow cytometry. The bar graph summary of three cell cytometric analyses shows the percentages of cells with highly fluorescent intensity according to treatments. Results are shown as mean ± SD of three separate experiments. Differences exist between columns labeled with different letters at the level of 0.05.

3. Discussion

A number of studies in the literature have indicated that oversulfated fucoidans exhibit greater anti-angiogenic activity compared to native fucoidans, and therefore by mitigating angiogenesis they can inhibit the growth of tumor cell growth more efficiently [6]. The wide range of anticancer activity seen among the various oversulfated fucoidan derivatives can probably be explained by differences in sulfate content [7]. The present study is an extension of our previous work on a native fucoidan (SC, extracted from *Sargassum aquifolium*) and three fucoidan hydrolysates, which we developed, termed SCA (degradation of SC by ascorbic acid), SCH (degradation of SC by hydrogen peroxide), and SCAH (degradation of SC by ascorbic acid + hydrogen peroxide). Our analyses determined that SCA was a suitable candidate for further development as an adjuvant therapy for lung cancer [8]. In the current study, we oversulfated SCA and developed two oversulfated fucoidans termed SCA-S1 and SCA-S2. The sulfate contents of SCA, SCA-S1, and SCA-S2 were 13.67 ± 2.19%, 34.67 ± 3.73%, and 60.63 ± 3.69%, respectively (Table 1). In a study by Cho et al. [7], the addition of sulfate groups increased the sulfate content of the low molecular weight fucoidan (F_{5-30K} fraction) up to 56.8%. The sulfate content of oversulfated F_{5-30K} fraction was similar to that of SCA-S2, indicating that oversulfation of fucoidan is capable of yielding a sulfate content reaching as high as 60% (approx.). A summary of the chemical properties of SCA, SCA-S1, and SCA-S2 is presented in Table 1. Increases in sulfate content may result in a proportional decrease in the fucose content of fucoidan, suggesting that oversulfation may modify the fundamental structure of fucoidan. The FTIR spectra for SCA, SCA-S1, and SCA-S2 (Figure 1) depict broader peak areas at 1243 (the asymmetric stretching of S=O), 840 (C–O–S bending vibration of sulfate substituents at the axial C-4 position), and 620/580 (the symmetric and anti-symmetric O=S=O deformations) cm^{-1} in SCA-S1 and SCA-S2, which are indicative of higher sulfate contents in SCA-S1 and SCA-S2. Moreover, Partankar et al. [33] reported that the sulfate peaks at around 820 and 840 cm^{-1} correspond to the equatorial C-2 and axial C-4 positions, respectively. In Figure 1, SCA showed a strong peak at around 840 cm^{-1}, which indicates that the sulfates had largely been substituted at the C-4 position. In contrast, the oversulfated SCA-S1 and SCA-S2 both showed a pronounced peak at 840 cm^{-1} with a shoulder at 820 cm^{-1} (Figure 1), providing evidence of a 2,4 disubstitution of the sulfate groups. These findings are in line with previously reported studies [7], showing that sulfation resulted in the emergence of a shoulder at 820 cm^{-1} alongside the main peak at 840 cm^{-1} in the IR spectra, indicative of 2,4 disulfation. NMR spectra can be used to further evaluate the structural characteristics of oversulfated fucoidans. After oversulfation, the ^{1}H-NMR and ^{13}C-NMR spectra of SCA, SCA-S1, and SCA-S2 (Figure 2) were found to be different. Nonetheless, the characteristic peaks of fucoidan were also detected in SCA, SCA-S1, and SCA-S2. Sulfur trioxide N,N-dimethylformamide complex (SO$_3$-DMF) (sulfating agents) in formamide (FA) solution was used to sulfate SCA-S1 and SCA-S2. Of note, the specific ^{1}H-NMR and ^{13}C-NMR signals representing DMF were detected in SCA-S1 and SCA-S2 (Figure 2), demonstrating the presence of sulfate groups in the fucoidan backbones.

In a previous study, we showed that the native fucoidan (SC) and fucoidan hydrolysates (SCA, SCH, and SCAH) lowered the ratios of live A-549 cells, and SCA, SCH, and SCAH conferred stronger cytotoxic effects on A-549 cells compared with SC [8]. However, all of the tested fucoidans (SC, SCA, SCH, and SCAH) showed less potent cytotoxic effects against normal BEAS-2B cells compared with that of A-549 cells [8]. Although there are a number of available human lung cancer cell lines that can be used to establish a tumor model, such as A-549, H-460, H-1299, H-1650, H-358, and HCC-827 [34], A-549 cells are adenocarcinomic human alveolar basal epithelial cells, which are widely used in models for the study of lung cancer and the development of drug therapies against it [8,35]. Moreover, A-549 cells are easy to maintain and grow faster compared with other lung cancer cells. Thus, A-549 cells were utilized in the present study to evaluate the anticancer effect of fucoidan extracts. In the current study, the most potent cytotoxic effects on A-549 cells were observed in SCA-S1 among the tested fucoidans (Figure 3A). The analyses of the cytotoxicities of SCA-S1 to A-549 cells and BEAS-2B cells at the concentration of 500 µg/mL revealed a survival rate of 19.3 ± 1.0% in A-549 cells, but in BEAS-2B cells the survival rate was 55.5 ± 1.0%, showing that SCA-S1 had a toxic effect on normal cells that was 2.9-fold (55.5/19.3 = 2.9) lower (Figure 3). Likewise, SCA-S2 was shown to have an approximately 3.0-fold (72.4/24.2 = 3.0) lower toxic effect on normal cells (Figure 3). In a study by Cho et al. [7], it was found that fucoidan (F$_{>30K}$ fraction, sulfate content = 41.2%) exhibited 50% anticancer activity against AGS, a human stomach cancer cell line, at a concentration exceeding 800 µg/mL. SCA-S1 possessed a sulfate content of 34.7%, which was similar to that in the F$_{>30K}$ fraction, but it showed a 50% anticancer activity against A-549 cells at a concentration of 74.4 µg/mL. While the cancer cell lines examined in the two aforementioned studies were different, the results still show that SCA-S1 confers a strongly potent effect against cancer cells.

Cell cycle analysis can be employed to assess the growth inhibitory effects of SCA, SCA-S1, and SCA-S2 on A-549 cells. Flow cytometry is a rapid technique that can be used to identify compounds capable of selective or preferential eradication of cancer cells by altering regulation of the cell cycle and/or inducing apoptosis. Treatment of cells with an apoptosis-inducing agent can lead to DNA fragmentation, which can also be analyzed by flow cytometry [24]. Small fragments of DNA can be eluted by washing with PBS. Any cells that have lost DNA will not be stained as obviously using PI stain and will appear to the left of the G_1 peak (the so-called sub-G_1 peak). Figure 4 shows that SCA-S2 had the highest percentage of cells in the sub-G_1 phase, followed by SCA-S1 and SCA. In Table 1, SCA-S2 had the greatest amount of sulfate, followed by SCA-S1 and SCA. Hence, increases in the sulfate content of fucoidan may promote the induction of sub-G_1 cell cycle arrest in a proportional manner.

MMP plays a vital role in cellular energy production (ATP) and in maintaining homeostasis within the cell [36]. MMP disruption is indicative of mitochondria dysfunction in the transduction of an apoptotic signal [37]. In Figure 5, SCA-S2 exerted the strongest effect in terms of induction of mitochondrial dysfunction in A-549 cells, followed by SCA-S1 and SCA. This trend was correlated with sulfate contents (Table 1). Bcl-2, an anti-apoptotic protein, has been postulated to block MMP depolarization, which in turn mitigates the activation of downstream apoptotic molecules, such as cytochrome *c*, AIF, and Smac/Diablo [26]. Moreover, suppression of Bcl-2 expression leads to cellular apoptosis. Figure 6 shows that all of the fucoidans were capable of suppressing the expression of Bcl-2, compared with the control. Release of cytochrome *c* from the mitochondria is a nearly apoptotic event in the mitochondria-dependent apoptotic pathway [38,39]. According to Figure 7, SCA-S2 showed the greatest cytochrome *c* release in A-549 cells, followed by SCA-S1 and SCA. This trend was in proportion to the sulfate contents of the fucoidans (Table 1). Taken together, these results indicate that induction of apoptosis by SCA, SCA-S1, and SCA-S2 was largely via a mitochondria-dependent apoptotic pathway. The sulfate content of fucoidan appears to play a key role in apoptotic cell death. The intrinsic pathway (mitochondria pathway) comprises a serial process involving loss of MMP, release of cytochrome *c* into the cytoplasm, formation of an apoptosome complex, culminating in the activation of caspase-3 [40,41]. Furthermore, the activation of caspase-3 plays a pivotal role in DNA fragmentation, which occurs in late phase apoptosis [31]. All of the fucoidans promoted the activation of caspase-3, as compared to the control, as shown in Figure 8. In Figure 9, the results show that the degree of DNA fragmentation in A-549 cells was enhanced following treatment with SCA, SCA-S1, and SCA-S2. In short, the oversulfated fucoidans exhibited greater DNA fragmentation compared with SCA and the control. Moreover, Annexin V-FITC/PI double staining revealed these fucoidans were likely responsible for A-549 cell death (largely involving late apoptosis), and compared with SCA and the control, oversulfated fucoidans had greater numbers of late apoptotic cells (Figure 10).

Activation of the Akt/mTOR/S6 signaling is common in a wide range of cancers [42,43]. It has been shown that commercialized fucoidan extract from *Fucus vesiculosus* suppressed p-Akt and p-mTOR in A-549 cells in a dose- and time-dependent manner [44]. In the current investigation, we found that SCA, SCA-S1, and SCA-S2 suppressed levels of p-Akt, p-mTOR, and p-S6 in comparison with the untreated control. Moreover, the results indicated that SCA-S1 and SCA-S2 showed greater effectiveness with respect to reducing expressions of p-Akt, p-mTOR, and p-S6 compared with SCA. These results provide clear evidence that the oversulfated fucoidan enhances the anticancer activity (particularly against lung cancer) and the underlying mechanism involves the Akt/mTOR/S6 pathway. These encouraging findings could be useful in the future development of fucoidans with extensive sulfate substitution with a view to boosting their anticancer properties. While the precise mechanism has yet to be fully elucidated, it is reasonable to postulate that the elevated negative charge induced by oversulfation enhances the interaction with particular proteins, including plasmatic proteins, adhesion proteins, and growth factors that play a role in cell proliferation, thereby facilitating cell growth suppression [7,45]. Further research is required to gain a complete understanding of the underlying mechanism of action of oversulfated fucoidans using other lung cancer cell lines, and to conduct in vivo models to investigate the upstream and downstream targeting molecules of signaling pathways in lung cancer.

4. Materials and Methods

4.1. Materials

Samples of *Sargassum aquifolium* were collected from Kenting (Pingtung, Taiwan). After washing and drying, samples were sealed in aluminum foil bags and kept at 4 °C until use. L-fucose, D-galactose, D-glucuronic acid, D-galacturonic acid, D-xylose, D-mannose, dimethyl sulfoxide (DMSO), potassium bromide (KBr), 2,2,2-Trifluoroacetic acid (TFA), and 3-(4,5-dimethylthiazol-2-yl)-2,5-diphenyltetrazolium bromide (MTT) were obtained from Sigma-Aldrich (St. Louis, MO, USA). Ham's F12K medium, DMEM medium, trypsin/EDTA, fetal bovine serum (FBS), penicillin, and streptomycin were purchased from Gibco Laboratories (Grand Island, NY, USA). TMRE was obtained from Molecular Probes, Invitrogen Corp. (Carlsbad, CA, USA). Unless otherwise stated, other reagents were purchased from Sigma-Aldrich (St. Louis, MO, USA).

4.2. Sulfation of Fucoidan

SCA was produced in accordance with the methods described in our previous studies [8]. Sulfation of SCA was performed according to the method described by Wang et al. [22]. The sulfation reagent, SO_3-DMF, was obtained by dropping 20 mL of chlorosulfonic acid into 100 mL of N,N-dimethylformamide under cooling in an ice-water bath. Dry SCA (0.1 g) was added to 10 mL formamide (FA), and the mixture was stirred at RT for 30 min in order to disperse it into the solvent. Then 10 mL SO_3-DMF reagent (for SCA-S1) or 20 mL SO_3-DMF reagent (for SCA-S2) was added. After reaction at RT for 4 h, the solution was neutralized to pH = 7.0 with 1 mol/L NaOH solution and dialyzed against distilled water for 24 h using 1000 Da MW cutoff dialysis membranes. The remnant was concentrated and lyophilized to obtain SCA-S1 and SCA-S2.

4.3. Analytical Methods

The fucose content was estimated using the protocol described by Huang et al. [46] and L-fucose was used as the standard. For the determination of the sulfate content, the sample was firstly hydrolyzed with 1 N HCl solution for 5 h at 105 °C. The hydrolysate was quantified to determine the percentage of sulfate composition using Dionex ICS-1500 Ion Chromatography with IonPac AS9-HC column at a flow rate of 1 mL/min at 30 °C with conductometric detection. The eluent was 9 mM Na_2CO_3, and K_2SO_4 was utilized as standard. Total sugar content was assayed using a phenol-sulfuric acid method using L-fucose as the standard.

4.4. Monosaccharide Composition Analysis

For the determination of monosaccharide composition, the sample was first hydrolyzed with 2 M trifluoroacetic acid (TFA) for 4 h at 110 °C. After removing the residual acid, the standard sugars and sample were pre-column derivatized with 1-phenyl-3-methyl-5-pyrazolone (PMP) for 100 min at 70 °C. The resulting solutions were extracted with chloroform three times. Then the PMP derivatives were eluted with a mixture of 0.1 M phosphate buffer (pH 6.7) and acetonitrile in a ratio of 83:17 (v/v, %) at a flow rate of 1 mL/min on a reversed-phase Inspire™ C18 (250 × 4.6 mm, 5 µm) column with detection at 245 nm. L-fucose, D-galactose, D-glucuronic acid, D-galacturonic acid, D-xylose, and D-mannose were used as standards.

4.5. FTIR Spectroscopy

The FTIR spectra were analyzed according to a protocol described in Huang et al. [47]. In brief, the sample was ground evenly with KBr (1:50, w/w, %) until particles measured less than 2.5 µm in size. The transparent KBr pellets were prepared at 500 kg/cm^2 under vacuum conditions. The FTIR spectra were obtained using an FT-730 spectrometer (Horiba, Kyoto, Japan). The signals were automatically collected using 60 scans over the range of 4000–400 cm^{-1} at a resolution of 16 cm^{-1} and were compared to a background spectrum collected from the KBr alone.

4.6. NMR Spectroscopy

The fucoidan sample was dissolved with 99.9% D_2O in an NMR tube and the NMR spectra were recorded using a Varian VNMRS-700 NMR spectrometer (Varian, Lexington, MA, USA).

4.7. Cell Culture

A-549 (human lung carcinoma, BCRC 60074, cultured in complete Ham's F12K medium) and BEAS-2B (human bronchial epithelial cells, ATCC CRL-9609, cultured in complete DMEM medium) were obtained from the BCRC (Bioresource Collection and Research Center, Hsinchu, Taiwan) and the ATCC (American Type Culture Collection, Manassas, VA, USA), respectively. All cells were cultured in a 37 °C humidified 5% CO_2 atmosphere, and the medium was changed every two to three days.

4.8. Evaluation of Cytotoxic Activity

The cytotoxic activity of the fucoidan derivatives was measured using the MTT assay. Cells were cultured in medium at 37 °C in a humidified atmosphere with 5% CO_2 for 24 h. The stock solution of fucoidan extract was prepared by dissolving it in phosphate-buffered saline (PBS) to a concentration of 20 mg/mL. The medium was then removed and the cells were treated with different concentrations of fucoidan extracts by diluting the stock solution with serum-free medium. After 48 h treatment, cells were washed with PBS once, and MTT reagent (0.1 mg/mL) was added. After a 4 h incubation, isopropanol was added and thoroughly mixed by pipetting to dissolve the formazan. The resultant solution was measured by absorption at 560 nm using a spectrophotometer. The cell viability was expressed as a percentage of MTT reduction.

4.9. Flow Cytometry-Based Analyses

In all flow cytometry-based analyses, cells (4×10^4 cells/mL) were incubated without (as a non-treated control) and with 200 µg/mL tested samples for 48 h, and then cells were trypsinized and rinsed with PBS to obtain cell samples. Then, each flow cytometry-based analysis was performed according to the following procedures.

The cell cycle analysis was performed according to the method described previously [48]. Briefly, A-549 cells were collected, washed twice with PBS, resuspended in 70% (v/v) ethanol, and stored at 4 °C for at least 2 h. The cells were then washed with staining buffer twice, and stained with 25 µg/mL RNase A. After staining with RNase A for 15 min, the cells were stained with 50 µg/mL PI solution, and flow cytometry-based analysis was performed.

For the MMP analysis, the assay was performed using the method of Yang et al. [49]. Briefly, single cell suspensions were washed twice with PBS and incubated, in the dark, for 20 min at 37 °C with TMRE (100 nM). After labeling, cells were washed and resuspended for flow-cytometric measurement in staining solution.

The Bcl-2 assay was done according to the method described by Yang et al. [49]. In brief, single-cell suspensions were fixed using fixation buffer at 37 °C for 20 min. The cells were subsequently permeabilized using permeabilization buffer, and incubated, in the dark, for 1 h at RT with FITC (fluorescein isothiocyanate)-labeled anti-Bcl-2 antibody (1:25, v/v). After labeling, cells were washed and resuspended for flow-cytometric measurement in staining solution.

The analysis of cytochrome c release was conducted according to the protocol described by Huang et al. [12]. Briefly, single-cell suspensions were fixed using fixation buffer at 37 °C for 20 min. The cells were subsequently permeabilized using permeabilization buffer and incubated in the dark for 1 h at RT with FITC-labeled anti-cytochrome c antibody (1:10, v/v). After labeling, cells were washed and resuspended for flow-cytometric measurement in staining solution.

For activated caspase-3 analysis, the method of Huang et al. [12] was employed. Briefly, single-cell suspensions were incubated, in the dark, for 1 h at 37 °C with FITC-DEVD-FMK solution. After labeling, cells were washed and resuspended for flow-cytometric measurement in staining solution.

For DNA fragmentation analysis, the procedure was conducted using the method described by Shiao et al. [50]. Briefly, A-549 cells were harvested and fixed with 4% paraformaldehyde, washed, and then incubated with 70% ice-cold ethanol at −20 °C overnight. Cells were washed with wash buffer, followed by the addition of BrdU, and then incubated with FITC-conjugated anti-BrdU antibody at RT for 30 min in the dark. After staining, the cells were resuspended in staining buffer for flow analysis.

The Annexin V-FITC/PI staining analysis was performed with an Annexin V-FITC apoptosis detection kit following the protocol described by Yang et al. [49]. Briefly, single-cell suspensions were incubated for 15 min at RT in the dark with Annexin V-FITC (1:20, v/v) and PI (1:20, v/v). After labeling, cells were washed and resuspended for flow-cytometric measurement in staining solution.

For phosphorylated Akt, mTOR, and S6 analyses, as well as Akt1, were done using the techniques described by Huang et al. [51]. In brief, single-cell suspensions were fixed using fixation buffer at 37 °C for 1 h. The cells were then incubated at RT for 1 h in the dark with APC (allophycocyanin)-conjugated anti-Akt1 antibody (1:50, v/v), FITC-conjugated anti-phospho-Akt (Ser473) antibody (1:20, v/v), PE (phycoerythrin)-conjugated anti-phospho-mTOR (Ser2448) antibody (1:20, v/v), or PE-conjugated anti-phospho-S6 (Ser235, Ser236) antibody (1:20, v/v). After labeling, cells were washed and resuspended for flow-cytometric measurement in staining solution. All of the abovementioned flow cytometric analyses were performed with a BD Accuri C6 flow cytometer (San Jose, CA, USA). All of the flow data were analyzed using BD Accuri C6 software.

4.10. Statistical Analysis

All data are expressed as mean ± SD (n = 3). Comparisons between different groups were performed by ANOVA followed by Duncan's multiple range test. A p-value less than 0.05 was considered statistically significant.

5. Conclusions

In this investigation, we successfully produced three fucoidans (SCA, SCA-S1, and SCA-S2) from *Sargassum aquifolium*, which contained different levels of sulfate content. Comparisons of SCA, SCA-S1, and SCA-S2 revealed differences in chemical compositions and structural features as a result of oversulfation treatment. The mitochondrion-dependent pathway was predominant in SCA-, SCA-S1-, and SCA-S2-induced apoptosis of A-549 cells as evidenced by the analyses of mitochondrial membrane potential (MMP), cytochrome c release, Bcl-2 expression, activation of caspase-3, and DNA fragmentation. Moreover, we demonstrated that oversulfation of fucoidan enhanced its activity against lung cancer cells and determined that the underlying mechanism likely involves the Akt/mTOR/S6 pathway. Our results indicate that oversulfated fucoidans hold considerable promise for further development for application as an adjuvant therapy in the treatment of cancer, especially lung cancer.

Author Contributions: Conceptualization, T.-C.W. and H.-H.H.; methodology, Y.-H.T.; software, H.-H.H.; validation, R.-H.H., Y.-H.H., and C.-Y.H.; formal analysis, H.-H.H., R.-H.H., and Y.-H.H.; investigation, Y.-H.T., C.-H.K., and Y.-H.H.; resources, C.-H.K., H.-H.H.; data curation, R.-H.H. and T.-C.W.; writing—original draft preparation, H.-H.H., Y.-H.H., and C.-H.K.; writing—review and editing, C.-H.K. and C.-Y.H.; supervision, Y.-H.H.; project administration, C.-Y.H.; funding acquisition, H.-H.H., Y.-H.H., and C.-Y.H. All authors have read and agreed to the published version of the manuscript.

Funding: This research was funded by a grant provided by Kaohsiung Medical University Hospital (KMUH109-9R19) to Hui-Hua Hsiao. This work was also supported by the Ministry of Science and Technology, Taiwan (grant number MOST 109-2221-E-992-052) and National Kaohsiung University of Science and Technology, Taiwan (grant number 110G07), which were awarded to Chun-Yung Huang. The authors thank the Ministry of Education, Taiwan, for supporting this study (grant number MOE-RSC-108RSN0005), awarded to Yong-Han Hong.

Institutional Review Board Statement: Not applicable.

Informed Consent Statement: Not applicable.

Data Availability Statement: Data is contained within the article.

Conflicts of Interest: The authors declare no conflict of interest.

References

1. Frión-Herrera, Y.; Díaz-García, A.; Ruiz-Fuentes, J.; Rodríguez-Sánchez, H.; Sforcin, J.M. Brazilian green propolis induced apoptosis in human lung cancer A549 cells through mitochondrial-mediated pathway. *J. Pharm. Pharmacol.* **2015**, *67*, 1448–1456. [CrossRef]
2. Islami, F.; Torre, L.A.; Jemal, A. Global trends of lung cancer mortality and smoking prevalence. *Transl. Lung Cancer Res.* **2015**, *4*, 327–338.

3. Ministry of Health and Welfare. Taiwan, Statistics of Causes of Death. Available online: https://dep.mohw.gov.tw/DOS/lp-4927-113.html (accessed on 15 March 2021).
4. Wang, J.; Zhang, Q.; Li, S.; Chen, Z.; Tan, J.; Yao, J.; Duan, D. Low molecular weight fucoidan alleviates diabetic nephropathy by binding fibronectin and inhibiting ECM-receptor interaction in human renal mesangial cells. *Int. J. Biol. Macromol.* **2020**, *150*, 304–314. [CrossRef]
5. Soeda, S.; Sakaguchi, S.; Shimeno, H.; Nagamatsu, A. Fibrinolytic and anticoagulant activities of highly sulfated fucoidan. *Biochem. Pharmacol.* **1992**, *43*, 1853–1858. [CrossRef]
6. Koyanagi, S.; Tanigawa, N.; Nakagawa, H.; Soeda, S.; Shimeno, H. Oversulfation of fucoidan enhances its anti-angiogenic and antitumor activities. *Biochem. Pharmacol.* **2003**, *65*, 173–179. [CrossRef]
7. Cho, M.L.; Lee, B.Y.; You, S.G. Relationship between oversulfation and conformation of low and high molecular weight fucoidans and evaluation of their in vitro anticancer activity. *Molecules* **2011**, *16*, 291–297. [CrossRef] [PubMed]
8. Wu, T.C.; Hong, Y.H.; Tsai, Y.H.; Hsieh, S.L.; Huang, R.H.; Kuo, C.H.; Huang, C.Y. Degradation of *Sargassum crassifolium* fucoidan by ascorbic acid and hydrogen peroxide, and compositional, structural, and in vitro anti-Lung cancer analyses of the degradation products. *Mar. Drugs* **2020**, *18*, 334. [CrossRef]
9. Movasaghi, Z.; Rehman, S.; Ur Rehman, D.I. Fourier transform infrared (FTIR) spectroscopy of biological tissues. *Appl. Spectrosc. Rev.* **2008**, *43*, 134–179. [CrossRef]
10. Shao, P.; Pei, Y.P.; Fang, Z.X.; Sun, P.L. Effects of partial desulfation on antioxidant and inhibition of DLD cancer cell of *Ulva fasciata* polysaccharide. *Int. J. Biol. Macromol.* **2014**, *65*, 307–313. [CrossRef] [PubMed]
11. Palanisamy, S.; Vinosha, M.; Marudhupandi, T.; Rajasekar, P.; Prabhu, N.M. Isolation of fucoidan from *Sargassum polycystum* brown algae: Structural characterization, in vitro antioxidant and anticancer activity. *Int. J. Biol. Macromol.* **2017**, *102*, 405–412. [CrossRef] [PubMed]
12. Huang, C.Y.; Kuo, C.H.; Chen, P.W. Compressional-puffing pretreatment enhances neuroprotective effects of fucoidans from the brown seaweed *Sargassum hemiphyllum* on 6-hydroxydopamine-induced apoptosis in SH-SY5Y cells. *Molecules* **2018**, *23*, 78. [CrossRef] [PubMed]
13. Synytsya, A.; Bleha, R.; Synytsya, A.; Pohl, R.; Hayashi, K.; Yoshinaga, K.; Nakano, T.; Hayashi, T. Mekabu fucoidan: Structural complexity and defensive effects against avian influenza A viruses. *Carbohydr. Polym.* **2014**, *111*, 633–644. [CrossRef] [PubMed]
14. Tako, M.; Nakada, T.; Hongou, F. Chemical characterization of fucoidan from commercially cultured *Nemacystus decipiens* (Itomozuku). *Biosci. Biotechnol. Biochem.* **1999**, *63*, 1813–1815. [CrossRef] [PubMed]
15. Immanuel, G.; Sivagnanavelmurugan, M.; Marudhupandi, T.; Radhakrishnan, S.; Palavesam, A. The effect of fucoidan from brown seaweed *Sargassum wightii* on WSSV resistance and immune activity in shrimp *Penaeus monodon* (Fab). *Fish Shellfish Immunol.* **2012**, *32*, 551–564. [CrossRef] [PubMed]
16. Jégou, C.; Kervarec, N.; Cérantola, S.; Bihannic, I.; Stiger-Pouvreau, V. NMR use to quantify phlorotannins: The case of *Cystoseira tamariscifolia*, a phloroglucinol-producing brown macroalga in Brittany (France). *Talanta* **2015**, *135*, 1–6. [CrossRef] [PubMed]
17. Ermakova, S.; Sokolova, R.; Kim, S.M.; Um, B.H.; Isakov, V.; Zvyagintseva, T. Fucoidans from brown seaweeds *Sargassum hornery*, *Eclonia cava*, *Costaria costata*: Structural characteristics and anticancer activity. *Appl. Biochem. Biotechnol.* **2011**, *164*, 841–850. [CrossRef] [PubMed]
18. Bilan, M.I.; Grachev, A.A.; Ustuzhanina, N.E.; Shashkov, A.S.; Nifantiev, N.E.; Usov, A.I. A highly regular fraction of a fucoidan from the brown seaweed *Fucus distichus* L. *Carbohydr. Res.* **2004**, *339*, 511–517. [CrossRef] [PubMed]
19. Kumar, T.V.; Lakshmanasenthil, S.; Geetharamani, D.; Marudhupandi, T.; Suja, G.; Suganya, P. Fucoidan—A α-D-glucosidase inhibitor from *Sargassum wightii* with relevance to type 2 diabetes mellitus therapy. *Int. J. Biol. Macromol.* **2015**, *72*, 1044–1047. [CrossRef] [PubMed]
20. Vishchuk, O.S.; Ermakova, S.P.; Zvyagintseva, T.N. Sulfated polysaccharides from brown seaweeds *Saccharina japonica* and *Undaria pinnatifida*: Isolation, structural characteristics, and antitumor activity. *Carbohydr. Res.* **2011**, *346*, 2769–2776. [CrossRef]
21. Imbs, T.I.; Ermakova, S.P.; Malyarenko, O.S.; Isakov, V.V.; Zvyagintseva, T.N. Structural elucidation of polysaccharide fractions from the brown alga *Coccophora langsdorfii* and in vitro investigation of their anticancer activity. *Carbohydr. Polym.* **2016**, *135*, 162–168. [CrossRef]
22. Wang, J.; Wang, F.; Zhang, Q.; Zhang, Z.; Shi, X.; Li, P. Synthesized different derivatives of low molecular fucoidan extracted from *Laminaria japonica* and their potential antioxidant activity in vitro. *Int. J. Biol. Macromol.* **2009**, *44*, 379–384. [CrossRef]
23. Chen, H.M.; Lee, M.J.; Kuo, C.Y.; Tsai, P.L.; Liu, J.Y.; Kao, S.H. *Ocimum gratissimum* aqueous extract induces apoptotic signalling in lung adenocarcinoma cell A549. *Evid. Based Complement. Altern. Med.* **2011**, *2011*, 739093. [CrossRef]
24. Ma, L.; Qin, C.; Wang, M.; Gan, D.; Cao, L.; Ye, H.; Zeng, X. Preparation, preliminary characterization and inhibitory effect on human colon cancer HT-29 cells of an acidic polysaccharide fraction from *Stachys floridana* Schuttl. ex Benth. *Food Chem. Toxicol.* **2013**, *60*, 269–276. [CrossRef]
25. Green, D.R.; Kroemer, G. The pathophysiology of mitochondrial cell death. *Science* **2004**, *305*, 626–629. [CrossRef]
26. Penninger, J.M.; Kroemer, G. Mitochondria, AIF and caspases—Rivaling for cell death execution. *Nat. Cell Biol.* **2003**, *5*, 97–99. [CrossRef] [PubMed]
27. Tissot, B.; Salpin, J.-Y.; Martinez, M.; Gaigeot, M.-P.; Daniel, R. Differentiation of the fucoidan sulfated L-fucose isomers constituents by CE-ESIMS and molecular modeling. *Carbohydr. Res.* **2006**, *341*, 598–609. [CrossRef]

8. Wang, C.Y.; Wu, T.C.; Hsieh, S.L.; Tsai, Y.H.; Yeh, C.W.; Huang, C.Y. Antioxidant activity and growth inhibition of human colon cancer cells by crude and purified fucoidan preparations extracted from *Sargassum cristaefolium*. *J. Food Drug Anal.* **2015**, *23*, 766–777. [CrossRef] [PubMed]
9. Jiang, X.; Wang, X. Cytochrome-c-mediated apoptosis. *Annu. Rev. Biochem.* **2004**, *73*, 87–106. [CrossRef] [PubMed]
10. Enari, M.; Sakahira, H.; Yokoyama, H.; Okawa, K.; Iwamatsu, A.; Nagata, S. A caspase-activated DNase that degrades DNA during apoptosis, and its inhibitor ICAD. *Nature* **1998**, *391*, 43–50. [CrossRef]
11. Liu, X.S.; Li, P.; Widlak, P.; Zou, H.; Luo, X.; Garrard, W.T.; Wang, X.D. The 40-kDa subunit of DNA fragmentation factor induces DNA fragmentation and chromatin condensation during apoptosis. *Proc. Natl. Acad. Sci. USA* **1998**, *95*, 8461–8466. [CrossRef] [PubMed]
12. Van Engeland, M.; Nieland, L.J.; Ramaekers, F.C.; Schutte, B.; Reutelingsperger, C.P. Annexin V-affinity assay: A review on an apoptosis detection system based on phosphatidylserine exposure. *Cytometry* **1998**, *31*, 1–9. [CrossRef]
13. Patankar, M.S.; Oehninger, S.; Barnett, T.; Williams, R.L.; Clark, G.F. A revised structure for fucoidan may explain some of its biological activities. *J. Biol. Chem.* **1993**, *268*, 21770–21776. [CrossRef]
14. Wang, J.; Wang, L.; Ho, C.-T.; Zhang, K.; Liu, Q.; Zhao, H. Garcinol from *Garcinia indica* downregulates cancer stem-like cell biomarker ALDH1A1 in nonsmall cell lung cancer A549 cells through DDIT3 activation. *J. Agric. Food Chem.* **2017**, *65*, 3675–3683. [CrossRef] [PubMed]
15. Foster, K.A.; Oster, C.G.; Mayer, M.M.; Avery, M.L.; Audus, K.L. Characterization of the A549 cell line as a type II pulmonary epithelial cell model for drug metabolism. *Exp. Cell Res.* **1998**, *243*, 359–366. [CrossRef] [PubMed]
16. Tang, X.Q.; Feng, J.Q.; Chen, J.; Chen, P.X.; Zhi, J.L.; Cui, Y.; Guo, R.X.; Yu, H.M. Protection of oxidative preconditioning against apoptosis induced by H_2O_2 in PC12 cells: Mechanisms via MMP, ROS, and Bcl-2. *Brain Res.* **2005**, *1057*, 57–64. [CrossRef] [PubMed]
17. Weng, D.; Lu, Y.; Wei, Y.; Liu, Y.; Shen, P. The role of ROS in microcystin-LR-induced hepatocyte apoptosis and liver injury in mice. *Toxicology* **2007**, *232*, 15–23. [CrossRef]
18. Gogvadze, V.; Orrenius, S.; Zhivotovsky, B. Multiple pathways of cytochrome c release from mitochondria in apoptosis. *Biochim. Biophys. Acta Bioenergy* **2006**, *1757*, 639–647. [CrossRef]
19. Campos, C.B.; Paim, B.A.; Cosso, R.G.; Castilho, R.F.; Rottenberg, H.; Vercesi, A.E. Method for monitoring of mitochondrial cytochrome c release during cell death: Immunodetection of cytochrome c by flow cytometry after selective permeabilization of the plasma membrane. *Cytom. Part A J. Int. Soc. Anal. Cytol.* **2006**, *69*, 515–523. [CrossRef] [PubMed]
20. Fox, R.; Aubert, M. Flow cytometric detection of activated caspase. In *Apoptosis and Cancer: Methods and Protocols*, 2008 ed.; Mor, G., Alvero, A.B., Eds.; Humana Press Inc.: Totowa, NJ, USA, 2008; pp. 47–56.
21. Robertson, J.D.; Orrenius, S.; Zhivotovsky, B. Nuclear events in apoptosis. *J. Struct. Biol.* **2000**, *129*, 346–358. [CrossRef]
22. Dienstmann, R.; Rodon, J.; Serra, V.; Tabernero, J. Picking the point of inhibition: A comparative review of PI3K/AKT/mTOR pathway inhibitors. *Mol. Cancer Ther.* **2014**, *13*, 1021–1031. [CrossRef]
23. Polivka, J., Jr.; Janku, F. Molecular targets for cancer therapy in the PI3K/AKT/mTOR pathway. *Pharmacol. Ther.* **2014**, *142*, 164–175. [CrossRef] [PubMed]
24. Lee, H.; Kim, J.-S.; Kim, E. Fucoidan from seaweed *Fucus vesiculosus* inhibits migration and invasion of human lung cancer cell via PI3K-Akt-mTOR pathways. *PLoS ONE* **2012**, *7*, e50624. [CrossRef] [PubMed]
25. Haroun-Bouhedja, F.; Ellouali, M.; Sinquin, C.; Boisson-Vidal, C. Relationship between sulfate groups and biological activities of fucans. *Thromb. Res.* **2000**, *100*, 453–459. [CrossRef]
26. Huang, C.Y.; Wu, S.J.; Yang, W.N.; Kuan, A.W.; Chen, C.Y. Antioxidant activities of crude extracts of fucoidan extracted from *Sargassum glaucescens* by a compressional-puffing-hydrothermal extraction process. *Food Chem.* **2016**, *197*, 1121–1129. [CrossRef]
27. Huang, C.Y.; Kuo, C.H.; Lee, C.H. Antibacterial and antioxidant capacities and attenuation of lipid accumulation in 3T3-L1 adipocytes by low-molecular-weight fucoidans prepared from compressional-puffing-pretreated *Sargassum crassifolium*. *Mar. Drugs* **2018**, *16*, 24. [CrossRef] [PubMed]
28. Wang, C.Y.; Wu, T.C.; Wu, C.H.; Tsai, Y.H.; Chung, S.M.; Hong, Y.H.; Huang, C.Y. Antioxidant, anti-inflammatory, and HEP G2 cell growth-inhibitory effects of aqueous-ethanol extracts obtained from non-puffed and compressional-puffed *Sargassum crassifolium*. *J. Mar. Sci. Technol.* **2020**, *28*, 200–210.
29. Yang, W.N.; Chen, P.W.; Huang, C.Y. Compositional characteristics and in vitro evaluations of antioxidant and neuroprotective properties of crude extracts of fucoidan prepared from compressional puffing-pretreated *Sargassum crassifolium*. *Mar. Drugs* **2017**, *15*, 183. [CrossRef] [PubMed]
30. Shiao, W.C.; Kuo, C.H.; Tsai, Y.H.; Hsieh, S.L.; Kuan, A.W.; Hong, Y.H.; Huang, C.Y. In vitro evaluation of anti-colon cancer potential of crude extracts of fucoidan obtained from *Sargassum glaucescens* pretreated by compressional-puffing. *Appl. Sci.* **2020**, *10*, 3058. [CrossRef]
31. Huang, C.Y.; Wu, T.C.; Hong, Y.H.; Hsieh, S.L.; Guo, H.R.; Huang, R.H. Enhancement of cell adhesion, cell growth, wound healing, and oxidative protection by gelatins extracted from extrusion-pretreated tilapia (*Oreochromis* sp.) fish scale. *Molecules* **2018**, *23*, 2406. [CrossRef] [PubMed]

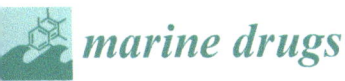

Review

Antifungal and Larvicidal Activities of Phlorotannins from Brown Seaweeds

Bertoka Fajar Surya Perwira Negara [1,2], Jae-Hak Sohn [1,2], Jin-Soo Kim [3,*] and Jae-Suk Choi [1,2,*]

1 Seafood Research Center, Industry-Academic Cooperation Foundation, Silla University, 606, Advanced Seafood Processing Complex, Wonyang-ro, Amnam-dong, Seo-gu, Busan 49277, Korea; ftrnd12@silla.ac.kr (B.F.S.P.N.); jhsohn@silla.ac.kr (J.-H.S.)
2 Department of Food Biotechnology, College of Medical and Life Sciences, Silla University, 140, Baegyang-daero 700beon-gil, Sasang-gu, Busan 46958, Korea
3 Department of Seafood and Aquaculture Science, Gyeongsang National University, 38 Cheondaegukchi-gil, Tongyeong-si, Gyeongsangnam-do 53064, Korea
* Correspondence: jinsukim@gnu.ac.kr (J.-S.K.); jsc1008@silla.ac.kr (J.-S.C.); Tel.: +82-55-772-9146 (J.-S.K.); +82-51-248-7789 (J.-S.C.)

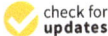

Citation: Negara, B.F.S.P.; Sohn, J.-H.; Kim, J.-S.; Choi, J.-S. Antifungal and Larvicidal Activities of Phlorotannins from Brown Seaweeds. *Mar. Drugs* **2021**, *19*, 223. https://doi.org/10.3390/md19040223

Academic Editor: Roland Ulber

Received: 22 March 2021
Accepted: 15 April 2021
Published: 16 April 2021

Publisher's Note: MDPI stays neutral with regard to jurisdictional claims in published maps and institutional affiliations.

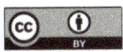

Copyright: © 2021 by the authors. Licensee MDPI, Basel, Switzerland. This article is an open access article distributed under the terms and conditions of the Creative Commons Attribution (CC BY) license (https://creativecommons.org/licenses/by/4.0/).

Abstract: Phlorotannins are secondary metabolites produced by brown seaweeds with antiviral, antibacterial, antifungal, and larvicidal activities. Phlorotannins' structures are formed by dibenzodioxin, ether and phenyl, ether, or phenyl linkages. The polymerization of phlorotannins is used to classify and characterize. The structural diversity of phlorotannins grows as polymerization increases. They have been characterized extensively with respect to chemical properties and functionality. However, review papers of the biological activities of phlorotannins have focused on their antibacterial and antiviral effects, and reviews of their broad antifungal and larvicidal effects are lacking. Accordingly, evidence for the effectiveness of phlorotannins as antifungal and larvicidal agents is discussed in this review. Online databases (ScienceDirect, PubMed, MEDLINE, and Web of Science) were used to identify relevant articles. In total, 11 articles were retrieved after duplicates were removed and exclusion criteria were applied. Phlorotannins from brown seaweeds show antifungal activity against dermal and plant fungi, and larvicidal activity against mosquitos and marine invertebrate larvae. However, further studies of the biological activity of phlorotannins against fungal and parasitic infections in aquaculture fish, livestock, and companion animals are needed for systematic analyses of their effectiveness. The research described in this review emphasizes the potential applications of phlorotannins as pharmaceutical, functional food, pesticide, and antifouling agents.

Keywords: phlorotannins; antifungal; larvicidal; brown seaweeds; biological activities

1. Introduction

Seaweeds are abundant in coastal regions and have become valuable sources of biologically active compounds and secondary metabolites, such as agar, carrageenan, alginate, alkaloids, phenolics, and phlorotannins, with extensive practical applications [1]. Phlorotannins are highly hydrophilic compounds formed by the acetate–malonate pathway. They contain phloroglucinol (Figure 1) (1,3,5-tryhydroxybenzene) units and have molecular sizes of 126 Da–650 kDa [2].

Ishige okamurae, Ecklonia cava, E. kurome, E. stolonifera, Pelvetia siliquosa, Eisenia arborea, and *E. bicyclis* as well as species in the genera *Cystophora* and *Fucus* have been reported to contain phlorotannins. Purified phlorotannins from these brown algae have antioxidant, antitumor, anticancer, anti-inflammatory, antiviral, antimicrobial, antifungal, and larvicidal activities, which are beneficial properties for the development of new functional agents [3–7].

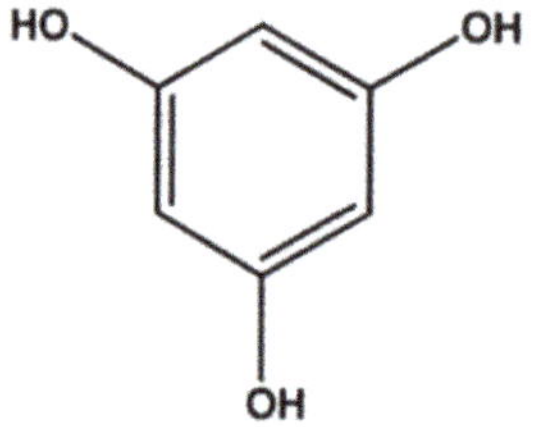

Figure 1. The basic structure of phlorotannins isolated from brown seaweeds [3].

Increasing antibiotic resistance and the spread of new variants of viruses are growing global problems [8]. Additionally, increases in mosquito larvae causing malaria, dengue hemorrhagic fever, filariasis, and chikungunya as well as biofouling marine invertebrate larvae have become major issues. Accordingly, the search for novel natural compounds to resolve these issues has been a major focus of research. Bioactive phlorotannins derived from brown algae have promising pharmacological and inhibitory effects [5,9–13] and, as described previously [10,14–16], may be valuable compounds for resolving these growing issues.

The five review papers on biological activities of phlorotannins reported by Eom et al. [5] focused on the antimicrobial activity of phlorotannins. Besednova et al. [17] and Zaporozhets and Besednova [18] have reviewed antiviral activities of phlorotannins. Nonetheless, reviews of their other biological activities, such as antifungal and larvicidal activities, are lacking. Accordingly, this review provides a comprehensive overview of antifungal and larvicidal activities of phlorotannins, providing a strong basis for their development as new functional agents. The biological activities of phlorotannins further support the utility of brown seaweeds as sources of novel functional agents derived from natural compounds.

2. Phlorotannins

Phlorotannins are produced and found in physodes, which are located in cells' periphery and perinuclear regions [19]. Phlorotannins belong to phloroglucinol's oligomers that can act as both primary and secondary metabolites. They are only found in brown seaweed and formed by the acetate–malonate (polyketide) pathway in the Golgi apparatus [20]. A combination of ether and phenyl, ether, dibenzodioxin, or phenyl linkages form the structures of phlorotannins (Figure 2). As a result, based on the structural linkage, phlorotannins can be divided into six groups. Eckols contain dibenzo-1,4-dioxin linkages, carmalols contain dibenzodioxin moiety, fucols contain aryl–aryl bonds, phloretols contain aryl–ether bonds, fucophloretols contain ether or phenyl linage, and fuhalols contain ortho-/para-arranged ether bridges containing an additional hydroxyl group on one unit [21].

Phlorotannins have been isolated from brown seaweed such as *Ecklonia cava*, *E. stolonifera*, *Sargassum ringgoldianum*, *Ishige okamurae*, *Fucus vesiculosus*, and *Eisenia bicyclis*, as well as species in the genera *Cystophora* and *Fucus*. Eckol, phloroglucinol, dieckol, diphlorethohydroxycarmalol, 6,6′-bieckol, phlorofucofuroeckol A, dioxinodehydroeckol, and 7-phloroeckol have been extracted from these seaweeds. Table 1 summarize the phlorotannins that were extracted from brown seaweeds.

Ether linkages

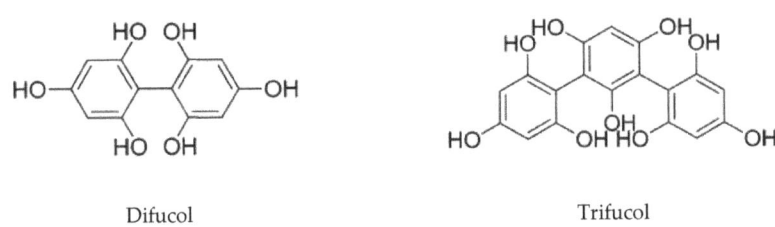

Diphlorethol   Bifuhalol   Trifuhalol C

Phenyl linkages

Difucol   Trifucol

Ether and phenyl linkages

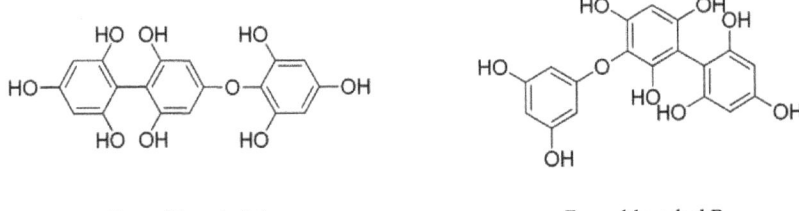

Fucophlorethol A   Fucophlorethol B

Dibenzodioxin linkages

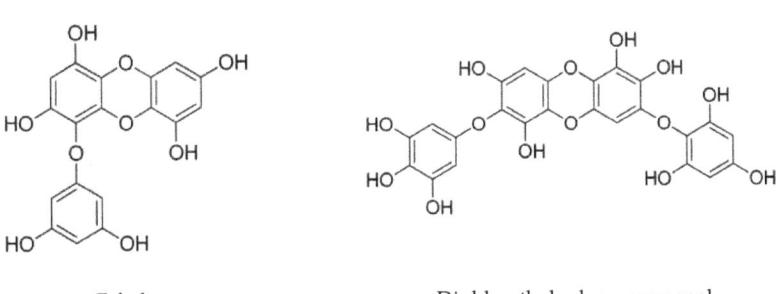

Eckol   Diphlorethohydroxycarmanol

Figure 2. Structure of phlorotannins contain ether and phenyl-, ether-, dibenzodioxin-, or phenyl-linkages [22].

Table 1. Phlorothannin compounds extracted from brown seaweeds.

Brown Seaweed	Compound	Ref.
Ecklonia cava	Eckol	[19–21]
	Phloroglucinol	[20–23]
	Dieckol	[20,21]
Ecklonia stolonifera	Phlorofucofuroeckol A	[24]
	Dieckol	
	Dioxinodehydroeckol	
Eisenia bicyclis	Phloroglucinol	[25]
	Eckol	
	7-phloroeckol	
	Phlorofucofuroeckol A	
	Dioxinodehydroeckol	
Sargassum ringgoldianum	Phlorotannins extract	[26]
Ishige okamurae	Phloroglucinol	[27]
	Diphlorethohydroxycarmalol	
	6,6'-bieckol	
Fucus vesiculosus	Phlorotannins extract	[28]

3. Antifungal Activity of Phlorotannins

The antifungal activity of phlorotannins has been evaluated by Kim et al. [29], Lopes et al. [30], Lee et al. [31], and Corato et al. [32]. These studies have reported the antifungal activity of phlorotannins against dermal fungi, such as *Candida albicans*, *Epidermophyton floccosum*, *Trichophyton rubrum*, and *Trichophyton mentagrophytes*, and plant fungi, such as *Botrytis cinerea* and *Monilinia laxa*, as summarized in Table 2.

Table 2. Antifungal activities of phlorotannins extracted from brown seaweeds.

Fungi	Extract/Chemical	Source	Activities	Ref.
Dermal fungi				
Candida albicans	Fucofuroeckol-A	Eisenia bicyclis	MIC [a] of 512 µg/mL	[29]
Candida albicans	Phlorotannins extract	Cystoseira nodicaulis	MIC of 15.6 mg/mL	[30]
Candida albicans		Crassiphycus usneoides	MIC of 31.3 mg/mL	
Candida albicans		Fucus spiralis	MIC of 31.3 mg/mL	
Epidermophyton floccosum		Cystoseira nodicaulis	MIC of 3.9 mg/mL	
Epidermophyton floccosum		Crassiphycus usneoides	MIC of 15.6 mg/mL	
Epidermophyton floccosum		Fucus spiralis	MIC of 7.8 mg/mL	
Trichophyton rubrum		Cystoseira nodicaulis	MIC of 3.9 mg/mL	
Trichophyton rubrum		Crassiphycus usneoides	MIC of 15.6 mg/mL	
Trichophyton rubrum		Fucus spiralis	MIC of 3.9 mg/mL	
Trichophyton mentagrophytes		Cystoseira nodicaulis	MIC of 7.8 mg/mL	
Trichophyton mentagrophytes		Crassiphycus usneoides	MIC of 31.3 mg/mL	
Trichophyton mentagrophytes		Fucus spiralis	MIC of 15.6 mg/mL	
Trichophyton rubrum	Dieckol	Ecklonia cava	MIC of 200 µM	[31]

Table 2. Cont.

Fungi	Extract/Chemical	Source	Activities	Ref.
		Plant fungi		
Botrytis cinerea	Phlorethols	Laminaria digitata	MGI [b] of 100%	[32]
	Fucophloretols			
Monilinia laxa	Phlorethols			
	Fucophloretols			

[a] MIC: Minimum inhibitory concentration. [b] MGI: Mycelia growth inhibition.

The effects of phlorotannins against dermal fungal pathogens have been evaluated. Lopes et al. [30] extracted phlorotannins from *Cystoseira nodicaulis*, *Crassiphycus usneoides*, and *Fucus spiralis* using *n*-hexane and then extracted using acetone:water (7:3). These phlorotannins exhibit antifungal activity against *C. albicans*, *E. floccosum*, and *T. mentagrophytes*. The MIC values of phlorotannins against these fungi range from 3.9 to 31.3 mg/mL. Fucofuroeckol-A, isolated from *Eisenia bicyclis*, and dieckol, isolated from *Ecklonia cava*, have antifungal activities [29,31]. Fucofuroeckol-A shows an MIC of 512 µg/mL against *C. albicans* [29], whereas dieckol exhibits a MIC of 200 µM against *Trichophyton rubrum* [31]. Although dieckol has shown antifungal activity, the concentration was extremely high. A general lack of selectivity of new drugs candidate should have >50% inhibition at a concentration less than 30 µM [33]. Corato et al. [32] have shown that phlorethols and fucophloretols extracted from *Laminaria digitata* are effective against plant fungal pathogens, such as *B. cinerea* and *M. laxa*, with 100% mycelial growth inhibition.

In fungal cell, phlorotannins block dimorphic complexes, resulting in the appearance of pseudohyphae with decreasing surface adhesive properties. The virulence and capacity to invade fungal host cells are also decreased by phlorotannins. On the other hand, phlorotannins induced reactive oxygen species (ROS) production and triggered early apoptosis, resulting in the activation of the CaMCA1 gene (Metacaspase 1) and membrane disruption. These inhibitory effects promote phlorotannins as new antifungal agents [29,30,32].

The effectiveness of phlorotannins as antifungal agents depends on numerous factors, such as the complex interactions between chemical compounds and the host and rates of degradation, hydrolysis, and polymerization. In the first step of nature compound discovery as new drug candidate, MICs are usually the starting point for larger preclinical evaluations of novel drug agents, and to ensure that compounds efficiently increase the success of treatment [31,32].

Increased rates of fungal infections in humans, animals, and plants necessitate the development of new antifungal agents. The antifungal effects of phlorotannin extracts, phlorethols, fucophloretols, fucofuroeckol-A, and dieckol have been evaluated. However, other subclasses of phlorotannins remain to be explored and should be a focus of further research aimed at the identification of novel antifungals.

4. Larvicidal Activity of Phlorotannins

The larvicidal activity of phlorotannins has been reported by Thangam and Kathiresan [34], Ravikumar et al. [35], Manilal et al. [36], Birrell et al. [37], Brock et al. [38], Lau and Qian [39], and Tsukamoto et al. [40]. These studies evaluated effects against mosquito larvae, such as *Aedes aegypti* and *Culex quinquefasciatus*, and against marine invertebrate larvae, such as *Acropora millepora*, *Balanus improvises*, *Hydroides elegans*, *Halocynthia roretzi*, and *Ciona savignyi*, as summarized in Table 3.

Table 3. Larvicidal activities of phlorotannins extracted from brown seaweeds.

Larvae	Extract/Chemical	Sources	Activities	Ref.
Mosquitos				
Aedes aegypti	Phlorotannins extract	*Dictyota dichotoma*	LC_{50} [a] of 61.66 mg/L	[34]
Aedes aegypti	Phlorotannins extract	*Dictyota dichotoma*	LC_{50} of 0.0683 µg/mL	[35]
Aedes aegypti	Phlorotannins extract	*Lobophora variegata*	LC_{50} of 70.38 µg/mL	[36]
Aedesaegypti		*Stoechospermum marginatum*	LC_{50} of 82.95 µg/mL	
Aedesaegypti		*Sargassum wightii*	LC_{50} of 84.82 µg/mL	
Culex quinquefasciatus		*Lobophora variegata*	LC_{50} of 79.43 µg/mL	
Culex quinquefasciatus		*Stoechospermum marginatum*	LC_{50} of 85.11 µg/mL	
Culex quinquefasciatus		*Sargassum wightii*	LC_{50} of 87.09 µg/mL	
Marine invertebrate				
Acropora millepora	Phlorotannins extract	*Padina* sp.	30% of coral settlement was reduced	[37]
Balanus improvisus	Phlorotannins extract	*Fucus vesiculosus*	Larvae settlement was deterred at 31.5 µg/mL of concentration	[38]
Hydroides elegans	Phlorotannins extract	*Sargassum tenerrimum*	LC_{50} of 13.98 µg/mL	[39]
Ciona savignyi	Phlorotannins extract	*Sargassum thunbergii*	33% of larval metamorphosis were inhibited at 25 µg/mL	[40]
Halocynthia roretzi			27% of larval metamorphosis were inhibited at 25 µg/mL	

[a] LC_{50}: Lethal concentration.

Phlorotannins show potential activity against mosquito larvae. Thangam and Kathiresan [34], Ravikumar et al. [35], and Manilal et al. [36] have reported that phlorotannins extracted from brown seaweeds, such as *Dictyota dichotoma*, *Lobophora variegata*, *Stoechospermum marginatum*, and *Sargassum wightii*, exhibit LC_{50} values ranging from 0.0683 to 85.11 µg/mL against mosquito larvae—namely, *A. aegypti* and *C. quinquefasciatus*.

Birrell et al. [37] reported that phlorotannins from *Padina* sp. reduce the settlement of *Acropora millepora* larvae by 30%. Furthermore, phlorotannins from *Fucus vesiculosus* inhibit the larval settlement of *Balanus improvises* [38].

Study by Lau and Qian [39] reported that phlorotannins extract from *Sargassum tenerrimum* showed larvicidal activity in *Hydroides elegans* with an LC_{50} of 13.98 µg/mL. Tsukamoto et al. [40] demonstrated that phlorotannins extract inhibit 33% and 27% larval metamorphosis of *Ciona savignyi* and *Halocynthia roretzi* at low concentrations (25 µg/mL).

In mosquito larvae, acute mortality and sublethality are the two main effects observed. With respect to sublethal effects, morphogenetic and external structural changes occur during the exposure period [41]. Other toxic effects, such as effects on growth, development, fecundity, fertility, and adult longevity in mosquitoes, have also been recorded [42,43]. Moreover, inhibitory effects on the cholinesterase enzymes cholinergic and gamma-aminobutyric acid (GABA) as well as mitochondrial and octopaminergic systems have also been recorded [44,45].

As larvae settlement inhibition agents, phlorotannins can influence the coral larval settlement process. In nature, phlorotannins delay the settlement process before larvae attach to substrates, even in areas free of macroalgae or with suitable substrates [37]. Furthermore, phlorotannins can inhibit settlement process of cyprids larvae. These findings indicate that phlorotannins from brown seaweeds might serve an essential ecological role as inhibitors of fouling. The larvicidal effects of phlorotannins might be mediated by various mechanisms, including the direct inhibition of the settlement and/or survival of larvae and regulation of the growth of bacterial microfoulers, affecting larval settlement. On the other hand, phlorotannins can quicken the metamorphosis of *Ciona savignyi* and *Halocynthia roretzi* compared to sulfoquinovosyl diacylglycerol at the same concentrations [40]. These findings suggest that phlorotannins can act as an antifouling agent without causing disruption to other organisms.

However, most studies of the larvicidal activity of phlorotannins have focused on crude phlorotannins. To the best of our knowledge, other subclasses of phlorotannins, such as fuhalols, phlorethols, fucols, and fucophloroethols, have not been tested. These phlorotannins have a wide range of biological activities and further studies should evaluate their larvicidal effects and underlying mechanisms.

5. Extraction of Phlorotannins from Brown Seaweeds

Solid–liquid extraction using organic solvents is the most common method for obtaining phlorotannins from brown seaweeds. Phlorotannins can be extracted using polar solvents, including acetone, ethanol, and methanol. A mixture of polar solvents and water is often used to extract phlorotannins [46–51]. During the extraction procedure, the temperature is set to no more than 52 °C (and commonly to room temperature) to minimize the degradation of polyphenolic compounds [46,47]. The amount of phlorotannins extracted depends on the type of seaweed and the solvent used. Table 4 show phlorotannin yields obtained using organic solvents. Extraction of phlorotannins using both methanol:water (60%:40%) and methanol yielded phlorotannins ranging from 2 to 370 mg/g. Methanol solvent yielded the most phlorotannins but needs further processing to purify the compounds.

Table 4. Yield of phlorotannins extracted from brown seaweeds using organic solvent.

Sources	Solvent	Yield	Ref.
Ascophyllum nodosum	Methanol:Water (60%:40%)	2 mg/g	[52]
Fucus serratus		2.6 mg/g	
Fucus vesiculosus		2.92 mg/g	
Laminaria hyperborean		2.46 mg/g	
Pelvetia canaliculata		2.2 mg/g	
Ascophyllum nodosum	Methanol:Water (60%:40%)	6.66 mg/g	[53]
Himanthalia elongata		2.79 mg/g	
Ecklonia kurome	Methanol	370 mg/g	[54]
Ishige okamurae	Methanol	190 mg/g	[55]

Naturally, concentration of phlorotannins in brown seaweeds is affected by biological factors, such as the species, tissue type, size, and age, as well as environmental conditions, such as nutrient levels, water temperature, season, herbivore intensity, and light intensity [46,47]. The extraction method also affects the yield.

Although solid–liquid extraction has been used to obtain phlorotannins from brown seaweeds, this method has a number of weaknesses, such as long extraction times for high yields, a lack of specificity, and the need to purify the extract [46–48]. Supercritical fluid extraction, microwave extraction, liquid extraction under pressure, ultrasonic extraction, and enzymatic extraction are alternative methods for phlorotannins extraction. These methods can increase yield, increase purity, and reduce extraction times [47–49,51,56].

Enzymatic extraction offers high yield values by the destruction of the cell wall. Puspita et al. [51] obtained a higher phlorotannins yield from *Sargassum polycystum* by the enzymatic method (21–38% phlorotannins) than by the solid solid–liquid method (3–15%). Similar to the enzymatic extraction method, the ultrasonic extraction method enables a high yield by destroying cell walls using mass transfer during the process [48]. Furthermore, the low time requirement is the greatest advantage of high-pressure liquid extraction and microwave methods [46–49,51].

6. Future Prospects for Phlorotannins

Since phlorotannins possess many biological activities, these compounds have attracted substantial research attention. The high effectiveness and low toxicity of these compounds support their utilization as components of pharmaceuticals, cosmetics, and food products (Figure 3).

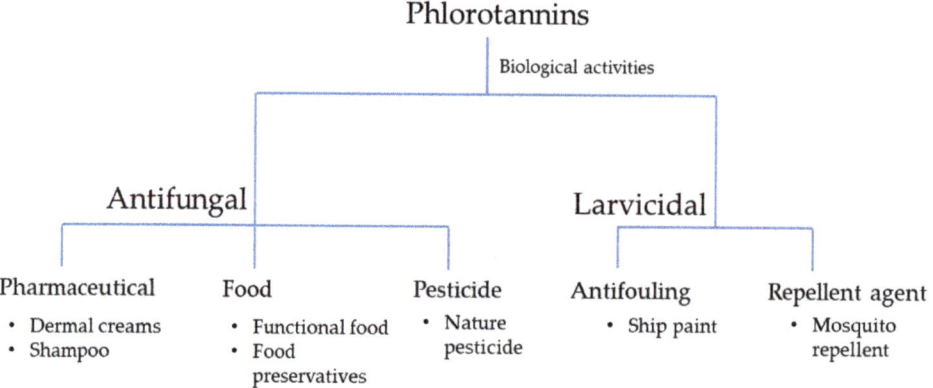

Figure 3. Application of phlorotannins as pharmaceutical, food, pesticide, antifouling, and repellent agents.

According to Paradis et al. [57], Baldrick et al. [58], and Shin et al. [59], no side effects of phlorotannins have been recorded after testing in humans. Negara et al. [60] further reported that phlorotannins exhibit biological activities with low toxic effects on humans and animals. Phlorotannins successfully decrease the incremental areas under the curve in plasma insulin, cholesterol (both low-density and high-density lipoprotein levels), DNA damage, body fat ratio, and waist/hip ratio. Um et al. [61] reported no serious side effects, such as nausea, mild fatigue, abdominal distension, and dizziness. Thus, phlorotannins are new candidates for applications as pharmaceutical, food, pesticide, antibiofouling, and repellent agents.

Kim et al. [29], Lopes et al. [30], and Lee et al. [31] have shown that phlorotannins exhibit antifungal activities against dermatophytic fungi, such as *Candida albicans*, *Epidermophyton floccosum*, *Trichophyton rubrum*, and *Trichophyton mentagrophytes*, which cause skin infections. Accordingly, phlorotannins are promising compounds for the development of dermal creams with antifungal effects. In addition, Corato et al. [32] reported that phlorotannins successfully inhibit the mycelia of plant fungal pathogens, suggesting that they are potentially new natural pesticides. In food, antifungal activities exhibited by phlorotannins could be developed as food preservatives.

The larvicidal activity of phlorotannins in mosquitos reported by Thangam and Kathiresan [34], Ravikumar et al. [35], and Manilal et al. [36] suggests that they may be effective mosquito repellent agents. Phlorotannins have shown effects against marine invertebrate larvae [37–40], suggesting that they are natural antifouling agents. Unlike heavy metals, which act as broad-spectrum toxins to both targeted and nontargeted marine organisms [62], the natural antifouling effects of phlorotannins showed specificity to the target organism.

Therefore, recent research clearly supports the use of phlorotannins as pharmaceutical, cosmetic, antifouling, and food preservation agents. However, in-depth studies of phlorotannins are needed to determine their precise effects.

7. Method

Following Systematic Reviews and Meta-Analyses (PRISMA) guidelines, various online databases (Web of Science, ScienceDirect, MEDLINE, and PubMed) were used for literature searches [63]. "Phlorotannins OR antifungal OR larvicidal OR activity OR biological OR in vitro" was used as the search strategy. English language and effectiveness were applied as filters. In total, 85 articles were collected. After filtering, 11 articles were reviewed.

8. Conclusions

Our review revealed that phlorotannins from brown seaweeds exhibit activities against dermal and plant fungi, and mosquito and marine organism larvae. These findings provide a basis for the development of phlorotannins as new functional foods, feeds, pharmaceuticals, and larvicidal agents. To the best of our knowledge, their effects against viral, microbial, and parasitic infections have not been evaluated in fish, livestock, and companion animals; further studies on the biological activities of phlorotannins in these organisms are needed.

Author Contributions: Conceptualization, J.-S.C.; methodology, B.F.S.P.N.; formal analysis, J.H.S.; data curation, J.H.S.; writing—original draft preparation, B.F.S.P.N.; writing—review and editing, J.-S.C.; visualization, J.-S.K.; supervision, J.-S.C., J.-S.K. All authors have read and agreed to the published version of the manuscript.

Funding: This study was funded by the Ministry of Oceans and Fisheries, Republic of Korea, under Project no. PJT201277.

Institutional Review Board Statement: Not applicable.

Conflicts of Interest: The authors declare no conflict of interest.

References

1. Arnold, T.M.; Targett, N.M. Quantifying in situ rates of phlorotannin synthesis and polymerization in marine brown algae. *J. Chem. Ecol.* **1998**, *24*, 577–595. [CrossRef]
2. Li, Y.X.; Wijesekara, I.; Li, Y.; Kim, S.K. Phlorotannins as bioactive agents from brown algae. *Process Biochem.* **2011**, *46*, 2219–2224. [CrossRef]
3. Kang, M.C.; Cha, S.H.; Wijesinghe, W.A.J.P.; Kang, S.M.; Lee, S.H.; Kim, E.A.; Song, C.B.; Jeon, Y.J. Protective effect of marine algae phlorotannins against AAPH-induced oxidative stress in zebrafish embryo. *Food Chem.* **2013**, *138*, 950–955. [CrossRef] [PubMed]
4. Cha, J.Y.; Lee, B.J.; Je, J.Y.; Kang, Y.M.; Kim, Y.M.; Cho, Y.S. GABA-enriched fermented *Laminaria japonica* protects against alcoholic hepatotoxicity in sprague-dawley rats. *Fish. Aquat. Sci.* **2011**, *14*, 79–88. [CrossRef]
5. Eom, S.H.; Kim, Y.M.; Kim, S.K. Antimicrobial effect of phlorotannins from marine brown algae. *Food Chem. Toxicol.* **2012**, *50*, 3251–3255. [CrossRef]
6. Gupta, S.; Abu-Ghannam, N. Recent developments in the application of seaweeds or seaweed extracts as a means for enhancing the safety and quality attributes of foods. *Innov. Food Sci. Emerg. Technol.* **2011**, *12*, 600–609. [CrossRef]
7. Kim, K.H.; Yu, D.; Eom, S.H.; Kim, H.J.; Kim, D.H.; Song, H.S.; Kim, D.M.; Kim, Y.M. Fucofuroeckol-A from edible marine alga *Eisenia bicyclis* to restore antifungal activity of fluconazole against fluconazole-resistant *Candida albicans*. *J. Appl. Phycol.* **2018**, *30*, 605–609. [CrossRef]
8. Kaplan, S.L.; Mason, E.O. Management of infections due to antibiotic-resistant *Streptococcus pneumonia*. *Clin. Microbiol. Rev.* **1998**, *11*, 628–644. [CrossRef] [PubMed]
9. Choi, J.S.; Lee, K.; Lee, B.B.; Kim, Y.C.; Kim, Y.D.; Hong, Y.K.; Cho, K.K.; Choi, I.S. Antibacterial activity of the phlorotannins dieckol and phlorofucofuroeckol-a from *Ecklonia cava* against propionibacterium acnes. *Bot. Sci.* **2014**, *92*, 425–431. [CrossRef]
10. Lee, J.H.; Eom, S.H.; Lee, E.H.; Jung, Y.J.; Kim, H.J.; Jo, M.R.; Son, K.T.; Lee, H.J.; Kim, J.H.; Lee, M.S.; et al. In vitro antibacterial and synergistic effect of phlorotannins isolated from edible brown seaweed *Eisenia bicyclis* against acne-related bacteria. *Algae* **2014**, *29*, 47–55. [CrossRef]
11. Karadeniz, F.; Kang, K.H.; Park, J.W.; Park, S.J.; Kim, S.K. Anti-HIV-1 activity of phlorotannin derivative 8,4"-dieckol from korean brown alga *Ecklonia cava*. *Biosci. Biotechnol. Biochem.* **2014**, *78*, 1151–1158. [CrossRef]
12. Morán-Santibañez, K.; Peña-Hernández, M.A.; Cruz-Suárez, L.E.; Ricque-Marie, D.; Skouta, R.; Vasquez, A.H.; Rodríguez-Padilla, C.; Trejo-Avila, L.M. Virucidal and synergistic activity of polyphenol-rich extracts of seaweeds against measles virus. *Viruses* **2018**, *10*, 465. [CrossRef] [PubMed]
13. Park, J.Y.; Kim, J.H.; Kwon, J.M.; Kwon, H.J.; Jeong, H.J.; Kim, Y.M.; Kim, D.; Lee, W.S.; Ryu, Y.B. Dieckol, a SARS-CoV 3CL(pro) inhibitor, isolated from the edible brown algae *Ecklonia cava*. *Bioorg. Med. Chem.* **2013**, *21*, 3730–3737. [CrossRef]

14. Lopes, G.; Sousa, C.; Silva, L.R.; Pinto, E.; Andrade, P.B.; Bernardo, J.; Mouga, T.; Valentão, P. Can phlorotannins purified extracts constitute a novel pharmacological alternative for microbial infections with associated inflammatory conditions? *PLoS ONE* **2012**, *7*, e31145. [CrossRef]
15. Nagayama, K.; Iwamura, Y.; Shibata, T.; Hirayama, I.; Nakamura, T. Bactericidal activity of phlorotannins from the brown alga *Ecklonia kurome*. *J. Antimicrob. Chemother.* **2002**, *50*, 889–893. [CrossRef] [PubMed]
16. Wang, Y.; Xu, Z.; Bach, S.J.; McAllister, T.A. Sensitivity of *Escherichia coli* to seaweed (*Ascophyllum nodosum*) phlorotannins and terrestrial tannins. *Asian-Australas. J. Anim. Sci.* **2009**, *22*, 238–425. [CrossRef]
17. Besednova, N.N.; Andryukov, B.G.; Zaporozhets, T.S.; Kryzhanovsky, S.P.; Fedyanina, L.N.; Kuznetsova, T.A.; Zvyagintseva, T.N.; Shchelkanov, M.Y. Antiviral Effects of Polyphenols from Marine Algae. *Biomedicines* **2021**, *9*, 200. [CrossRef] [PubMed]
18. Zaporozhets, T.S.; Besednova, N.N. Biologically active compounds from marine organisms in the strategies for combating coronaviruses. *AIMS Microbiol.* **2020**, *6*, 470–494. [CrossRef]
19. Santos, S.A.O.; Félix, R.; Pais, A.C.S.; Rocha, S.M.; Silvestre, A.J.D. The quest for phenolic compounds from macroalgae: A review of extraction and identification methodologies. *Biomolecules* **2019**, *9*, 847. [CrossRef]
20. Stengel, D.B.; Connan, S.; Popper, Z.A. Algal chemodiversity and bioactivity: Sources of natural variability and implications for commercial application. *Biotechnol. Adv.* **2011**, *29*, 483–501. [CrossRef]
21. Heo, S.J.; Ko, S.C.; Cha, S.H.; Kang, D.H.; Park, H.S.; Choi, Y.U.; Kim, D.; Jung, W.-K.; Jeon, Y.J. Effect of phlorotannins isolated from *Ecklonia cava* on melanogenesis and their protective effect against photo-oxidative stress induced by UV-B radiation. *Toxicol. In Vitro* **2009**, *23*, 1123–1130. [CrossRef] [PubMed]
22. Arbenz, A.; Avérous, L. Chemical modification of tannins to elaborate aromatic biobased macromolecular architectures. *Green Chem.* **2015**, *17*, 2626–2646. [CrossRef]
23. Kang, K.A.; Lee, K.H.; Chae, S.; Zhang, R.; Jung, M.S.; Ham, Y.M.; Baik, J.S.; Lee, N.H.; Hyun, J.W. Cytoprotective effect of phloroglucinol on oxidative stress induced cell damage via catalase activation. *J. Cell. Biochem.* **2006**, *97*, 609–620. [CrossRef] [PubMed]
24. Kim, A.R.; Shin, T.S.; Lee, M.S.; Park, J.Y.; Park, K.E.; Yoon, N.Y.; Kim, J.S.; Choi, J.S.; Jang, B.C.; Byun, D.S.; et al. Isolation and identification of phlorotannins from *Ecklonia stolonifera* with antioxidant and anti-inflammatory properties. *J. Agric. Food Chem.* **2009**, *57*, 3483–3489. [CrossRef]
25. Jung, H.A.; Jin, S.E.; Ahn, B.R.; Lee, C.M.; Choi, J.S. Anti-inflammatory activity of edible brown alga Eisenia bicyclis and its constituents fucosterol and phlorotannins in LPS-stimulated RAW264.7 macrophages. *Food Chem. Toxicol.* **2013**, *59*, 199–206. [CrossRef]
26. Nakai, M.; Kageyama, N.; Nakahara, K.; Miki, W. Phlorotannins as radical scavengers from the extract of *Sargassum ringgoldianum*. *Mar. Biotechnol.* **2006**, *8*, 409–414. [CrossRef]
27. Cruces, E.; Huovinen, P.; Gómez, I. Interactive effects of UV radiation and enhanced temperature on photosynthesis, phlorotannin induction and antioxidant activities of two sub-Antarctic brown algae, *Mar. Biol.* **2013**, *160*, 1–13. [CrossRef]
28. Wang, T.; Jonsdottir, R.; Liu, H.; Gu, L.; Kristinsson, H.G.; Raghavan, S.; Olafsdottir, G. Antioxidant capacities of phlorotannins extracted from the brown algae *Fucus vesiculosus*. *J. Agric. Food Chem.* **2012**, *60*, 5874–5883. [CrossRef]
29. Kim, H.J.; Dasagrandhi, C.; Kim, S.H.; Kim, B.G.; Eom, S.H.; Kim, Y.M. In vitro antibacterial activity of phlorotannins from edible brown algae, *Eisenia bicyclis* against streptomycin-resistant *Listeria monocytogenes*. *Indian J. Microbiol.* **2018**, *58*, 105–108. [CrossRef]
30. Lopes, G.; Pinto, E.; Andrade, P.B.; Valentao, P. Antifungal activity of phlorotannins against dermatophytes and yeasts: Approaches to the mechanism of action and influence on *Candida albicans* virulence factor. *PLoS ONE* **2013**, *8*, e72203. [CrossRef]
31. Lee, M.H.; Lee, K.B.; Oh, S.M.; Lee, B.H.; Chee, H.Y. Antifungal Activities of Dieckol Isolated from the Marine Brown Alga *Ecklonia cava* against *Trichophyton rubrum*. *J. Korean Soc. Appl. Biol. Chem.* **2010**, *53*, 504–507. [CrossRef]
32. Coratoa, U.D.; Salimbenib, R.; Pretisb, A.D.; Avellab, N.; Patruno, G. Antifungal activity of crude extracts from brown and red seaweeds by a supercritical carbon dioxide technique against fruit postharvest fungal diseases. *Postharvest Biol. Technol.* **2017**, *131*, 16–30. [CrossRef]
33. Hefti, F.F. Requirements for a lead compound to become a clinical candidate. *BMC Neurosci.* **2008**, *9*, S7. [CrossRef]
34. Thangam, T.S.; Kathiresan, K. Mosquito larvicidal effect of seaweed extracts. *Bot. Mar.* **1991**, *34*, 433–435. [CrossRef]
35. Ravikumar, S.; Ali, M.S.; Beula, J.M. Mosquito larvicidal efficacy of seaweed extracts against dengue vector of *Aedes aegypti*. *Asian Pac. J. Trop Biomed.* **2011**, *1*, S143–S146.
36. Manilal, A.; Thajuddin, N.; Selvin, J.; Idhayadhulla, A.; Kumar, R.S.; Sujith, S. In vitro mosquito larvicidal activity of marine algae against the human vectors, *Culex quinquefasciatus* (Say) and *Aedes aegypti* (Linnaeus) (Diptera: Culicidae). *Int. J. Zool. Res.* **2011**, *7*, 272–278. [CrossRef]
37. Birrell, C.L.; McCook, L.J.; Willis, B.L.; Harrington, L. Chemical effects of macroalgae on larval settlement of the broadcast spawning coral *Acropora millepora*. *Mar. Ecol. Prog. Ser.* **2008**, *362*, 129–137. [CrossRef]
38. Brock, E.; Nylund, G.M.; Pavia, H. Chemical inhibition of barnacle larval settlement by the brown alga *Fucus vesiculosus*. *Mar. Ecol. Prog. Ser.* **2007**, *337*, 165–174. [CrossRef]
39. Lau, S.C.K.; Qian, P.Y. Phlorotannins and related compounds as larval settlement inhibitors of the tube-building polychaete *Hydroides elegans*. *Mar. Ecol. Prog. Ser.* **1997**, *159*, 219–227. [CrossRef]
40. Tsukamoto, S.; Hirota, H.; Kato, H.; Fusetani, N. Phlorotannins and Sulfoquinovosyl Diacylglycerols: Promoters of larval metamorphosis in ascidians, isolated from the brown alga *Sargassum thunbergii*. *Fish. Sci.* **1994**, *60*, 319–321. [CrossRef]

1. Arias, J.R.; Mulla, M.S. Morphogenetic aberrations induced by a juvenile hormone analogue in the mosquito *Culex tarsalis* (Diptera: Culicidae). *J. Med. Entomol.* **1975**, *12*, 309–318. [CrossRef] [PubMed]
2. Kumar, S.; Singh, A.P.; Nair, G.; Batra, S.; Seth, A.; Wahab, N.; Warikoo, R. Impact of *Parthenium hysterophorus* leaf extracts on the fecundity, fertility and behavioural response of *Aedes aegypti* L. *Parasitol. Res.* **2011**, *108*, 853–859. [CrossRef] [PubMed]
3. Asha, A.; Rathi, J.M.; Raja, D.P.; Sahayaraj, K. Biocidal activity of two marine green algal extracts against third instar nymph of *Dysdercus cingulatus* (Fab.) (Hemiptera: Pyrrhocoridae). *J. Biopest.* **2012**, *5*, 129–134.
4. Nathan, S.S.; Choi, M.Y.; Paik, C.H.; Seo, H.Y.; Kalaivani, K.; Kim, J.D. Effect of azadirachtin on acetylcholinesterase (AChE) activity and histology of the brown planthopper *Nilaparvata lugens* (Stål). *Ecotoxicol. Environ. Saf.* **2008**, *70*, 244–250. [CrossRef]
5. Kukel, C.F.; Jennings, K.R. Delphinium alkaloids as inhibitors of alpha-bungarotoxin binding to rat and insect neural membranes. *Can. J. Physiol. Pharmacol.* **1994**, *72*, 104–107. [CrossRef]
6. Machu, L.; Mišurcová, L.; Ambrozova, J.V.; Orsavová, J.; Mlcek, J.; Sochor, J.; Jurikova, T. Phenolic Content and Antioxidant Capacity in Algal Food Products. *Molecules* **2015**, *20*, 1118–1133. [CrossRef]
7. Imbs, T.I.; Zvyagintseva, T.N. Phlorotannins are polyphenolic metabolites of brown algae. *Russ. J. Mar. Biol.* **2018**, *44*, 217–227. [CrossRef]
8. Aminina, N.M.; Vishnevskaya, T.I.; Karaulova, E.P.; Epur, N.V.; Yakush, E.V. Prospects for the Use of Commercial and Potentially Commercial Brown Algae of the Far Eastern Seas as a Source of Polyphenols. *Russ. J. Mar. Biol.* **2020**, *46*, 34–41. [CrossRef]
9. Aminina, N.M.; Vishnevskaya, T.I.; Karaulova, E.P.; Epur, N.V.; Yakush, E.V. Content of polyphenols and antioxidant activity of extracts from certain species of seaweeds. *TINRO News* **2017**, *189*, 184–191.
10. Moizer, E.B.; Skerget, M.; Knez, S.; Epur, N.V.; Yakush, E.V. Polyphenols: Extraction methods, antioxidative action, bioavailability and anticancerogenic effects. *Molecules* **2016**, *21*, 901.
11. Puspita, M.; Déniel, M.; Widowati, I.; Radjasa, O.K.; Douzenel, P.; Marty, C.; Vandanjon, L.; Bedoux, G.; Bourgougnon, N. Total phenolic content and biological activities of enzymatic extracts from *Sargassum muticum* (Yendo) Fensholt. *Environ. Biol. Fishes* **2017**, *29*, 2521–2537. [CrossRef]
12. O'Sullivan, A.M.; O'Callaghan, Y.C.; O'Grady, M.N.; Queguineur, B.; Hanniffy, D.; Troy, D.J.; Kerry, J.P.; O'Brien, N.M. In vitro and cellular antioxidant activities of seaweed extracts prepared from five brown seaweeds harvested in spring from the West Coast of Ireland. *Food Chem.* **2011**, *126*, 1064–1070. [CrossRef]
13. Quéguineur, B.; Goya, L.; Ramos, S.; Martín, M.A.; Mateos, R.; Guiry, M.D.; Bravo, L. Effect of phlorotannin-rich extracts of *Ascophyllum nodosum* and *Himanthalia elongata* (phaeophyceae) on cellular oxidative markers in human HepG2 cells. *J. Appl. Phycol.* **2013**, *25*, 1–11. [CrossRef]
14. Nagayama, K.; Shibata, T.; Fujimoto, K.; Honjo, T.; Nakamura, T. Algicidal effect of phlorotannins from the brown alga *Ecklonia kurome* on red tide microalgae. *Aquaculture* **2003**, *218*, 601–611. [CrossRef]
15. Zou, Y.; Qian, Z.J.; Li, Y.; Kim, M.M.; Lee, S.H.; Kim, S.K. Antioxidant effects of phlorotannins isolated from *Ishige okamurae* in free radical mediated oxidative systems. *J. Agric. Food Chem.* **2008**, *56*, 7001–7009. [CrossRef] [PubMed]
16. Rajbhar, K.; Dawda, H.; Mucundan, U. Polyphenols: Methods of extraction. *Sci. Rev. Chem. Commun.* **2015**, *5*, 1–6.
17. Paradis, M.E.; Couture, P.; Lamarche, B. A randomised crossover placebo-controlled trial investigating the effect of brown seaweed (*Ascophyllum nodosum* and *Fucus vesiculosus*) on postchallenge plasma glucose and insulin levels in men and women. *Appl. Physiol. Nutr. Metab.* **2011**, *36*, 913–919. [CrossRef]
18. Baldrick, F.R.; McFadden, K.; Ibars, M.; Sung, C.; Moffatt, T.; Megarry, K.; Thomas, K.; Mitchell, P.; Wallace, J.M.W.; Pourshahidi, L.K.; et al. Impact of a (poly)phenol-rich extract from the brown algae *Ascophyllum nodosum* on DNA damage and antioxidant activity in an overweight or obese population: A randomized controlled trial. *Am. J. Clin. Nutr.* **2018**, *108*, 688–700. [CrossRef]
19. Shin, H.C.; Kim, S.H.; Park, Y.; Lee, B.H.; Hwang, H.J. Effects of 12-week oral supplementation of *Ecklonia cava* polyphenols on anthropometric and blood lipid parameters in overweight korean individuals: A double-blind randomized clinical trial. *Phytother. Res.* **2012**, *26*, 363–368. [CrossRef]
20. Negara, B.F.S.P.; Sohn, J.H.; Kim, J.S.; Choi, J.S. Effects of phlorotannins on organisms: Focus on the safety, toxicity, and availability of phlorotannins. *Foods* **2021**, *10*, 452. [CrossRef]
21. Um, M.Y.; Kim, J.Y.; Han, J.K.; Kim, J.; Yang, H.; Yoon, M.; Kim, J.; Kang, S.W.; Cho, S. Phlorotannin supplement decreases wake after sleep onset in adults with self-reported sleep disturbance: A randomized, controlled, double-blind clinical and polysomnographic study. *Phytother. Res.* **2018**, *32*, 698–704. [CrossRef]
22. Cho, J.Y.; Kwon, E.H.; Choi, J.S.; Hong, S.Y.; Shin, H.W.; Hong, Y.K. Antifouling activity of seaweed extracts on the green alga *Enteromorpha prolifera* and the mussel *Mytilus edulis*. *J. Appl. Phycol.* **2001**, *13*, 117–125.
23. Liberati, A.; Altman, D.G.; Tetzlaff, J.; Mulrow, C.; Gøtzsche, P.C.; Ioannidis, J.P.; Clarke, M.; Devereaux, P.J.; Kleijnen, J.; Moher, D. The PRISMA statement for reporting systematic reviews and meta-analyses of studies that evaluate health care interventions: Explanation and elaboration. *PLoS Med.* **2009**, *6*, e1000100. [CrossRef]

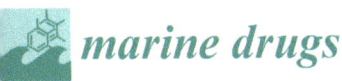

Article

Screening of In-Vitro Anti-Inflammatory and Antioxidant Activity of *Sargassum ilicifolium* Crude Lipid Extracts from Different Coastal Areas in Indonesia

Saraswati [1], Puspo Edi Giriwono [1,2], Diah Iskandriati [3] and Nuri Andarwulan [1,2,*]

1. Department of Food Science and Technology, Faculty of Agricultural Engineering and Technology, IPB University (Bogor Agricultural University), West Java 16680, Indonesia; saraswati_231@apps.ipb.ac.id (S.); pegiriwono@apps.ipb.ac.id (P.E.G.)
2. Southeast Asian Food and Agricultural Science Technology (SEAFAST) Center, IPB University (Bogor Agricultural University), West Java 16680, Indonesia
3. Primate Research Center, IPB University (Bogor Agricultural University), West Java 16151, Indonesia; atie@indo.net.id
* Correspondence: andarwulan@apps.ipb.ac.id; Tel.: +62-251-8626-7252

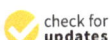

Citation: Saraswati; Giriwono, P.E.; Iskandriati, D.; Andarwulan, N. Screening of In-Vitro Anti-Inflammatory and Antioxidant Activity of *Sargassum ilicifolium* Crude Lipid Extracts from Different Coastal Areas in Indonesia. *Mar. Drugs* **2021**, *19*, 252. https://doi.org/10.3390/md19050252

Academic Editor: Roland Ulber

Received: 24 March 2021
Accepted: 26 April 2021
Published: 28 April 2021

Publisher's Note: MDPI stays neutral with regard to jurisdictional claims in published maps and institutional affiliations.

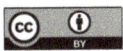

Copyright: © 2021 by the authors. Licensee MDPI, Basel, Switzerland. This article is an open access article distributed under the terms and conditions of the Creative Commons Attribution (CC BY) license (https://creativecommons.org/licenses/by/4.0/).

Abstract: *Sargassum* brown seaweed is reported to exhibit several biological activities which promote human health, such as anticancer, antimicrobial, antidiabetic, anti-inflammatory, and antioxidant activity. This study aimed to investigate the anti-inflammatory and antioxidant activity of crude lipid extracts of *Sargassum ilicifolium* obtained from four different coastal areas in Indonesia, namely Awur Bay–Jepara (AB), Pari Island–Seribu Islands (PI), Sayang Heulang Beach–Garut (SHB), and Ujung Genteng Beach–Sukabumi (UGB). Results showed that treatment of RAW 264.7 macrophage cells with UGB and AB crude lipid extracts (12.5–50 µg/mL) significantly suppressed the nitric oxide production after lipopolysaccharide stimulation, both in pre-incubated and co-incubated cell culture model. The anti-inflammatory effect was most marked in the pre-incubated cell culture model. Both two crude lipid extracts showed 2,2-diphenyl-1-picrylhydrazyl radical scavenging activity and high ferric reducing antioxidant power, which were amounted to 36.93–37.87 µmol Trolox equivalent/g lipid extract and 681.58–969.81 µmol FeSO$_4$/g lipid extract, respectively. From this study, we can conclude that crude lipid extract of tropical *S. ilicifolium* can be further developed as a source of anti-inflammatory and antioxidant agent.

Keywords: anti-inflammatory; antioxidant; coastal area; crude lipid extract; *Sargassum ilicifolium*

1. Introduction

As one of the countries with the longest coastline in the world, Indonesia's seaweed-producing potential is very high. Indonesia was able to produce up to 10.4 million tons of fresh seaweed in 2017. In international trade, Indonesia is one of the main players, with an export volume reaching 212,962 tons in 2018 [1]. Of the global production of cultured seaweed, Indonesia contributed almost 38% to the total production, which made Indonesia the second-largest seaweed producer in the world after China [2]. Among hundreds of seaweed species found in Indonesian waters, only a few species have been optimally cultivated, especially from agar- and carrageen-producing groups such as *Gracilaria* sp., *Kappaphycus alvarezii*, and *E. denticulatum*. The utilization of brown seaweed in Indonesia is still limited, even though its health benefits have been empirically and scientifically recognized [3].

Brown seaweed, especially *Sargassum* species, has become one of the important ingredients in the traditional medicine of East Asian communities. Some *Sargassum* species have been utilized for generations by Chinese and Korean people to treat several inflammation-associated health problems, such as the painful scrotum, edema, liver organ swelling, chronic bronchitis, etc. [4,5]. Several studies on *Sargassum* summarized by Saraswati et al. [6] indicated the promising anti-inflammatory effect of this seaweed genus, for both acute and chronic conditions. Although several screening studies demonstrated the predominance of *Sargassum* lipid-soluble fractions which are responsible for inflammatory activity [7–10], the potency of the lipid-soluble compounds of tropical *Sargassum* has not been fully explored. To date of our knowledge, the sulfated polysaccharides of tropical *Sargassum* are the most studied compounds for their anti-inflammatory activity [5]. The utilization of tropical *Sargassum* lipid-soluble fractions/compounds as a source of anti-inflammatory and antioxidant agents can be one of the valorization efforts of seaweed metabolites [11].

One of the *Sargassum* species which is widely distributed in Indonesian waters with promising biomass is *S. ilicifolium*. Together with other species from *Sargassum* subgenus, this seaweed is included as one of the most abundant species distributed in the Pacific basin, primarily southwestern Pacific regions such as North Australia, Fiji, Guam, Indonesia, Malaysia, Micronesia, New Caledonia, Papua New Guinea, Philippines, Singapore, Solomon Islands, and Taiwan [12,13]. *S. ilicifolium* was first described by Agardh in 1820, and this seaweed is known from not only the tropical Pacific region, but also the Indian ocean region [14]. In addition, *S. cristaefolium*, *S. duplicatum*, *S. berberifolium*, and *Fucus latifolius* are all recognized as synonyms of *S. ilicifolium*, according to Guiry and Guiry [12]. Wu et al. [15] have reported the anti-inflammatory effect of crude sulfated polysaccharides derived from *S. ilicifolium* (as *S. cristaefolium*) in lipopolysaccharide (LPS)-induced murine macrophage RAW 264.7 cells. The anti-inflammatory studies of *S. ilicifolium* and *S. duplicatum* have been previously investigated by several research groups on different models, such as carrageenan-induced rat paw edema [16], 12-O-techanoyl-13-myristate-induced polymorphonuclear leukocyte [17], LPS-induced RAW 264.7 cells [18,19], and indomethacin-induced rat inflammatory bowel disease [20].

In the present study, we aimed to investigate the anti-inflammatory and antioxidant activity of crude lipid extracts of *S. ilicifolium* obtained from four different coastal areas around Java Island–Indonesia, namely Sayang Heulang Beach/SHB, Ujung Genteng Beach/UGB, Pari Island/PI, and Awur Bay/AB-Jepara. SHB and UGB are located at the southern waters of Java Island, while PI and AB are in the northern waters of Java. The anti-inflammatory effect of brown seaweed crude lipid extracts was assayed on LPS-induced RAW 264.7 cells under two different experimental models, i.e., pre-incubated and co-incubated model. While the antioxidant activity was examined through 2,2-diphenyl-1-picrylhydrazyl (DPPH) radical scavenging method and ferric reducing antioxidant power (FRAP) method. These study results are expected to provide baseline information for further development of Indonesian *S. ilicifolium* as a source of anti-inflammatory and antioxidant ingredients.

2. Results

2.1. Cell Viability after Treatment of S. ilicifolium Crude Lipid Extract

Cell viability assay was carried out to determine doses of samples for anti-inflammatory activity assay. Figure 1 shows RAW 264.7 cells viability after brown seaweed lipid extract treatment for 24 h. Because decreased viability was most marked at 100 µg/mL, doses of samples ranging from 12.5–50 µg/mL were chosen for further anti-inflammatory assay. Treatment of RAW 264.7 cells with crude lipid extract from Pari Island (PI) samples exhibited the highest cytotoxicity. PI extract yielded 63.9% viability at 12.5 µg/mL, while 100 µg/mL of PI extract caused a significant cytotoxic effect with viability value at 22.6%. The weakest cytotoxic effect was found in Awur Bay (AB) sample treatment with cell viability at 12.5, 25, and 50 µg/mL were 90.0, 88.8, and 74.6%, respectively. When excluding PI treatment due to its highest cytotoxic effect, UGB treatment showed a sharp decrease in viability at a dose range of 12.5–50 µg/mL. At 50 µg/mL, viability of the UGB-treated group only reached 48.22%, while the viability of SHB and AB treatment group at a dose of 50 µg/mL were 69.01 and 74.64%, respectively. Determination of cell viability becomes important, so the observed anti-inflammatory effect is deemed not to be attributable to cytotoxic effects [21,22].

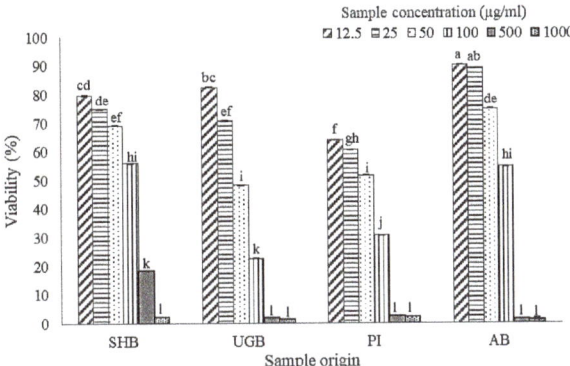

Figure 1. Viability of RAW 264.7 cells after incubated by *Sargassum ilicifolium* crude lipid extracts (12.5–1000 µg/mL) for 24 h. Note: SHB = Sayang Heulang Beach, UGB = Ujung Genteng Beach, PI = Pari Island, AB = Awur Bay. Means with at least one same letter are not significantly different based on Duncan's test ($p > 0.05$). Error bars indicate the value of standard deviation.

2.2. Anti-Inflammatory Activity of S. ilicifolium Crude Lipid Extract

In this study, lipopolysaccharide (LPS) from *Escherichia coli* O111:B4 was used to stimulate an inflammatory response in RAW 264.7 macrophage cells. It was proven by the significant increase of nitric oxide (NO) production in the LPS-treated group (control +) if compared to the non-LPS treatment group (control-). Nitric oxide (NO) is a signaling molecule that plays a key role in the pathogenesis of inflammation. The impaired production of NO is associated with tissue damage, neurodegeneration, and inflammatory disorders in joint, gut, and lung since it acts as pro-inflammatory mediator which can amplify the inflammatory response. Hence, an effort to find selective NO inhibitors becomes a therapeutic advance in the management of inflammatory diseases [23].

Effects of brown seaweed lipid extract treatment on NO production of LPS-induced RAW 264.7 macrophage cells are shown in Figures 2 and 3. UGB sample provided the strongest NO inhibition activity. In the pre-incubated cell culture model, level of NO inhibition by UGB treatment reached 83.21% at a dose of 50 µg/mL and 26.10% at 12.5 µg/mL. While NO inhibition level by UGB treatment in the co-incubation model ranged from 28.07–61.81%. Treatment of RAW 264.7 cells by SHB samples in the pre-incubated cell culture model exhibited no significant reversion of LPS-induced NO production. In the co-incubation model, SHB treatment gave lowest NO inhibition activity, only ranging from 10.15–25.38%. AB treatment showed a promising NO inhibition activity with a more acceptable cytotoxic effect. Level of NO inhibition by AB treatment was ranging from 11.29–65.76% in pre-incubated cell culture model and 13.44–41.80% in co-incubation model. Jaswir et al. [18] found that treatment of RAW 264.7 cells with water extracts (50 µg/mL) of three different Malaysian *Sargassum* species could inhibit LPS-induced NO production around 40–52%. A study by Jayawardena et al. [9] reported that LPS-induced NO production in RAW 264.7 cells was inhibited by treatment of Korean *S. horneri* ethanolic extract through suppression of nuclear factor (NF)-kappa B transactivation, decreased mitogen-activated protein kinases (MAPKs) phosphorylation, and increased expression of nuclear factor E2-related factor 2 (Nrf2) and heme oxygenase 1 (HO-1). The activation of NF-kB transcription factor and MAPKs (i.e., extracellular-signal regulated kinase (ERK), Jun N-terminal kinase (JNK), and p38) are known to play a critical role in the regulation of inflammatory response, whilst the activation Nrf2/HO-1 pathway induce the cytoprotective effect against oxidative stress due to inflammatory stimulation.

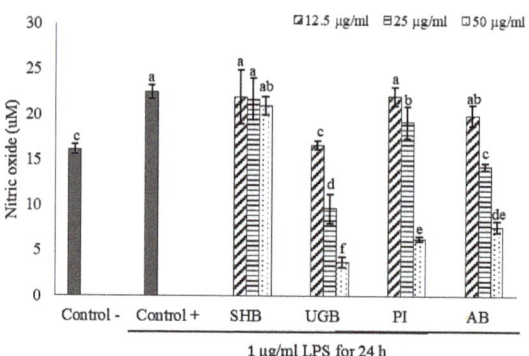

Figure 2. Effect of *Sargassum ilicifolium* crude lipid extracts (12.5–50 µg/mL) on LPS-induced NO production in pre-incubated cell culture model. RAW 264.7 cells (10^4 cells/well in 96-well culture plates) were incubated by sample for 24 h before LPS stimulation. Note: SHB = Sayang Heulang Beach, UGB = Ujung Genteng Beach, PI = Pari Island, AB = Awur Bay. Means with at least one same letter are not significantly different based on Duncan's test ($p > 0.05$). Error bars indicate the value of standard deviation.

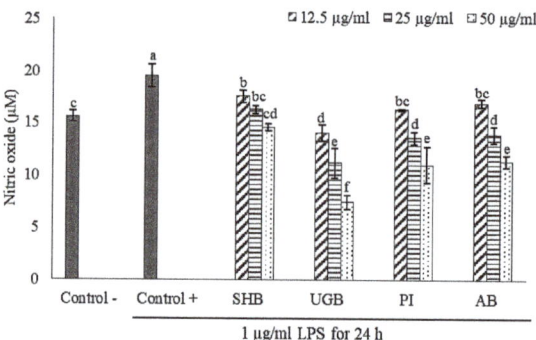

Figure 3. Effect of *Sargassum ilicifolium* crude lipid extracts (12.5–50 µg/mL) on LPS-induced NO production in co-incubated cell culture model. RAW 264.7 cells (10^4 cells/well in 96-well culture plates) were incubated by sample and LPS for 24 h simultaneously. Note: SHB = Sayang Heulang Beach, UGB = Ujung Genteng Beach, PI = Pari Island, AB = Awur Bay. Means with at least one same letter are not significantly different based on Duncan's test ($p > 0.05$). Error bars indicate the value of standard deviation.

Pre-incubation of RAW 264.7 cells with *S. ilicifolium* lipid extracts before LPS stimulation exerted a stronger anti-inflammatory effect than in co-incubation mode. This indicated that bioactive compounds contained in the tested extracts could counter the inflammatory response through intracellular actions due to their capability in permeating cell membranes. Thus, the outcome of pre-incubation may reflect a preventive action [24]. Gany et al. [25] revealed that pre-incubation of C8B4 microglia cells for 3 h with lipid-soluble extract (0.4 mg/mL) of *Padina australis* was able to significantly reduce LPS-induced NO production up to 75.67%. Moreover, LPS-induced pro-inflammatory cytokines production (e.g., tumor necrosis factor (TNF)-α, interleukin (IL)-6, and IL-1β) of those cells were also reversed by the aforementioned treatment. On the contrary of our results, Hidalgo et al. [26] found that co-incubation of RAW 264.7 macrophages cells with protocatechuic acid (phenolic compound) and inflammatory stimulant (LPS and/or IFN-γ) gave stronger NO inhibition than in the pre-incubation model. The anti-inflammatory effect of phenolic compounds might be generated from their radicals scavenging activity in the surrounding environment of inflamed cells [27] and direct interaction of phenolic compounds with inflammatory stimulants [26].

2.3. DPPH Radical Scavenging and Ferric Reducing Ability of S. ilicifolium Crude Lipid Extract

Since oxidative stress and inflammation are closely linked and affecting each other, exploring anti-inflammatory and antioxidant properties of natural compounds becomes an interesting research topic [28]. Anti-inflammatory and antioxidant activity of natural compounds may contribute to the prevention of chronic diseases, e.g., cardiovascular diseases, cancer, diabetes, Alzheimer's, etc. [29]. In the present study, the antioxidant activity of brown seaweed lipid extract was assessed through the DPPH radical scavenging and FRAP assay (Table 1).

Table 1. Total lipid and antioxidant activity of *Sargassum ilicifolium* from different coastal areas.

Observed Parameters	Sample Origin			
	SHB	UGB	PI	AB
Total lipid (g/100 g seaweed db) [1]	3.55 ± 0.29 [b 2]	2.76 ± 0.28 [a]	2.73 ± 0.19 [a]	4.32 ± 0.09 [c]
Antioxidant activity (µmol TE/g seaweed db) [1]	1.27 ± 0.01 [c]	1.01 ± 0.00 [b]	0.96 ± 0.03 [a]	1.58 ± 0.001 [d]
Antioxidant activity (µmol TE/g lipid extract) [1]	34.61 ± 0.17 [a]	37.87 ± 0.08 [b]	37.24 ± 1.15 [b]	36.93 ± 0.18 [b]
DPPH scavenging effect (%) with extract concentration of 500 ppm [1]	39.6 ± 0.15 [a]	42.57 ± 0.08 [b]	42.00 ± 1.05 [b]	41.71 ± 0.17 [b]
FRAP (µmol FeSO$_4$/g seaweed db) [1]	23.44 ± 0.41 [d]	25.98 ± 1.28 [b]	16.32 ± 0.04 [c]	29.24 ± 0.32 [a]
FRAP (µmol FeSO$_4$/g lipid extract) [1]	637.06 ± 11.12 [a]	969.31 ± 47.88 [c]	634.88 ± 1.50 [a]	681.58 ± 7.48 [b]

[1] All observed parameters values are given as mean ± SD. [2] Means in the same row with different superscripts differ significantly by Duncan's test ($p < 0.05$). Note: SHB = Sayang Heulang Beach, UGB = Ujung Genteng Beach, PI = Pari Island, AB = Awur Bay, db = dry basis.

SHB sample showed the lowest DPPH scavenging activity, while PI and SHB sample exhibited the lowest ferric reducing antioxidant power per gram dry lipid extract. On the other hand, AB and SHB samples had the higher DPPH scavenging activity per gram seaweed (dry basis) as those samples had higher yield of dry lipid extract than UGB and PI samples. Fu et al. [30] found that the DPPH scavenging activities of Malaysian *S. polycystum* ethanolic extracts derived from different extraction parameters (solvent percentage, solid to solvent ratio, temperature, and time) were around 0.1–0.9 µmol Trolox equivalent (TE)/g dry weight of seaweed. Those were still lower than the DPPH scavenging activities observed in this study (0.96–1.58 µmol TE/g seaweed on a dry basis). Moreover, Ummat et al. [31] reported that the DPPH radical scavenging activities of the ethanolic extracts derived from 11 different brown seaweed species through conventional extraction process ranged from 9.98–82.70 µmol TE/g extract. They also found that ultrasound-assisted extraction could enhance the DPPH scavenging activities which reached 20.78–116.26 µmol TE/g extract. According to the reports of Budhiyanti et al. [32], different extracts (membrane-bound and cytoplasmic extracts) from *Sargassum* sp. (450 ppm) provided DPPH radical scavenging effects in the range of 0.17–48.71%, similar to data found in this work. Nevertheless, the antioxidant effects of the *Sargassum* sp. extracts were much lower than that of the synthetic BHT (butylated hydroxytoluene) since a lower concentration (100 ppm) provided a 90% DPPH scavenging effect. Synthetic antioxidants have been widely used because of their higher stability, performance, and wide availability, but their safety issues have been raised over timer. Synthetic antioxidants, including BHT and BHA, are reported to be responsible for several side effects such as carcinogenesis and liver damage [33,34]. In addition, the worldwide trend toward the usage of natural compounds encourages massive exploration of natural antioxidants as replacements for synthetic ones. In this regard, seaweed has been largely studied as one of the richest sources of natural antioxidants [34].

The differences in DPPH scavenging activities shown by various studies could be due to differences in species, extraction methods, and environmental conditions [30–32]. A study by Silva et al. [35] showed that ferric reducing antioxidant power of different lipid-soluble fractions derived from brown seaweed *Bifurcaria bifurcata* were ranging from

7.64–1128.20 µmol FeSO$_4$/g fraction, while the FRAP values found in this study were about 634.88–969.31 µmol FeSO$_4$/g lipid extract. Those observed values were still within the range found in the aforementioned study.

According to Pearson's correlation analysis (Table 2), there is a positive correlation between antioxidant activity (DPPH and FRAP assay) and anti-inflammatory activity (both pre-incubated and co-incubated cell culture model). The antioxidant capacity of the bioactive compounds in *Sargassum* extract might contribute to suppressing oxidative stress status in the inflamed cells [36], so the positive reciprocal feedback loop between inflammation and oxidative stress could be interrupted. UGB was found to show the strongest NO-inhibition capacity in the two indicated models. Moreover, UGB also gave the highest ferric reducing antioxidant power which reached 969.31 ± 47.88 µmol FeSO$_4$/g lipid extract, while its DPPH radical scavenging activity per tested lipid extract was not significantly different ($p > 0.05$) from PI and AB samples. It could indicate that the reducing power of the tested extract might greatly contribute to interfere with inflammatory response in LPS-induced RAW 264.7 cells.

Table 2. Relationship between antioxidant and anti-inflammatory activity of crude lipid extract of *S. ilicifolium*.

Treatment	Pearson's Correlation Coefficient
DPPH vs. FRAP	0.484
DPPH vs. NO Inhibition in Pre-incubated Model	0.758 **
FRAP vs. NO Inhibition in Pre-incubated Model	0.749 **
DPPH vs. NO Inhibition in Co-incubated Model	0.794 **
FRAP vs. NO Inhibition in Co-incubated Model	0.819 **
NO Inhibition in Pre-incubated Model vs NO Inhibition in Co-incubated Model	0.865 **

Note: Data were statistically analyzed using Pearson's correlation coefficient test. ** indicate correlation is significant at 0.01 level (2-tailed). DPPH means 2,2-diphenyl-1-picrylhydrazyl radical scavenging activity of crude lipid extract, while FRAP means ferric reducing antioxidant power.

The FRAP method is known as the most putative method which reflects the electron-donating capacity of the bioactive compounds or food components. The transferred electron will then reduce any compound, including metals, carbonyl groups, and radicals [37]. Although the ability of bioactive compounds to reduce iron has little relationship to the radical quenching processes (hydrogen atom transfer) mediated by most antioxidants, the oxidation or reduction of radicals into ions still stops radical chains. Furthermore, DPPH radical scavenging activity of bioactive compound delineates the electron-donating capacity as the main reaction and hydrogen-atom abstraction as a marginal reaction [38]. Rajauria [39] reported that the ferric reducing antioxidant power and DPPH radical scavenging activity of brown seaweeds (*Himanthalia elongata, Saccharina latissima*-formerly *Laminaria saccharina* and *Laminaria digitata*) lipophilic extracts were positively correlated with their total phenol, flavonoid, carotenoid, and chlorophyll contents. Syad et al. [40] found that the presence of a high amount of terpenoid compounds in non-polar extract of brown seaweed *S. wightii* could be the possible reason for its potential antioxidant activity, characterized by its strong DPPH, OH·, and H$_2$O$_2$ radical scavenging activity, and the high ferric reducing antioxidant power.

Several compounds that are potentially responsible for the anti-inflammatory activity of *Sargassum* non-polar fraction include fucosterol or other steroid compounds, fucoxanthin and its derivatives, fatty acids and simple organic compounds such as hexadecanoic acid, neophytadiene, tetradecanoic, 8-heptadecene, and 3,7,11,15-tetramethyl-2-hexadecen-1-ol, omega-3 fatty acids (C20:5n3 and C18:4n3), some phenolic compounds, and other pigment compounds contained in *Sargassum* [6]. According to our study results, UGB and AB samples exhibited the most promising anti-inflammatory and antioxidant effects. Although PI sample also showed a strong NO-inhibition effect on RAW 264.7 cells after LPS stimulation, this sample was not considered as potential anti-inflammatory sources because it gave the highest cytotoxicity to the cells. Both cytotoxic and biological activities of bioactive components need to be considered because they provide an overview of the safety and efficacy of the tested compound [41–43]. In the anti-inflammatory screening studies, Adebayo et al. [41] and Somchit et al. [42] used the selectivity index (SI) to ascertain that the observed anti-inflammatory effect of the tested compound was not due to a general metabolic toxic effect on the RAW 264.7 cell lines. A higher SI value is indicative of selective anti-inflammatory activity while a low SI value indicates higher cellular toxicity. SI is calculated by dividing the half-maximal cytotoxic concentration (CC50) by the half-maximal inhibitory concentration (IC_{50}). When comparing between AB and UGB treatment (Table S1), AB treatment was found to have higher selectivity index (3.19 in pre-incubated model and 2.03 in co-incubated model) than UGB (2.17 in pre-incubated model and 1.54 in co-incubated model).

The biological activity of tested samples will be strongly influenced by their bioactive content. Furthermore, the bioactive content of seaweed, especially lipid-soluble component, is affected by several factors, such as genetic, algal life stage, physiological status, light intensity, season, hydrodynamic condition, and other environmental parameters like temperature, pH, salinity, dissolved oxygen, total nitrogen, total phosphorus, etc [44,45]. Our previous preliminary study on chemical profiling of *S. ilicifolium* (as *S. cristaefolium*) from different coastal areas showed that all tested samples have distinct lipid-soluble profiles with different morphological characteristics [46]. According to the principal component analysis (PCA) results on lipid-soluble components in that study, SHB and AB samples were clustered together at close proximity, whilst PI and UGB samples are located in the opposite F1 score range (positive factor score). SHB and AB were characterized by larger blade size, higher content of chlorophyll, fucoxanthin, carotenoid, polyunsaturated fatty acids (PUFA), total n-3 fatty acids, total n-6 fatty acids, and also a lower ratio of n-6 to n-3. While PI and UGB were characterized by smaller blade size, higher content of saturated fatty acids/SFA (C14:0, C15:0, C16:0, C18:0, C20:0), some monounsaturated fatty acids/MUFA (C16:1, C17:1, C18:1n9, C22:1n9), C20:2, and C22:6n3. When comparing PI and UGB samples, UGB were found to have higher content of C12:0, C18:2n6, C18:3n6, C20:1n9, C20:5n3, and total PUFA than PI. The results of gas chromatography-flame ionization detector (GC-FID) analysis on samples' FAME are attached in the supplementary materials (Figures S1–S5).

In the present study, we found that differences in water groups (southern or northern water of Java) did not appear to affect the tendency of anti-inflammatory and antioxidant activity. UGB and AB samples, which represented two distinctive water groups, exhibited a promising anti-inflammatory and antioxidant effects. Both of them have a distinct lipid-soluble profile as previously described. Based on morphological observation of fresh seaweeds, UGB had a narrow blade size (0.7 ± 0.2 cm width and 1.6 ± 0.3 cm length) with green color, while AB had a wide blade size (1.8 ± 0.2 cm width and 4.5 ± 0.3 length) with a dark-brown color [46]. The different morphological appearances might indicate different developmental stages [47]. However, the thallus size and morphological appearance can also be greatly influenced by the natural environmental condition [12,14]. Koivikko [48] stated that the degree of polymerization of phlorotannins, a typical phenolic compound in brown seaweed, will be different among developmental stages, young thallus tends to contain a high amount of short oligomers, while adult thallus will accumulate longer and more complex forms of phlorotannins, which are more difficult to degrade or exude. Actually, data regarding the content and composition of lipid-soluble phenolic compounds were not available in this study, but this group of compounds may also be responsible for the anti-inflammatory and antioxidant activity of the lipid-soluble/non-polar fraction of *Sargassum* as summarized by Saraswati et al. [6]. Although lipid class composition (neutral lipid, glycolipid, and phospholipid) of UGB and AB samples were not significantly different [46], their qualitative composition would strongly influence their bioactivity. Tasende [49] revealed that the distribution of sterols composition (part of neutral lipid fraction) was greatly affected by the algal life cycle and this would have an implication to the bioactivity of algal lipid.

Based on the facts found in this study, the single compound responsible for providing anti-inflammatory and antioxidant effects could not be well defined. According to the results of Pearson's correlation analysis on lipid-soluble components from our previous study [46] and the bioactivities (anti-inflammatory and antioxidant) from our present study (Table S2), the lipid-soluble components which were found to be positively correlated with anti-inflammatory activity (both models), DPPH scavenging activity, and ferric reducing antioxidant power in a consistent manner were only chlorophyll a, neutral lipid content, total SFA, and total MUFA content. However, this is not sufficient to draw conclusions, because the metabolite information contained in the crude lipid extract was not comprehensive enough. For example, the qualitative composition of neutral lipid which could influence the observed bioactivity was not available in this study.

A high-throughput approach using mass spectroscopy (MS) or nuclear magnetic resonance (NMR) methods may provide a clearer picture of the responsible compounds for bioactivity. The study of Saraswati et al. [50] reported that there were several putative compounds in the lipid-soluble fraction of S. *ilicofolium* (as S. *cristaefolium*) that had a strong correlation with NO inhibition activity in LPS-induced RAW 264.7, DPPH scavenging activity, and ferric reducing antioxidant power. These compounds included porphyrin derivatives (pheophytin a, 13^2-hydroxypheophytin a, pheophorbide a), all-trans fucoxanthin, and some monogalactosyldiacylglycerols (MGDG), such as MGDG (16:0/18:1), MGDG (20:5/18:3), and MGDG (18:3/18:4). That study used a metabolomic approach to determine the responsible compounds for bioactivity. Metabolite profiling in that study was performed using ultra-high performance liquid chromatography-electrospray ionization orbitrap tandem mass spectrometry (UHPLC-MS/MS).

Although the results of the Pearson's correlation analysis between omega-3 PUFA or fucoxanthin content and anti-inflammatory activity in this study did not show a positive association, the high content of omega-3 PUFA and fucoxanthin in AB samples might contribute to the reported anti-inflammatory activity according to the facts reported by Saraswati et al. [50]. Ahmad et al. [51] stated that a complex mixture of saturated, monounsaturated, and polyunsaturated fatty acids may all impact the anti-inflammatory activity of marine lipid extracts. Eventually, we can conclude that the observed anti-inflammatory and antioxidant effect in this study might be generated from the cumulative effect of all lipid-soluble constituents contained in the brown seaweed lipid extract.

3. Materials and Methods

3.1. Materials

Murine macrophage RAW 264.7 cells (TIB-71™, ATCC, Manassas, VA, USA) were used as a cell culture model for anti-inflammatory activity screening. Other materials used in this study included powdered Roswell Park Memorial Institute (RPMI) 1640 medium, 6-hydroxy-2,5,7,8-tetramethylchroman-2-carboxylic acid or Trolox, 2,2-diphenyl-1-picrylhydrazyl (DPPH), 2,4,6-tris(2-pyridyl)-s-triazine (TPTZ), lipopolysaccharides (LPS) of *Escherichia coli* O111:B4, sodium nitrite, and Griess reagent from Sigma UK (Gillingham, UK), penicillin-streptomycin and fetal bovine serum (FBS) (Gibco™ Life Technologies Corporation, Gaithersbug, MD, USA), chloroform and methanol from Merck KGaA (Darmstadt, Germany), and other reagents used for anti-inflammatory and antioxidant activity assay.

3.2. Brown Seaweed Sampling and Sample Preparation

Brown seaweed samples were harvested from four different coastal areas, i.e., Awur Bay, Jepara, Central Java (6°36′54″ S, 110°38′55″ E) and Pari Island, Seribu Islands, DKI Jakarta (5°51′48″ S, 106°36′29″ E), Sayang Heulang Beach, Garut, West Java (7°40′12″ S, 107°41′50″ E) and Ujung Genteng Beach, Sukabumi, West Java (7°21′39″ S, 106°24′10″ E) in the same monsoon season (March–April 2017). Awur Bay and Pari Island are located in the northern waters of Java Island, while Sayang Heulang Beach and Ujung Genteng Beach are included as southern parts of Java Island. Seaweed identification was conducted at Marine Hydrobiology Division, Department of Marine Science and Technology, Bogor Agricultural University.

Fresh seaweed was firstly cleaned from physical impurities (e.g., sand and gravel) and dried before the extraction step. Drying was carried out using an oven dryer at 50 °C until seaweed moisture content reached <10%. The dried seaweed was ground to yield seaweed powder (18 mesh particle size). Dried seaweed powder was then stored at 4 °C.

3.3. Preparation of Crude Lipid Extract and The Chemical Characterization

A crude lipid extract was prepared by referring to the method of Bligh and Dyer [52] with modification as described by Susanto et al. [53]. The modification applied was rehydration of dried seaweed using distilled water (1:9, w/v) for one hour. Maceration of rehydrated seaweed was performed at room temperature for two hours using the mixture of chloroform (C) and methanol (M) at a ratio of 1:2 (v/v). A lipid extract was subsequently filtered by Buchner funnel with Whatman filter paper No. 1. The resulted filtrate was added using chloroform and distilled water to get the final ratio of C/M/W at 1:1:0.9. The chloroform layer containing crude lipid extract was separated and the solvent was evaporated using a rotary vacuum evaporator (R-300, Büchi, Flawil, Switzerland) with water bath temperature and vacuum pressure set to 50 °C and 332 bar, respectively. The remaining solvent in crude lipid extract was then evaporated by nitrogen flushing. The dried crude lipid extract was stored at −20 °C until further analysis. Crude lipid extraction procedure was performed in triplicate. Chemical characterization of crude lipid extract had been performed in our previous study [46]. The observed chemical characteristic parameters included total lipid, pigment profile (chlorophyll a, chlorophyll c, fucoxanthin, β-carotene), lipid class composition (neutral lipid, glycolipid, phospholipid), and fatty acid profile.

3.4. Bioactivity Examination

3.4.1. Cell Culture and Cell Viability Assay

Murine macrophage RAW 264.7 cells were grown in the RPMI 1640 medium with inactivated FBS 10%, $NaHCO_3$ 2%, and penicillin-streptomycin 100 U/mL in a humidified incubator (CO_2 5%, 37 °C). The cells were grown to 80–90% confluence, harvested by scraping, and diluted in fresh medium to the desired concentration of cells per ml. Cell viability was determined by methylthiazolyl tetrazolium (MTT) reduction assay [54]. The medium containing RAW 264.7 cells was cultured in a 96-well plate at a density of 10^5 cells per mL. The plate was incubated overnight and then treated by 100 µL medium containing crude lipid extract at different concentrations (12.5–1000 µg/mL). After 24 h of incubation and cells rinsing by phosphate buffer saline (PBS), about 50 µg MTT reagent was added to each well and the plate was incubated for another 4 h at 37 °C. Formazan crystal was dissolved by 100 µL ethanol 96%. Optical density was measured at 595 nm using a microplate reader (BioRad, Hercules, CA, USA). The optical density of formazan formed by untreated cells (control) was taken as 100% viability.

3.4.2. Anti-Inflammatory Activity Assay

Anti-inflammatory activity of brown seaweed crude lipid extract was observed through nitric oxide (NO) inhibition level in lipopolysaccharide (LPS)-induced RAW 264.7 cells. Cells were firstly seeded at a density of 10^4 cells/well in a 96-microwell plate overnight. After cell adherence, cells were treated by crude lipid extracts and LPS under two different models, namely pre-incubated and co-incubated cell culture models as previously described by Wen et al. [55]. The doses of samples given to the cells were 12.5, 25, and 50 µg/mL. In pre-incubated cell culture model, cells were firstly treated by crude lipid extract at different concentrations for 24 h and followed by LPS stimulation (1 µg/mL) for another 24 h. Before LPS stimulation, the culture medium was discarded to remove samples and cells were rinsed by phosphate buffer saline thrice. In co-incubated cell culture model, cells were treated by crude lipid extract and LPS (1 µg/mL) simultaneously for

24 h in a humidified atmosphere (CO_2 5%, 37 °C). Cell culture supernatant was harvested and stored at −80 °C until further analysis. Anti-inflammatory assay was performed in triplicate. Medium in the anti-inflammatory assay was similar to the medium used in the cell culture preparation, i.e., RPMI 1640 with inactivated FBS 10%, $NaHCO_3$ 2%, and penicillin-streptomycin 100 U/mL.

NO detection was performed according to the study of Rao et al. [56]. The amount of accumulated nitrite was used as an indicator of NO production in the culture medium. About 50 µL cell culture medium was mixed with 50 µL of the Griess reagent. Subsequently, the mixture was incubated at room temperature for 15 min in the dim light. The absorbance was measured at 540 nm using a UV-Vis microplate spectrophotometer (BioTek, Winooski, VT, USA). The standard calibration curve was prepared using sodium nitrite solution (1.56 to 100 mM). Fresh culture medium was used as a blank in every experiment.

3.4.3. 2,2-Diphenyl-1-Picrylhydrazyl (DPPH) Scavenging Assay

The seaweed extract in methanol (1 mL, 500 ppm) was mixed with 2 mL of 0.08 mM methanolic solution of DPPH in a test tube [32]. Then, the mixture was vortexed and left for 30 min at room temperature in the dark. The absorbance was measured at 517 nm using a UV-Vis spectrophotometer. A calibration curve was made using Trolox as a standard. Antioxidant activity was expressed as µmol Trolox equivalent (TE)/g fraction. A blank was made by mixing 1 mL of methanol with 2 mL of 0.08 mM methanolic solution of DPPH. DPPH radical scavenging effect (RSE) was calculated using the following formula:

RSE (%) = 1 − (Absorbance of sample/Absorbance of blank) × 100%.

3.4.4. Ferric Reducing Antioxidant Power (FRAP) Assay

FRAP reagent was prepared from 2.5 mL of 10 mM 2,4,6-tris(2-pyridyl)-s-triazine (TPTZ) solution in 40 mM hydrochloric acid with 2.5 mL of 20 mM iron (III) chloride and 25 mL of 300 mM acetate buffers at pH 3.6. The FRAP reagent was prepared fresh daily and warmed to 37 °C in a water bath. 200 µL of sample extract (500 ppm) was added to 1.3 mL of FRAP reagent and was allowed to react for 30 min in a 37 °C water bath. The absorbance of the reaction mixture was recorded at 593 nm using a UV-Vis spectrophotometer. The standard curve was constructed using ferrous sulfate and the result was expressed in µmol ferrous equivalent (FE)/g fraction [57].

3.5. Statistical Analysis

Data are presented as mean ± standard deviation (SD). The effects of different samples to observed parameters were analyzed by one-way analysis of variance (ANOVA) and followed by Duncan posthoc test by IBM SPSS 20 (IBM, North Castle, NY, USA).

4. Conclusions

Crude lipid extracts of UGB and AB samples gave a promising anti-inflammatory effect in the in vitro model of LPS-induced RAW 264.7 cells. Intracellular action is thought to greatly contribute to the anti-inflammatory effect observed in this study, as the stronger NO-inhibition effect was found in the pre-incubated cell culture model than in co-incubated model. AB treatment showed a promising NO inhibition activity with a more acceptable cytotoxic effect at the indicated dose range. The anti-inflammatory activity of brown seaweed lipid extracts was positively correlated with their antioxidant activity (both DPPH and FRAP). These reported biological activities can be the basis for further development of *S. ilicifolium* as a source of functional ingredient.

Supplementary Materials: The following are available online at https://www.mdpi.com/article/10.3390/md19050252/s1, Figure S1: GC-FID chromatogram of fatty acid methyl ester (FAME) mix C4-24 (external standard) according to study of Saraswati et al. [38], Figure S2: GC-FID chromatogram of SHB's FAME according to study of Saraswati et al. [38], Figure S3: GC-FID chromatogram of UGB's FAME according to study of Saraswati et al. [38], Figure S4: GC-FID chromatogram of PI's FAME according to study of Saraswati et al. [38], Figure S5: GC-FID chromatogram of AB's FAME according to study of Saraswati et al. [38]. Table S1: Selectivity index (SI) of UGB and AB treatment on RAW 264.7 cells, Table S2: The results of Pearson's correlation analysis between lipid-soluble compounds and bioactivities (anti-inflammatory and antioxidant).

Author Contributions: Conceptualization, S., P.E.G., D.I., N.A.; methodology, S., P.E.G., D.I.; formal analysis, S.; investigation, S.; writing—original draft preparation, S.; writing—review and editing, P.E.G., D.I., N.A.; supervision, P.E.G., D.I., N.A.; funding acquisition, N.A. All authors have read and agreed to the published version of the manuscript.

Funding: This research was funded by Directorate General of Research Empowerment and Development, Ministry of Research, Technology and Higher Education of Republic Indonesia through PMDSU program (Grant No. 025/E3/2017). The APC was funded by Bogor Agricultural University (N.A.).

Data Availability Statement: Not applicable.

Acknowledgments: Acknowledgements are due to Ministry of Research, Technology, and Higher Education of Republic Indonesia for providing scholarship in the PMDSU study program, and to Tropical Biopharmaca Research Center of IPB University for microplate spectrophotometer analysis.

Conflicts of Interest: The authors declare no conflict of interest.

References

1. Ministry of Marine and Fisheries, Republic of Indonesia. *Marine and Fisheries in Figures 2018*; The Center for Data, Statistics, and Information of Ministry of Marine and Fisheries: Jakarta, Indonesia, 2018.
2. Ferdouse, F.; Holdt, L.S.; Smith, R.; Murua, P.; Yang, Z. *The Global Status of Seaweed Production, Trade and Utilization*; Food and Agriculture Organization of The United Nations: Rome, Italy, 2018.
3. Brown, E.M.; Allsopp, P.J.; Magee, P.J.; Gill, C.I.; Nitecki, S.; Strain, C.R.; Mcsorley, E.M. Seaweed and human health. *Nutr. Rev.* **2014**, *72*, 205–216. [CrossRef] [PubMed]
4. Vo, T.-S.; Ngo, D.-H.; Kim, S.-K. Potential targets for anti-inflammatory and anti-allergic activities of marine algae: An overview. *Inflamm. Allergy Drug Targets* **2012**, *11*, 90–101. [CrossRef]
5. Liu, L.; Heinrich, M.; Myers, S.; Dworjanyn, S.A. Towards a better understanding of medicinal uses of the brown seaweed *Sargassum* in traditional chinese medicine: A phytochemical and pharmacological review. *J. Ethnopharmacol.* **2012**, *142*, 591–619. [CrossRef] [PubMed]
6. Saraswati; Giriwono, P.E.; Iskandriati, D.; Tan, C.P.; Andarwulan, N. *Sargassum* seaweed as a source of anti-inflammatory substances and the potential insight of the tropical species: A review. *Mar. Drugs* **2019**, *17*, 590. [CrossRef] [PubMed]
7. Karadeniz, F.; Lee, S.G.; Oh, J.H.; Kim, J.A.; Kong, C.S. Inhibition of MMP-2 and MMP-9 activities by solvent-partitioned *Sargassum horneri* extracts. *Fish. Aquat. Sci.* **2018**, *21*, 1–7. [CrossRef]
8. Gwon, W.G.; Lee, S.G.; Kim, J.I.; Kim, Y.M.; Kim, S.B.; Kim, H.R. Hexane fraction from the ethanolic extract of *Sargassum serratifolium* suppresses cell adhesion molecules via regulation of NF-κB and Nrf2 pathway in human umbilical vein endothelial cells. *Fish. Aquat. Sci.* **2019**, *22*, 1–10. [CrossRef]
9. Jayawardena, T.U.; Kim, H.S.; Sanjeewa, K.K.A.; Kim, S.Y.; Rho, J.R.; Jee, Y.; Ahn, G.; Jeon, Y.J. *Sargassum horneri* and isolated 6-hydroxy-4,4,7a-trimethyl-5,6,7,7a-tetrahydrobenzofuran-2(4H)-one (HTT); LPS-induced inflammation attenuation via suppressing NF-κB, MAPK and oxidative stress through Nrf2/HO-1 pathways in RAW 264.7 macrophages. *Algal Res.* **2019**, *40*, 101513. [CrossRef]
10. Mun, O.J.; Kwon, M.S.; Karadeniz, F.; Kim, M.; Lee, S.H.; Kim, Y.Y.; Seo, Y.; Jang, M.S.; Nam, K.H.; Kong, C.S. Fermentation of *Sargassum thunbergii* by kimchi-derived *Lactobacillus* sp. SH-1 attenuates LPS-stimulated inflammatory response via downregulation of JNK. *J. Food Biochem.* **2017**, *41*, 1–9. [CrossRef]
11. Torres, M.D.; Kraan, S.; Domínguez, H. Seaweed biorefinery. *Rev. Environ. Sci. Biotechnol.* **2019**, *18*, 335–388. [CrossRef]
12. Guiry, M.D.; Guiry, G.M. *Sargassum Ilicifolium* (Turner) C. Agardh 1820. 2021. Available online: https://www.algaebase.org/search/species/detail/?species_id=4580 (accessed on 16 April 2020).
13. Coppejans, E.; De Clerck, O.; Leliaert, F. Marine brown algae (Phaeophyta) from the north coast of Papua New Guinea, with a description of *Dictyota magneana* sp. nov. *Cryptogam. Algol.* **2001**, *22*, 15–40. [CrossRef]
14. Soe-Htun, U.; Yoshida, T. Studies on morphological variations in *Sargassum cristaefolium* C. Agardh (Phaeophyta, Fucales). *Jpn. J. Phycol.* **1986**, *34*, 275–281.
15. Wu, G.J.; Shiu, S.M.; Hsieh, M.C.; Tsai, G.J. Anti-inflammatory activity of a sulfated polysaccharide from the brown alga *Sargassum cristaefolium*. *Food Hydrocoll.* **2016**, *53*, 16–23.
16. Simpi, C.; Nagathan, C.; Karajgi, S.; Kalyane, N. Evaluation of marine brown algae *Sargassum ilicifolium* extract for analgesic and anti-inflammatory activity. *Pharmacogn. Res.* **2013**, *5*, 146.
17. Lavanya, R.; Seethalakshmi, S.; Gopal, V.; Chamundeeswari, D. Effect of crude sulphated polysaccharide from marine brown algae in TPA induced inflammation on poly morphonuclear leukocytes. *Int. J. Pharm. Pharm. Sci.* **2015**, *7*, 100–102.

18. Jaswir, I.; Monsur, H.A.; Simsek, S.; Amid, A.; Alam, Z.; bin Salleh, M.N.; Tawakalit, A.-H.; Octavianti, F. Cytotoxicity and inhibition of nitric oxide in lipopolysaccharide-induced mammalian cell lines by aqueous extracts of brown seaweed. *J. Oleo Sci.* **2014**, *63*, 787–794. [PubMed]
19. Monsur, A.H.; Jaswir, I.; Simsek, S.; Amid, A.; Alam, Z.; Tawakalit, A.-H. Cytotoxicity and inhibition of nitric oxide syntheses in LPS induced macrophage by water soluble fractions of brown seaweed. *Food Hydrocoll.* **2014**, *42*, 269–274.
20. Rosdiana, A.; Rahmah, N.L. Potency of brown seaweed (*Sargassum duplicatum* Bory) ethanol and ethyl acetate fraction to malondialdehyde concentration decreasing and histological retrieval of IBD (inflammatory bowel disease) rat small intestinal jejunum. *Media Vet. Med.* **2011**, *4*, 57–64.
21. Heo, S.-J.; Yoon, W.-J.; Kim, K.-N.; Oh, C.; Choi, Y.-U.; Yoon, K.-T.; Kang, D.-H.; Qian, Z.-J.; Choi, I.-W.; Jung, W.-K. Anti-inflammatory effect of fucoxanthin derivatives isolated from *Sargassum siliquastrum* in lipopolysaccharide-stimulated RAW 264.7 macrophage. *Food Chem. Toxicol.* **2012**, *50*, 3336–3342.
22. Gallily, R.; Yekhtin, Z.; Hanuš, L.O. The anti-inflammatory properties of terpenoids from *Cannabis*. *Cannabis Cannabinoid Res.* **2018**, *3*, 282–290. [CrossRef]
23. Sharma, J.N.; Al-Omran, A.; Parvathy, S.S. Role of nitric oxide in inflammatory diseases. *Inflammopharmacology* **2007**, *15*, 252–259.
24. Matos, M.S.; Romero-Díez, R.; Álvarez, A.; Bronze, M.R.; Rodríguez-Rojo, S.; Mato, R.B.; Cocero, M.J.; Matias, A.A. Polyphenol-rich extracts obtained from winemakingwaste streams as natural ingredients with cosmeceutical potential. *Antioxidants* **2019**, *8*, 355. [CrossRef] [PubMed]
25. Gany, S.A.; Tan, S.C.; Gan, S.Y. Anti-neuroinflammatory properties of Malaysian brown and green seaweeds. *Int. J. Ind. Manuf. Eng.* **2014**, *8*, 1269–1275.
26. Hidalgo, M.; Martin-Santamaria, S.; Recio, I.; Sanchez-Moreno, C.; De Pascual-Teresa, B.; Rimbach, G.; De Pascual-Teresa, S. Potential anti-inflammatory, anti-adhesive, anti/estrogenic, and angiotensin-converting enzyme inhibitory activities of anthocyanins and their gut metabolites. *Genes Nutr.* **2012**, *7*, 295–306. [CrossRef]
27. Lopes, G.; Sousa, C.; Silva, L.R.; Pinto, E.; Andrade, P.B.; Bernardo, J.; Mouga, T.; Valentão, P. Can phlorotannins purified extracts constitute a novel pharmacological alternative for microbial infections with associated inflammatory conditions? *PLoS ONE* **2012**, *7*, e31145. [CrossRef]
28. Arulselvan, P.; Fard, M.T.; Tan, W.S.; Gothai, S.; Fakurazi, S.; Norhaizan, M.E.; Kumar, S.S. Role of antioxidants and natural products in inflammation. *Oxid. Med. Cell. Longev.* **2016**, *2016*. [CrossRef]
29. Chohan, M.; Naughton, D.P.; Jones, L.; Opara, E.I. An investigation of the relationship between the anti-inflammatory activity, polyphenolic content, and antioxidant activities of cooked and in vitro digested culinary herbs. *Oxid. Med. Cell. Longev.* **2012**, *2012*. [CrossRef]
30. Fu, C.W.F.; Ho, C.W.; Yong, W.T.L.; Abas, F.; Tan, T.B.; Tan, C.P. Extraction of phenolic antioxidants from four selected seaweeds obtained from Sabah. *Int. Food Res. J.* **2016**, *23*, 2363–2369.
31. Ummat, V.; Tiwari, B.K.; Jaiswal, A.K.; Condon, K.; Garcia-Vaquero, M.; O'Doherty, J.; O'Donnell, C.; Rajauria, G. Optimisation of ultrasound frequency, extraction time and solvent for the recovery of polyphenols, phlorotannins and associated antioxidant activity from brown seaweeds. *Mar Drugs.* **2020**, *18*, 250. [CrossRef] [PubMed]
32. Budhiyanti, S.A.; Raharjo, S.; Marseno, D.W.; Lelana, I.Y.B. Antioxidant activity of brown algae *Sargassum* species extract from the coastline of Java island. *Am. J. Agric. Biol. Sci.* **2012**, *7*, 337–346. [CrossRef]
33. Lourenço, S.C.; Moldão-Martins, M.; Alves, V.D. Antioxidants of natural plant origins: From sources to food industry applications. *Molecules* **2019**, *24*, 4132. [CrossRef]
34. Corsetto, P.A.; Montorfano, G.; Zava, S.; Colombo, I.; Ingadottir, B.; Jonsdottir, R.; Sveinsdottir, K.; Rizzo, A.M. Characterization of antioxidant potential of seaweed extracts for enrichment of convenience food. *Antioxidants* **2020**, *9*, 249. [CrossRef]
35. Silva, J.; Alves, C.; Freitas, R.; Martins, A.; Pinteus, S.; Ribeiro, J.; Gaspar, H.; Alfonso, A.; Pedrosa, R. Antioxidant and neuroprotective potential of the brown seaweed *Bifurcaria bifurcata* in an in vitro Parkinson's disease model. *Mar. Drugs* **2019**, *17*, 85. [CrossRef] [PubMed]
36. Nair, V.; Bang, W.Y.; Schreckinger, E.; Andarwulan, N.; Cisneros-Zevallos, L. Protective role of ternatin anthocyanins and quercetin glycosides from butterfly pea (*Clitoria ternatea* Leguminosae) blue flower petals against lipopolysaccharide (LPS)-induced inflammation in macrophage cells. *J. Agric. Food Chem.* **2015**, *63*, 6355–6365. [CrossRef] [PubMed]
37. Gulcin, I. Fe^{3+}–Fe^{2+} transformation method: An important antioxidant assay. In *Advanced Protocols in Oxidative Stress III, Methods in Molecular Biology, vol 1208*; Armstrong, D., Ed.; Springer Science+Business Media: New York, NY, USA, 2015; pp. 233–246.
38. Prior, R.L.; Wu, X.; Schaich, K. Standardized methods for the determination of antioxidant capacity and phenolics in foods and dietary supplements. *J. Agric. Food Chem.* **2005**, *53*, 4290–4302. [CrossRef] [PubMed]
39. Rajauria, G. In-vitro antioxidant properties of lipophilic antioxidant compounds from 3 brown seaweed. *Antioxidants* **2019**, *8*, 596. [CrossRef]
40. Syad, A.N.; Shunmugiah, K.P.; Kasi, P.D. Antioxidant and anti-cholinesterase activity of *Sargassum wightii*. *Pharm. Biol.* **2013**, *51*, 1401–1410. [CrossRef]
41. Adebayo, S.A.; Steel, H.C.; Shai, L.J.; Eloff, J.N. Investigation of the mechanism of anti-inflammatory action and cytotoxicity of a semipurified fraction and isolated compounds from the leaf of *Peltophorum africanum* (Fabaceae). *J. Evid. Based Complement. Altern. Med.* **2017**, *22*, 840–845. [CrossRef]

42. Somchit, N.; Kimseng, R.; Dhar, R.; Hiransai, P.; Changtam, C.; Suksamrarn, A.; Chunglok, W. Curcumin pyrazole blocks lipopolysaccharide-induced inflammation via suppression of JNK activation in RAW 264.7 macrophages. *Asian Pac. J. Allergy Immunol.* **2018**, *36*, 184–190.
43. Muller, P.Y.; Milton, M.N. The determination and interpretation of the therapeutic index in drug development. *Nat. Rev. Drug Discov.* **2012**, *11*, 751–761. [CrossRef] [PubMed]
44. Ismail, M.M.; Osman, M.E.H. Seasonal fluctuation of photosynthetic pigments of most common red seaweeds species collected from Abu Qir, Alexandria, Egypt. *Rev. Biol. Mar. Oceanogr.* **2016**, *51*, 515–525. [CrossRef]
45. Gosch, B.J.; Paul, N.A.; de Nys, R.; Magnusson, M. Spatial, seasonal, and within-plant variation in total fatty acid content and composition in the brown seaweeds *Dictyota bartayresii* and *Dictyopteris australis* (Dictyotales, Phaeophyceae). *J. Appl. Phycol.* **2015**, *27*, 1607–1622. [CrossRef]
46. Saraswati; Giantina, G.; Faridah, D.N.; Giriwono, P.E.; Iskandriati, D.; Andarwulan, N. Water and lipid-soluble component profile of *Sargassum cristaefolium* from different coastal areas in Indonesia with potential for developing functional ingredient. *J. Oleo Sci.* **2020**, *69*, 1517–1528. [CrossRef] [PubMed]
47. Foseid, L.; Devle, H.; Stenstrøm, Y.; Naess-andresen, C.F.; Ekeberg, D. Fatty acid profiles of stipe and blade from the Norwegian brown macroalgae *Laminaria hyperborea* with special reference to acyl glycerides, polar lipids, and free fatty acids. *J. Lipids* **2017**, *2017*, 102970. [CrossRef] [PubMed]
48. Koivikko, R. *Brown Algal Phlorotannins: Improving and Applying Chemical Methods*; University of Turku: Turku, Finland, 2008.
49. Tasende, M.G. Fatty acid and sterol composition of gametophytes and sporophytes of *Chondrus crispus* (Gigartinaceae, Rhodophyta). *Sci. Mar.* **2000**, *64*, 421–426. [CrossRef]
50. Saraswati; Giriwono, P.E.; Iskandriati, D.; Tan, C.P.; Andarwulan, N. In-vitro anti-inflammatory activity, free radical (DPPH) scavenging, and ferric reducing ability (FRAP) of *Sargassum cristaefolium* lipid-soluble fraction and putative identification of bioactive compounds using UHPLC-ESI-ORBITRAP-MS/MS. *Food Res. Int.* **2020**, *137*, 109702. [CrossRef] [PubMed]
51. Ahmad, T.B.; Rudd, D.; Kotiw, M.; Liu, L.; Benkendorff, K. Correlation between fatty acid profile and anti-inflammatory activity in common Australian seafood by-products. *Mar. Drugs* **2019**, *17*, 155. [CrossRef] [PubMed]
52. Bligh, E.G.; Dyer, W.J. A rapid method of total lipid extraction and purification. *Can. J. Biochem. Physiol.* **1959**, *37*, 911–917. [CrossRef]
53. Susanto, E.; Fahmi, A.S.; Hosokawa, M.; Abe, M.; Miyashita, K. Lipids, fatty acids, and fucoxanthin content from temperate and tropical brown seaweeds. *Aquat. Procedia* **2016**, *7*, 66–75. [CrossRef]
54. Kamal, A.F.; Iskandriati, D.; Dilogo, I.H.; Siregar, N.C.; Hutagalung, E.U.; Susworo, R.; Yusuf, A.A.; Bachtiar, A. Biocompatibility of various hydroxyapatite scaffolds evaluated by proliferation of rat's bone marrow mesenchymal stem cells: An in vitro study. *Med. J. Indones.* **2013**, *22*, 202–208. [CrossRef]
55. Wen, Z.-S.; Xiang, X.-W.; Jin, H.-X.; Guo, X.-Y.; Liu, L.-J.; Huang, Y.-N.; OuYang, X.-K.; Qu, Y.-L. Composition and anti-inflammatory effect of polysaccharides from *Sargassum horneri* in RAW264.7 macrophages. *Int. J. Biol. Macromol.* **2016**, *88*, 403–413. [CrossRef]
56. Rao, U.M.; Ahmad, B.A.; Mohd, K.S. In vitro nitric oxide scavenging and anti inflammatory activities of different solvent extract of various parts of Musa paradisiaca. *Malaysian J. Anal. Sci.* **2016**, *20*, 1191–1202. [CrossRef]
57. Benzie, I.; Strain, J. The ferric reducing ability of plasma (FRAP) as a measure of antioxidant power: The FRAP assay. *Biochem.* **1996**, *239*, 70–76. [CrossRef] [PubMed]

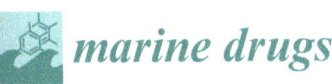

Article

Impact of Phlorotannin Extracts from *Fucus vesiculosus* on Human Gut Microbiota

Marcelo D. Catarino [1], Catarina Marçal [1], Teresa Bonifácio-Lopes [2], Débora Campos [2], Nuno Mateus [3], Artur M. S. Silva [1], Maria Manuela Pintado [2] and Susana M. Cardoso [1,*]

1. LAQV-REQUIMTE, Department of Chemistry, University of Aveiro, 3810-193 Aveiro, Portugal; mcatarino@ua.pt (M.D.C.); catarina.marcal@ua.pt (C.M.); artur.silva@ua.pt (A.M.S.S.)
2. CBQF-Centro de Biotecnologia e Química Fina–Laboratório Associado, Escola Superior de Biotecnologia, Universidade Católica Portuguesa, Rua Diogo Botelho 1327, 4169-005 Porto, Portugal; mvlopes@portu.ucp.pt (T.B.-L.); dcampos@porto.ucp.pt (D.C.); mpintado@porto.ucp.pt (M.M.P.)
3. REQUIMTE/LAQV, Department of Chemistry and Biochemistry, Faculty of Sciences, University of Porto, 4169-007 Porto, Portugal; nbmateus@fc.up.pt
* Correspondence: susanacardoso@ua.pt; Tel.: +351-234-370-360; Fax: +351-234-370-084

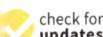

Citation: Catarino, M.D.; Marçal, C.; Bonifácio-Lopes, T.; Campos, D.; Mateus, N.; Silva, A.M.S.; Pintado, M.M.; Cardoso, S.M. Impact of Phlorotannin Extracts from *Fucus vesiculosus* on Human Gut Microbiota. *Mar. Drugs* 2021, *19*, 375. https://doi.org/10.3390/md19070375

Academic Editor: Roland Ulber

Received: 31 May 2021
Accepted: 21 June 2021
Published: 29 June 2021

Publisher's Note: MDPI stays neutral with regard to jurisdictional claims in published maps and institutional affiliations.

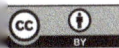

Copyright: © 2021 by the authors. Licensee MDPI, Basel, Switzerland. This article is an open access article distributed under the terms and conditions of the Creative Commons Attribution (CC BY) license (https://creativecommons.org/licenses/by/4.0/).

Abstract: Recent studies indicate that plant polyphenols could be pointed as potential prebiotic candidates since they may interact with the gut microbiota, stimulating its growth and the production of metabolites. However, little is known about the fate of brown seaweeds' phlorotannins during their passage throughout the gastrointestinal tract. This work aimed to evaluate the stability and bioaccessibility of *Fucus vesiculosus* phlorotannins after being submitted to a simulated digestive process, as well as their possible modulatory effects on gut microbiota and short-chain fatty acids production following a fermentation procedure using fecal inoculates to mimic the conditions of the large intestine. The stability of phlorotannins throughout the gastrointestinal tract was reduced, with a bioaccessibility index between 2 and 14%. Moreover, slight alterations in the growth of certain commensal bacteria were noticed, with *Enterococcus* spp. being the most enhanced group. Likewise, *F. vesiculosus* phlorotannins displayed striking capacity to enhance the levels of propionate and butyrate, which are two important short-chain fatty acids known for their role in intestinal homeostasis. In summary, this work provides valuable information regarding the behavior of *F. vesiculosus* phlorotannins along the gastrointestinal tract, presenting clear evidence that these compounds can positively contribute to the maintenance of a healthy gastrointestinal condition.

Keywords: phlorotannins; brown seaweeds; gut microbiota; bioaccessibility; short-chain fatty acids; prebiotics; gastrointestinal tract

1. Introduction

The human intestinal tract harbors a complex community of microorganisms, collectively termed as intestinal or gut microbiota. The microbial colonization of the gastrointestinal tract starts right after birth and undergoes a symbiotic co-evolution along with their host, importantly contributing to the maintenance of intestinal homeostasis, development and integrity of the mucosal barrier, production of various nutrients, protection against microbial pathogens, maturation of the immune system and many other functions [1]. Throughout adulthood, the intestinal microbiota is regarded as relatively stable, although it may be affected by several extrinsic factors including dietary habits, medication (especially with antibiotics), environmental pollution and exposure to xenobiotics, physical activity and hygiene [2]. When these factors cause significant changes in the composition and/or function of the gut microbiota, the whole microbial ecosystem is perturbed to an extent that exceeds its resistance and resilience capabilities, leading to a condition known as dysbiosis. Consequently, dysbiosis has been associated with an increasing list of diseases, which include inflammatory bowel disease (IBD), irritable bowel syndrome

(IBS), coeliac disease and colorectal cancer (CRC) [3]. Additionally, several extra-intestinal disorders such as asthma [4], systemic lupus erythematosus [5], cardiovascular disease [6] or even mental and neurodegenerative diseases including autism, anxiety, depression, chronic pain, Parkinson's, Alzheimer's or Huntington's can be linked to a dysfunctional gut microbiota [7–9].

Based on this evidence, it is clear that the manipulation of gut microbiota could be regarded as a promising strategy to treat disease and improve health. In this context, prebiotics appear as important tools capable of manipulating and modifying the gut microbiota composition and promoting the host's health status. They were first described in 1995 [10] and are currently defined as "a substrate that is selectively utilized by host microorganisms conferring a health benefit" [11]. In other terms, prebiotics are non-digestible dietary components that act as substrates that selectively stimulate the growth and/or biological activity of health-promoting bacteria residing in the host's colon. Common prebiotics include several non-digestible polysaccharides, such as resistant starch and pectin, as well as oligosaccharides such as fructo-oligosaccharides (FOSs), galacto-oligosaccharides (GOSs), lactulose and inulin, which are found mainly in several land-vegetables, fruits and milk [12]. More recently, increasing evidence has shown that other compounds such as polyphenols and polyunsaturated fatty acids may also display modulatory effects on gut microbiota populations through selective prebiotic effects and antimicrobial activities against gut pathogenic bacteria [13,14]. Indeed, animal studies have demonstrated that the consumption of polyphenols, especially catechins, anthocyanins and proanthocyanidins, not only favors the growth of probiotic bacteria, such as *Lactobacillus*, *Bifidobacterium*, *Akkermansia*, *Roseburia* and *Faecalibacterium* spp., but also increases the production of short-chain fatty acids (SCFAs), including butyrate, which is the major energy source for the colonic epithelium and profoundly influences intestinal homeostasis [15]. Likewise, clinical trials have also revealed that the consumption of anthocyanins and ellagic acid promotes increases in *Lactobacillus acidophilus*, *Bifidobacterium* and *Faecalibacterium* spp. abundance in the stool and a reduction of the lipopolysaccharide-binding protein in the plasma of volunteers [16,17].

In contrast, studies regarding the prebiotic potential of seaweeds (particularly brown) are still scarce and essentially focused on the in vitro effects of their polysaccharides, while the fate of phlorotannins when crossing the gastrointestinal tract, remains deeply unexplored subject [18]. These compounds are specific phenolics biosynthesized only by brown seaweeds consisting of polymeric structures composed of several phloroglucinol units [18], and, despite the fact that they have been reported in the literature for their promising and versatile bioactive health benefits, only a limited number of studies have addressed their behavior in the gastrointestinal tract. Recent works have shown that an *Ecklonia radiata* phlorotannin-enriched extract performed better than inulin as it promoted a higher increase in *Lactobacillus*, *F. prausnitzii*, *C. coccoides*, Firmicutes and *E. coli* in fermentations conducted with human fecal microbiota [19], while the administration of *Lessonia turbeculata* polyphenol-rich extract to streptozotocin-induced diabetic rats was found to significantly restore the relative abundance of the overall bacterial diversity and SCFAs to levels similar to the negative control [20]. Interestingly, to the authors knowledge, no studies addressing the stability and bioactivity of phlorotannins throughout the gastrointestinal tract has been performed yet.

In this context, the aim of this work was to evaluate the stability and bioaccessibility of *F. vesiculosus* phlorotannin-rich extracts when crossing the gastrointestinal tract and ultimately disclose their possible modulatory effects toward the gut microbiota and short-chain fatty acid production.

2. Results and Discussion

2.1. Stability, Bioaccessibility and Antioxidant Activity of F. vesiculosus Extracts throughout the Simulated GIT

To evaluate the stability of *F. vesiculosus* phlorotannins throughout the digestive tract, both crude (CRD) and ethyl acetate fraction (EtOAc) were submitted to a simulated gastrointestinal (GIT) digestion and evaluated for their total phlorotannin content and antioxidant activity after each gut compartment. The results presented in Table 1 clearly demonstrate that the total phlorotannin content of the EtOAc fraction progressively decreased after each step from the GIT simulation. Interestingly, in the case of CRD, after the initial decrease in the mouth, an increase in the phlorotannin levels was found after the stomach digestion, followed by another decrease in the intestine. The reduction in the total phlorotannin content (TPhC) of the samples after the mouth digestion could be explained by possible interactions occurring between phlorotannins and the salivary proteins. In fact, such interactions are very well described for plant tannins and very relevant for the development of important sensory characteristics of certain foods and beverages such as wine [21]. The extreme pH conditions in the stomach can also explain why the TPhC of the EtOAc kept decreasing in this compartment. However, in the case of CRD, because this sample is more complex and contains other non-phlorotannin compounds, it is possible that such compounds might be interacting with phlorotannins, protecting them from reacting with the mouth proteins and degrading with the low stomach pH. In turn, the stomach pH may also promote the degradation of those non-phlorotannin compounds, promoting the release of the phlorotannins, making them more available to react with the 2,4-dimethoxybenzaldehyde (DMBA). In fact, similar observations have been previously reported for plant phenolics [22,23] and are on the basis of the delivery strategies in which phenolic compounds are encapsulated in order to resist the gastrointestinal conditions and reach intact for absorption in the intestines [24]. Additionally, it was noticed that even though undigested EtOAc had higher TPhC compared to the undigested CRD, after the stomach and intestine digestion, the TPhC of the latter was slightly higher compared with the EtOAc, which is in agreement with the hypothesis that the EtOAc phlorotannins were more exposed to the GIT degradation than those of CRD.

Table 1. Total phlorotannin content and antioxidant activity of *F. vesiculosus* crude and ethyl acetate fraction through the different stages of gastrointestinal digestion.

Sample	GIT Stage	TPhC (mg PGE/g ext)	(1) NO• (IC$_{50}$ µg/mL)	(2) O$_2$•− (IC$_{50}$ µg/mL)
CRD	Undigested	9.93 ± 1.48 [a]	161 ± 8.8 [a]	417 ± 164.5 [a]
	Mouth	6.33 ± 2.96 [b]	309 ± 105.2 [b]	745 ± 88.2 [b]
	Stomach	8.52 ± 1.16 [a,b]	171 ± 27.1 [a]	378 ± 26.6 [a]
	Intestine	5.17 ± 0.70 [b]	287 ± 27.2 [a,b]	1105 ± 421.3 [b]
	Retentate *	4.60 ± 0.26 [b]	141 ± 9.1 [a]	294 ± 19.3 [a]
	Permeate *	1.40 ± 0.19 [c]	2551 ± 30.7 [c]	2580 ± 75.2 [c]
EtOAc	Undigested	17.39 ± 1.77 [a]	45 ± 2.5 [a]	118 ± 17.6 [a]
	Mouth	13.83 ± 0.74 [b]	73 ± 11.0 [a,b]	221 ± 1.1 [a,b]
	Stomach	5.67 ± 0.91 [c]	109 ± 7.1 [a,b]	244 ± 0.4 [a,b]
	Intestine	3.28 ± 0.55 [c]	195 ± 38.5 [b,c]	564 ± 19.9 [c]
	Retentate *	2.97 ± 0.62 [c,d]	281 ±16.1 [c]	383 ± 18.2 [b,c]
	Permeate *	0.37 ± 0.10 [d]	1531 ± 52.2 [d]	3074 ± 32.3 [d]
Standard compound		-	36 ± 0.9	6 ± 0.5

CRD—crude extract; EtOAc—ethyl acetate fraction; GIT—gastrointestinal tract; TPhC—total phlorotannin content. (1) Standard compound for NO• is ascorbic acid; (2) standard compound for O$_2$•− is gallic acid; * results for DMBA expressed in mg PGE/g intestine digest. Data represent the mean ± SD of at least three independent assays. For each sample, different letters indicate significant differences within the same column ($p < 0.05$).

At the end of the simulated GIT, only a small portion of the total phlorotannins loaded in the system was bioaccessible, which is in line with previous studies carried out on land plant tannins. At this point, it is important to clarify that the term "bioavailability" expresses the fraction of an ingested compound/nutrient that reaches the systemic circulation to be distributed to organs and tissues and to manifest its bioactivity. However, before becoming bioavailable, the target compound/nutrient must be released from the food matrix and made available for bloodstream absorption, which is what defines the term "bioaccessibility" [25]. Interestingly, despite the fact that the undigested CRD exhibited lower TPhC compared to the undigested EtOAc, the bioaccessibility index of the former was 14.1%, while the latter was only 2.0%. Once again, this outcome might be in part explained by the fact that EtOAc experienced higher phlorotannin degradation than CRD, and, therefore, when the compounds reach the intestine to be absorbed, the TPhC of the matrix is already lower.

Concerning the antioxidant activity of the samples after each step of the GIT simulation, both NO$^\bullet$ and SO$^{\bullet-}$ results were in line with the TPhC of the respective samples, i.e., the samples with higher phlorotannin concentrations exhibited the lowest IC$_{50}$ values and vice versa. Indeed, strong negative correlations were found between the TPhC and the antioxidant assays with CRD showing R^2 of -0.82 and -0.94 and EtOAc showing R^2 of -0.91 and -0.82 in NO$^\bullet$ and SO$^{\bullet-}$, respectively, thus indicating a clear association between the phlorotannin content after each step of the simulated digestion and the antioxidant activities observed.

2.2. Prebiotic Effect

The prebiotic activity of digested *F. vesiculosus* CRD and EtOAc was studied on four strains in basal Man–Rogosa–Sharpe (MRS) broth without glucose, at concentrations of 1–2% (w/v). Figure 1 presents the growth curves of the evaluated *Lactobacillus* and *Bifidobacteria* strains over 24 h, as no further alterations were observed between 24 and 48 h. All the probiotic microorganisms were affected by the presence of the *F. vesiculosus* samples in different manners. *Lactobacillus casei* exhibited a growth behavior identical for almost all the conditions tested, with no differences observed on the maximum optical density (OD), although the seaweed samples seemed to slightly delay their growth during the first 10 h. The only notable exception was EtOAc at 1%, which caused a slight decrease of the growth curve of this strain. In turn, the incubation of *L. acidophilus* with either CRD or EtOAc presented a growth curve considerably higher than that of FOS, for all the concentrations tested, thus indicating that both CRD and EtOAc stimulate the growth of this strain.

In contrast, *B. animalis* growth was the least pronounced of all the strains tested, in the presence of either CRD or EtOAc, suggesting that they might exert a bacteriostatic effect on this strain. The results for *B. animalis* spp. *lactis* demonstrated that the CRD at 1% displayed better stimulatory effects than FOS, although the bacterial growth was completely abolished for higher concentrations, indicating that, in such conditions, this extract impairs the growth of this strain. Positive stimulatory effects were noticed for EtOAc at 1 and 1.5% as well, which demonstrated growth curves identical to that of FOS. However, for the concentration of 2%, this sample also exhibited inhibitory effects toward this strain.

The potential prebiotic effect of seaweeds is a subject barely studied so far. Nevertheless, Martelli et al. [26] recently showed that four strains of probiotic bacteria (*L. casei*, *L. paracasei*, *L. rhamnosus* and *B. subtilis*) all exhibited good capacity to grow in a broth medium containing *Himanthalia elongata* flour (5%), which is in line with previous works that demonstrated the capacity of different brown algae species (*Sargassum siliquanstrum*, *Laminaria digitata*, *Laminaria saccharina*) to stimulate the growth of several probiotic bacteria including *Weissella* spp., *Lactobacillus* spp., *Leuconostoc* spp., *L. plantarum* and *L. rhamnosus* [27–29]. However, seaweeds have a very complex matrix and the contribution of phlorotannins for the effects observed by these authors are likely to be negligible. In fact, current knowledge regarding the fate of seaweed polyphenols in the human gastrointestinal tract is scarce. In the work developed by Corona et al. [30], after submitting a polyphenol-rich extract from *A. nodosum* to a simulated gastrointestinal digestion followed by fecal fermentation, they were able to find seven phlorotannin-derived metabolites, and, although the microbiota composition was not assessed, the presence of these metabolites suggests that phlorotannins might have been used by the colonic bacteria. In turn, in a 24 h in vitro fermentation carried out using *Ecklonia radiata* phlorotannin extract, a significant increase in the populations of Bacteroidetes, *Clostridium coccoides*, *E. coli* and *Faecalibacterium prausnitzii* was observed, although the levels of *Bifidobacterium* and *Lactobacillus* populations were found to be decreased [19]. With these results, we demonstrate for the first time that *F. vesiculosus* extract and phlorotannin-enriched fraction can stimulate the growth of some probiotic strains in a similar way to that of FOS.

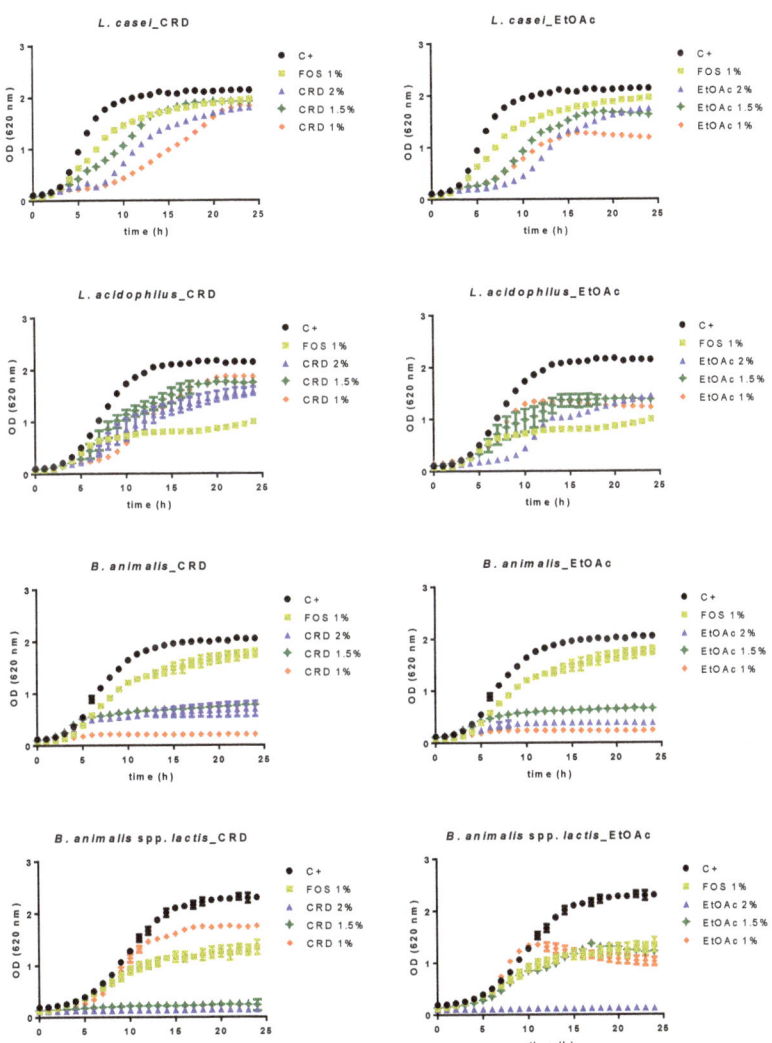

Figure 1. Growth curves of *L. casei*, *L. acidophilus*, *B. animalis* and *B. animalis* spp. *lactis* in the presence of different concentrations of digested crude extract (CRD) and ethyl acetate fraction (EtOAc). Data represent the mean ± SD of at least three independent assays.

2.3. Evolution of the Gut Microbiota Profile Groups

After GIT simulation, the digested *F. vesiculosus* CRD and EtOAc were submitted to human feces fermentation during 48 h, and aliquots were taken at 0, 12, 24 and 48 h to study their effect upon the human microbiota. Three of the four dominant phyla in the human gut were evaluated, namely Firmicutes (represented by *Clostridium leptum*, *Enterococcus* spp. and *Lactobacillus* spp.), Bacteroidetes (represented by *Bacteroides* spp.) and Actinobacteria (represented by *Bifidobacterium* spp.), and the compositional averages of the copy numbers obtained by real-time PCR of these main groups are depicted in the Table 2.

Table 2. Fecal microbiota composition of volunteer participants.

Division (Genus)	Number of Copies (n = 5) [a]
Universal	7.52 ± 0.38
Firmicutes	4.76 ± 0.20
Clostridium leptum	4.97 ± 0.26
Enterococcus spp.	2.07 ± 0.63
Lactobacillus spp.	3.27 ± 0.72
Bacteroidetes	5.46 ± 0.63
Bacteroides spp.	3.76 ± 0.55
Bifidobacterium spp.	4.42 ± 0.45
F:B ratio	0.97 ± 0.23

[a] Values are presented as mean ± SD of five independent assays and expressed as log10 16S rRNA gene copies per 20 ng of DNA.

The numbers were in agreement with those found in healthy volunteers' feces, with *Clostridium*, *Bacteroides* and *Bifidobacterium* comprising the dominant genera while *Lactobacillus* spp. and *Enterococcus* appeared as the subdominant genera [31–33]. Figure 2 depicts the relative differences (in %) between the microbiota groups of the tested samples and control feces, along 12, 24 and 48 h of fermentation. Overall, both CRD and EtOAc promoted a modest positive effect on gut microbiota growth, as noticed by the increment in the universal microorganisms compared to the control over time, while FOS exerted a positive effect on the initial 12 h that reversed for the following 24 and 48 h.

The EtOAc fraction caused a positive effect over time on the phyla Firmicutes and Bacteroidetes, which are representative of a healthy microbiota [34], while CRD and FOS exhibited a null or negative effect on these two groups. In turn, as expected, FOS exerted a very positive effect on *Lactobacillus* spp. and *Bifidobacterium* spp., two genera that are the markers of prebiosis par excellence. Likewise, despite not having an effect as sharp as FOS, EtOAc fraction also positively stimulated the growth of these two probiotic groups over time, although in the case of *Lactobacillus* spp., the effect lasted only until 24 h, becoming null at the end of the fermentation (48 h). Identical behavior was noticed for CRD on *Bifidobacterium* spp., promoting their growth only during the first 24 h. Curiously, no effect was observed on *Lactobacillus* spp., contrarily to what was expected since *L. casei* and *L. acidophilus* responded with a very positive growth behavior in the presence of this sample on the prebiotic studies (Section 2.2).

Interestingly, the group of *Enterococcus* spp. was the most beneficiated by CRD and EtOAc, although the levels of these organisms progressively decreased over time, contrarily to FOS which promoted their growth at each time point. Poor gut health outcomes have generally been linked to this genus [35], although this is a controversial subject since not all enterococcal strains cause health problems. In fact, strains such as *E. faecium* SF68® and *E. faecalis* Symbio-flor® have been marketed as probiotics for two decades without incidence and with very few reported adverse events [36]. Moreover, enterococcal probiotics have been shown to be effective in limiting gastrointestinal infectious burden and in the treatment of gastrointestinal infections and diarrhea [37].

On the contrary, *Clostridium leptum*, an important butyrate-producing strain, was the least affected by the studied samples, with only CRD causing a slight negative effect on its growth over time.

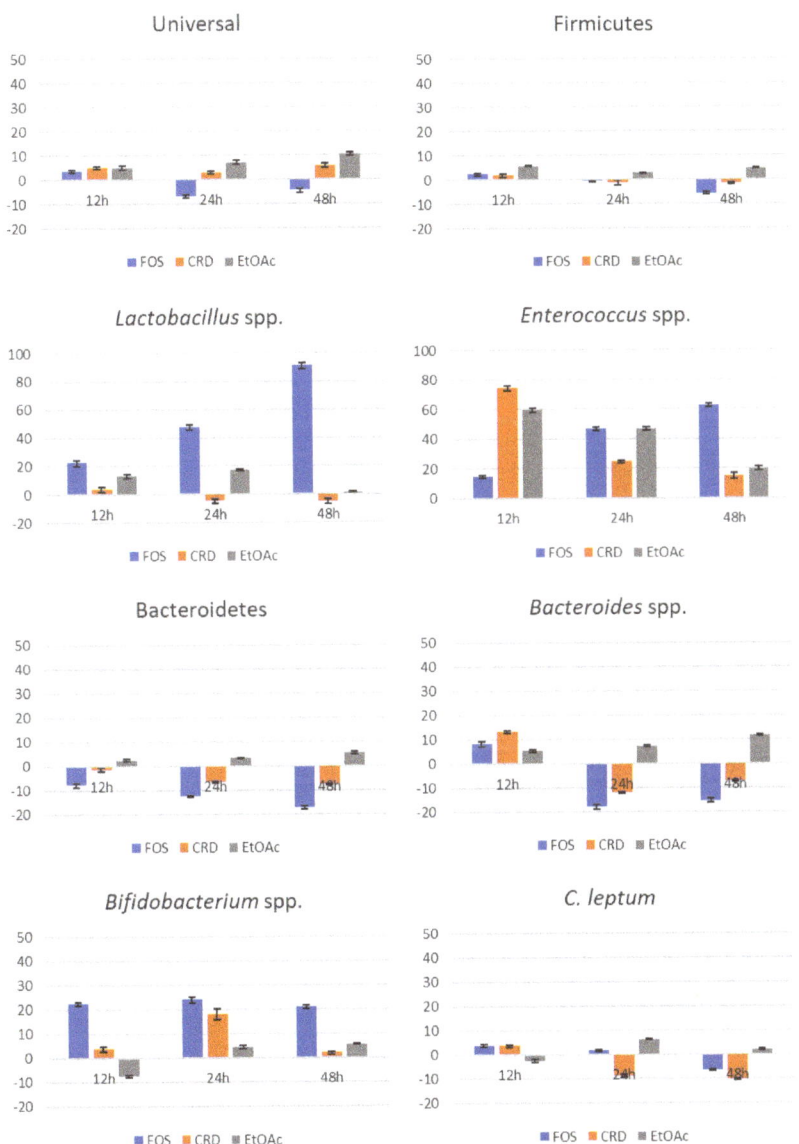

Figure 2. Evolution of the gut microbiota groups (relative differences to negative control in %) along the fermentation. Data represent the mean ± SD of five independent assays.

Regarding *Bacteroides* spp., the results demonstrated that even though all the samples promoted an increment in this group during the first 12 h, only EtOAc maintained this positive effect throughout the fermentation course. Instead, FOS and CRD turned out to negatively affect the growth of these bacteria after 24 h and until the end of the fermentation. Similar to *Enterococcus* spp., there is some controversy around the probiotic potential of the genus *Bacteroides*. On one hand, this group has been associated with the development of intestinal dysfunctions such as diarrhea, inflammatory bowel disease and colorectal cancer, and, on the other hand, it has been recently considered as a next generation probiotic candidate due to its potential role in promoting host health through the regulation of intestinal redox levels or the production of important short-chain fatty acids such as acetate, propionate and butyrate, which in turn can contribute to the regulation of toxin transport from the gut lumen to blood, the prevention of colon cancer and the prevention of inflammatory conditions [38].

Another important aspect to consider is the ratio between Firmicutes and Bacteroidetes (F:B), the most predominant phyla in the human colon. Together they comprise 90% of the total gut microbiota and, thus, their proportion can give us a global idea of the total effect of *F. vesiculosus* samples on the intestinal flora. Commonly, healthy individuals display a nearly 1:1 ratio of Firmicutes to Bacteroidetes, and significant alterations of this ratio have been associated with pathological states [39]. For instance, increased F:B ratios have been linked to the pathophysiology of obesity [40], while patients of type II diabetes mellitus were found to have their levels of Firmicutes significantly reduced compared to their non-diabetic counterparts and consequently had decreased F:B ratios [41]. In this work, a slight increase of the F:B ratio was noticed for FOS and EtOAc (1.36 ± 0.10 and 1.24 ± 0.14, respectively) compared to the control (1.09 ± 0.05) during the first 12 h of fermentation, which then returned to normal levels over the next 24 and 48 h (Figure 3A). On the contrary, CRD did not cause any significant alterations of this parameter maintaining the F:B ratio values stable and close to one over the course of the fermentation.

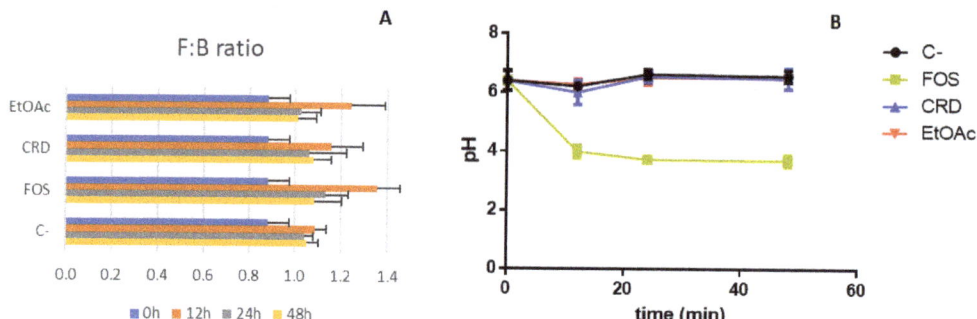

Figure 3. Firmicutes:Bacteroidetes (F:B) ratio (**A**) and variation of the pH (**B**) throughout the fermentation of digested FOS, CRD and EtOAC with human microbiota. Data represent the mean ± SD of five independent assays.

Very few studies focusing on the prebiotic potential of phlorotannin-rich extracts have been conducted so far, although there are already some insights on this matter. Interestingly, Charoensiddhi et al. [19] reported that, after the 24 h fermentation period of a phlorotannin-rich extract of *E. radiata* with human fecal samples, only the group of Bacteroidetes showed an increased growth compared to the negative control, while Firmicutes and *Bifidobacterium* spp. remained unchanged and *Lactobacillus* spp. and *Enterococcus* spp. actually decreased. However, these authors also observed a stimulation of the growth of *Faecalibacterium prausnitzii* and *Clostridium coccoides*, which were not analyzed in this study but are two important groups associated to SCFA production (particularly butyrate) and health-promoting effects [42,43]. In a different work, the administration of a polyphenol-rich extract from the brown algae *Lessonia trabeculata* to streptozotocin-induced diabetic rats under a high-fat diet significantly restored the levels of the three dominant phyla, i.e., Firmicutes, Bacteroidetes and Proteobacteria, as well as the F:B ratio to values identical of the negative control [20]. To the authors knowledge, this work was the first assessing the potential modulatory effects of *F. vesiculosus* phlorotannin extracts on human gut microbiota and allowed the disclosure of valuable information on how *F. vesiculosus* phlorotannins may impact on the human gastrointestinal microflora.

2.4. Organic Acids Profile and pH Variation

The changes in the concentration of short-chain fatty acids along the fermentation of FOS, CRD and EtOAc with human feces in basal media were analyzed by HPLC and are presented in Table 3. SCFAs such as acetate, propionate and butyrate are volatile fatty acids that are produced by the gut microbiota in the colon as a result of the fermentation and metabolization of food components that are undigested/unabsorbed in the upper GIT.

Table 3. Concentration of organic acids (succinic, lactic, acetic, propionic and butyric) throughout fermentation of digested FOS, CRD and EtOAC with human microbiota (mg/mL).

Organic Acids	Time (h)	Ctrl	FOS	CRD	EtOAc
Total	0	2.38 ± 0.63 [a;A]	2.38 ± 0.63 [a;A]	2.38 ± 0.63 [a;A]	2.38 ± 0.63 [a;A]
	12	5.24 ± 1.98 [a;A]	10.89 ± 2.79 [b;B]	7.43 ± 2.09 [b;A]	7.76 ± 1.92 [b;A,B]
	24	4.90 ± 1.59 [a;A]	12.63 ± 2.37 [b,c;B]	7.08 ± 2.45 [b;A]	7.55 ± 1.75 [b;A]
	48	4.10 ± 2.01 [a;A]	14.78 ± 4.00 [c;B]	5.04 ± 1.57 [a,b;A]	6.38 ± 1.98 [b;A]
Succinic acid	0	0.45 ± 0.20 [a;A]	0.45 ± 0.20 [a;A]	0.45 ± 0.20 [a;A]	0.45 ± 0.20 [a;A]
	12	0.77 ± 0.75 [a;A]	1.85 ± 0.92 [b;B]	2.29 ± 1.39 [c;B]	2.15 ± 1.15 [b;B]
	24	1.12 ± 0.53 [a;A]	1.97 ± 0.58 [b;B]	2.02 ± 0.93 [b,c;A,B]	1.35 ± 0.50 [a,b;A,B]
	48	0.74 ± 0.71 [a;A]	2.03 ± 0.85 [b;B]	1.12 ± 0.20 [a,b;A,B]	1.40 ± 0.89 [a,b;A,B]
Lactic acid	0	ND	ND	ND	ND
	12	1.21 ± 0.93 [a;A]	3.91 ± 1.94 [a;B]	0.87 ± 0.22 [a;A]	0.87 ± 0.23 [a;A]
	24	0.34 ± 0.14 [a;A]	4.81 ± 0.75 [a,b;B]	0.76 ± 0.58 [a;A]	0.26 ± 0.16 [a;A]
	48	ND	5.49 ± 2.14 [b]	ND	ND
Acetic acid	0	0.16 ± 0.04 [a;A]	0.16 ± 0.04 [a;A]	0.16 ± 0.04 [a;A]	0.16 ± 0.04 [a;A]
	12	0.81 ± 0.10 [b;A]	1.36 ± 0.75 [b;A]	1.03 ± 0.09 [b;A]	1.02 ± 0.19 [b;A]
	24	0.82 ± 0.17 [b;A]	1.65 ± 0.52 [b;B]	0.92 ± 0.22 [b;A]	0.96 ± 0.30 [b;A]
	48	0.78 ± 0.20 [b;A]	2.77 ± 1.21 [c;B]	0.78 ± 0.20 [b;A]	0.93 ± 0.28 [b;A]
Propionic acid	0	0.34 ± 0.09 [a;A]	0.34 ± 0.09 [a;A]	0.34 ± 0.09 [a;A]	0.34 ± 0.09 [a;A]
	12	0.53 ± 0.23 [a;A]	1.48 ± 0.32 [b;B]	1.14 ± 0.49 [b;B]	1.43 ± 0.87 [b;B]
	24	0.65 ± 0.35 [a;A]	1.89 ± 0.75 [b,c;C]	1.25 ± 0.58 [b;B]	0.85 ± 0.27 [a,b;A,B]
	48	0.50 ± 0.24 [a;A]	1.64 ± 0.60 [b;B]	0.77 ± 0.20 [a,b;A]	0.90 ± 0.24 [a,b;A]
Butyric acid	0	1.41 ± 0.25 [a;A]	1.41 ± 0.25 [a;A]	1.41 ± 0.25 [a;A]	1.41 ± 0.25 [a;A]
	12	1.92 ± 0.69 [a;A]	2.29 ± 0.99 [a;A]	2.10 ± 0.79 [a;A]	2.71 ± 0.94 [a;A]
	24	2.24 ± 0.67 [a;A]	2.23 ± 0.86 [a;A]	2.54 ± 1.05 [a;A]	4.12 ± 0.37 [b;B]
	48	2.23 ± 1.35 [a;A]	2.70 ± 1.43 [a;A]	2.31 ± 0.85 [a;A]	4.31 ± 0.62 [b;B]

Ctrl—negative control; FOS—fructo-oligosaccharides; CRD—crude extract; EtOAc—ethyl acetate fraction; ND—not detected. Different letters indicate significant differences ($p < 0.05$). The capital letters indicate the differences among the Ctrl, FOS, CRD and EtOAc for organic acid concentration at the same time (same row), and the lowercase letters indicate the differences for the same sample over time for each organic acid concentration (same column within an organic acid). Data represent the mean ± SD of five independent assays.

In this study, fermentation with FOS caused a remarkable increase in the production of total organic acids, while in the fermentations carried out with *F. vesiculosus* samples, a tendential increase in the total organic acid levels was noticed despite not being statistically significant when compared with the negative control. These results are also reflected in the pH changes registered during the fermentation (Figure 3B), with FOS producing a significant decrease in the pH values, while the pH registered for CRD and EtOAc remained similar to that of the control, at least for the time window tested. Differences in the SCFA profiles, however, were detected between samples. One of the most evident differences was noticed for lactate, which was the main metabolite produced over the entire fermentation of FOS. This outcome also relates with the high stimulatory effects that FOS produced on *Lactobacillus* spp. and *Bifidobacterium* spp. validated above with the 16S rRNA gene analysis (Section 2.3). On the other hand, similar to the negative control, the lactate production in fermentations carried out with CRD and EtOAc were nearly null, and even undetectable, at 48 h. An identical pattern was found for acetate production, which was remarkably stimulated in the presence of FOS but not affected by CRD or EtOAc. Under normal conditions this acid together with propionic and butyric acids comprise the three major SCFAs normally produced in the gut, which are important for the maintenance of intestinal homeostasis [44]. In particular, acetate plays a very important role in energy homeostasis, contributing to appetite regulation, promoting fat oxidation, improving insulin sensitivity and glucose homeostasis, and enhancing the inflammatory status [45].

Interestingly, all three samples promoted an increase in the succinate level, which reached its maximum at 12 h and was kept constant for FOS until the end of the fermentation, while for CRD and EtOAc it decreased over time. On one hand, the accumulation of this organic acid in the gut lumen is usually associated with microbiota disturbances commonly linked to poor gut health states such as antibiotic-induced dysbiosis, motility disturbances and specifically IBD [46]. On the other hand, succinate is also a key intermediate in the production of propionate, which in turn is responsible for modulating lipogenesis, controlling appetite and preventing colon cancer [47]. In fact, the levels of propionate production herein noted seem to follow an identical behavior compared with that of succinate, showing an accentuated increase during the initial phase of the fermentation and a decrease at the end, only for CRD and EtOAc. Indeed, high correlation coefficients between these two organic acids were obtained (R^2 = 0.99, 0.88 and 0.97 for FOS, CRD and EtOAc, respectively), which confirms that the production of propionate is indeed associated with the production of succinate.

One of the most important SCFAs produced in the gut is butyrate, which has been repeatedly reported for its positive health-promoting effects. In addition to its function as the primary energy source for colonocytes, butyrate also importantly contributes to the improvement of the gut barrier function, exerts anti-inflammatory and regenerative effects, prevents the formation of colon cancer and helps reduce both type II diabetes and obesity [39]. Therefore, stimulating the production of high levels of this SCFA is of great interest for promoting the healthy function of the gut. The results herein obtained revealed that only the EtOAc led to a significant increase in butyric acid, while, in CRD and FOS, the levels of this SCFA did not differ much from the negative control.

The main butyrate-producing bacteria are *Faecalibacterium prausnitzii*, *Clostridium* spp., *Eubacterium* spp., *Roseburia* spp. and *Anaerostipes* spp., which belong to the Firmicutes phylum [44], and, despite the fact that the *C. leptum* did not show significant positive growth in the presence of EtOAc, an increase in the group Firmicutes was noticed on the EtOAc-fermented samples, which might explain the increased levels of butyrate registered. In turn, the lack of production of butyrate, which was not expected, in the FOS fermentation could be possibly explained by the absence of the common cross-feeding effect among intestinal bacteria that produce acetate, propionate or butyrate as the final product of lactate metabolization [48]. Indeed, the fact that lactate has accumulated so much throughout the fermentation of FOS indicates that it has not been utilized as a substrate by other bacteria. Nevertheless, it must be considered that this experiment was performed without pH control, and, thus, it is likely that the sharp decrease in the pH may have impaired the growth of certain lactate-utilizing bacteria and favored the growth of the lactate-producing ones, therefore contributing to the increasing accumulation of this organic acid at the expense of other SCFAs [49].

When comparing these results with those previously reported by Charoensiddhi et al. [19], the stimulatory effects of *F. vesiculosus* phlorotannin samples herein tested on the production of SCFAs were much more promising than those of the *E. radiata* phlorotannin-rich extract used in their study. In fact, the authors reported that the fermentation of the phlorotannin extract caused a reduction on the levels of total SCFAs with a remarkable decrease in the concentration of acetic acid in comparison with the negative control. Contrarily, Yuan et al. [20] found that the administration of a polyphenol-rich extract from the brown algae *Lessonia trabeculata* to streptozotocin-induced diabetic rats, under a high-fat diet, significantly restored the levels of acetate and butyrate that were depleted in the diabetic control groups. Notably, the levels of butyrate in the treated rats were even higher than those of the control group, i.e., healthy rats. In our study, despite the fact that the total SCFA production was much lower than that observed for FOS, both CRD and EtOAc exhibited interesting alterations in the SCFA profiles stimulating the production of propionate and, in the case of EtOAc, butyrate as well. These SCFAs could exert interesting beneficial health properties not only in the colon and gut microbiota but also in other organs, which could partly explain the health benefits attributed to phlorotannins.

3. Materials and Methods

3.1. Chemicals

Grounded *Fucus vesiculosus* harvested in July 2017 was purchased from Algaplus Lda. Acetone, methanol, n-hexane, ethyl acetate, DMSO, glacial acetic acid, hydrochloric acid and sodium hydroxide were acquired from Fisher (Pittsburgh, PA, USA). Sodium nitroprusside and sulfanilamide were ordered from Acros Organics (Hampton, NH, USA). Ascorbic acid, gallic acid, NADH, NBT, PMS, FOS, DMBA, α-amylase, paraffin, bile salts, pancreatin, pepsin, sodium hydrogen carbonate, D-glucose, organic acids (succinate, lactate, propionate, butyrate and acetate) and sulfuric acid were obtained from Sigma (St. Louis, MO, USA). Man–Rogosa–Sharpe (MRS) medium and L-cysteine-HCl were purchased from Biokar (Allonne, France) and Merck (Darmstadt, Germany), respectively, while trypticase soya broth (TSB) without dextrose and bactopeptone were acquired from BBL (Cockeysville, Maryland, MD, USA) and Amersham (Buckinghamshire, UK), respectively. Salt solution A (100.0 g/L NH_4Cl, 10.0 g/L $MgCl_2 \cdot 6H_2O$, 10.0 g/L $CaCl_2 \cdot 2H_2O$), salt solution B (200.0 g/L $K_2HPO_4 \cdot 3H_2O$) and resazurin solution were ordered from ATCC (Manassas, VA, USA). Sodium di-hydrogen phosphate and potassium di-hydrogen phosphate were purchased from Panreac (Barcelona, Spain). Dinitrosalicylic acid and acarbose were purchased from Acros Organics (Hampton, NH, USA), calcium chloride from ChemLab (Eernegem, Belgium) and orlistat from AlfaAesar (Ward Hill, MA, USA). Finally, the *Bifidobacterium animalis* BB0 were acquired from CSK (Ede, The Netherlands), *Bifidobacterium animalis* spp. *lactis* Bb12 and *Lactobacillus casei* 01 from Chr. Hansen (Hørsholm, Denmark) and *Lactobacillus acidophilus* La-5 from Lallemand (MontReal, QC, Canada).

3.2. Extraction Procedure

The extracts were prepared following the optimal conditions determined through the response surface method as previously described [50]. For this, 30 g of dried algal powder was dispersed in 2100 mL of 70% acetone solution and incubated for 3 h at room temperature under constant agitation. The mixture was filtered through cotton to remove the solid residues and then through a G4 glass filter. Afterward the extract was concentrated in a rotary evaporator to about 250 mL. The concentrated extract was defatted using n-hexane (1:1, v/v) for several times (until a colorless non-polar fraction was obtained), and the aqueous phase was further submitted to liquid–liquid extraction with ethyl acetate (1:1, v/v) for three times to obtain a phlorotannin-purified fraction (EtOAc). Finally, the solvent was removed from the EtOAc fraction by rotary evaporation. Both CRD and EtOAc were then freeze dried and stored at $-20\,°C$ until further use.

3.3. Gastrointestinal Digestion Simulation

The simulation of the gastrointestinal digestion of the *F. vesiculosus* sample extracts was performed according to the method described by Campos et al. [33]. Oral digestion was started by suspending 1 g of dried sample (CRD or EtOAc) in 20 mL of distilled water followed by the adjustment of the pH between 5.6 and 6.9 with $NaHCO_3$ prior to the addition of 0.6 mL/min of α-amylase at 100 U/mL. Enzymatic digestion was carried out during 2 min of mastication, at 37 °C and 200 rpm. Before moving to the next compartment, the pH of mouth digest was adjusted to 2.0 using 1M HCl and then mixed with a simulated gastric juice consisting of pepsin 25 mg/mL added at a ratio of 0.05 mL/mL of mouth digest. Incubation was carried out over 60 min at 37 °C and 130 rpm. Finally, for intestinal digestion the pH of gastric digest was adjusted to 6.0 using 1M $NaHCO_3$ prior to the addition of a simulated intestinal juice consisting of 2 g/L of pancreatin and 12 g/L bile salts at a ratio of 0.25 mL/mL of gastric digest. The samples were then incubated during 120 min, at 37 °C and 45 rpm, to mimic a long intestine digestion process. In the final step of intestinal digestion, samples were submitted to a dialysis process during 48 h at room temperature using a membrane with a molecular pore size of 3 kDa to reproduce the natural absorption step in the small intestine. At the end of this process, the permeate represented the bioaccessible fraction, while the retentate represented the non-absorbable fraction, both of which were then used for the fermentation experiments. An aliquot of 2 mL was collected before the digestion simulation and after each step of digestion, i.e., mouth digest, gastric digest, intestinal digest, permeate and retentate, and stored at −80 °C until further use for phlorotannin quantification and antioxidant experiments.

3.4. Determination of the Phlorotannin Content and Antioxidant Activities

Quantification of the TPhC was carried out according to the 2,4-dimethoxybenzaldehyde (DMBA) colorimetric method [51]. For this, equal volumes of the stock solutions of DMBA (2%, m/v) and HCl (6%, v/v), both prepared in glacial acetic acid, were mixed prior to use (work solution). Afterwards, 250 µL of this solution was added to 50 µL of each extract in a 96-well plate and the reaction was incubated in the dark, at room temperature. After 60 min, the absorbance was read at 515 nm and the phlorotannin content was determined by using a regression equation of the phloroglucinol linear calibration curve (0.06–0.1 mg/mL). The results were expressed as mg phloroglucinol equivalents/g dry seaweed (mg PGE/g DW).

The NO$^\bullet$ scavenging method was adapted from Pereira et al. [52]. For this, 100 µL of six different sample concentrations (0–1 mg/mL) was mixed with 100 µL of sodium nitroprusside (3.33 mM in 100 mM sodium phosphate buffer pH 7.4) and incubated for 15 min under a fluorescent lamp (Tryun 26 W). Next, 100 µL of Griess reagent (0.5% sulfanilamide and 0.05% N-(1-naphthyl)ethylenediamine dihydrochloride in 2.5% H_3PO_4) was added to the mixture, which was incubated for another 10 min at RT in the dark. The absorbance was then measured at 562 nm, and the NO$^\bullet$ scavenging capacity was calculated as the concentration of the sample capable of scavenging 50% of the radical. Ascorbic acid was used as the reference compound.

The $O_2^{\bullet -}$ scavenging method was carried out according to the method described by Pereira et al. [53]. In a 96-well plate, 75 µL of six different sample concentrations (0.0–2.0 mg/mL) was mixed with 100 µL of β-NADH (300 µM), 75 µL of NBT (200 µM) and 50 µL of PMS (15 µM). After 5 min, the absorbances at 560 nm were recorded and the inhibition calculated as the concentration capable of scavenging 50% of $O_2^{\bullet -}$ (IC_{50}). Gallic acid was used as the reference compound.

3.5. Determination of the Phlorotannin Content and Antioxidant Activities

Potential prebiotic effects of *F. vesiculosus* phlorotannin-rich samples were determined for *Bifidobacterium animalis* B0, *Bifidobacterium animalis* spp. *lactis* BB12, *Lactobacillus casei* 01 and *Lactobacillus acidophilus* LA-5. Strains were stored at −80 °C in MRS broth with 30% (v/v) glycerol. *L. casei* 01 and *L. acidophilus* LA-5 inocula were prepared by suspending each bacterial colony into MRS broth, achieving a turbidity equivalent to 0.5 McFarland standard, and then diluting to reach the recommended concentration of probiotic bacteria in the wells, 5×10^5 CFU/mL. Twenty microliters of each inoculum were transferred to a 96-well microplate and every well was fulfilled (to the final volume of 200 µL) with each *F. vesiculosus* sample, diluted in basal MRS broth without glucose at concentrations of 1, 1.5 and 2% (w/v). The microplate was incubated at 37 °C for 48 h with agitation. Similarly, *B. animalis* B0 and *B. lactis* BB12 inocula were prepared under an anaerobic atmosphere, by suspending each bacterial colony into MRS broth supplemented with 0.05% (v/v) L-cysteine-HCl, achieving a final turbidity equivalent to 0.5 McFarland standard, and then diluted to reach the recommended concentration of probiotic bacteria in the wells, 5×10^5 CFU/mL. Twenty microliters of each inoculum were transferred to a 96-well microplate and every well was fulfilled (to the final volume of 200 µL) with each

F. vesiculosus sample, diluted in basal MRS broth without glucose at concentrations of 1, 1.5 and 2% (*w*/*v*). The microplate was sealed with paraffin and incubated at 37 °C for 48 h with agitation. In all plates, OD measurements at 620 nm were registered every hour. Three controls were also performed: the first one containing inoculum and MRS broth with glucose (positive control), the second one containing inoculum and FOS in MRS broth without glucose (FOS control) and the third one containing only inoculum and MRS broth (negative control).

3.6. In Vitro Fermentation Assays

The human feces were collected into sterile plastic vases and kept under anaerobic conditions, until further notice (maximum of 2 h after collection). The samples were obtained fresh, from healthy human donors, with the premises of not having any known metabolic or gastrointestinal disorder. Moreover, the donors confirmed that they were not taking any probiotic or prebiotic supplements, as well as any form of antibiotics for the previous 3 months. The basal medium was prepared as described previously [33], consisting of a nutrient base medium containing 5.0 g/L trypticase soya broth (TSB) without dextrose (BBL, Cockeysville, Maryland, MD, USA), 5.0 g/L bactopeptone (Amersham, Buckinghamshire, UK), 0.5 g/L L-cysteine-HCl (Merck, Germany), 1.0% (*v*/*v*) of salt solution A (100.0 g/L NH_4Cl, 10.0 g/L $MgCl_26H_2O$, 10.0 g/L $CaCl_22H_2O$), 0.2% (*v*/*v*) of salt solution B (200.0 g/L $K_2HPO_43H_2O$) and 0.2% (*v*/*v*) of 0.5 g/L resazurin solution, prepared in distilled water and with pH adjustment at 6.8. The basal medium was dispensed into airtight glass anaerobic bottles, sealed with aluminum caps before sterilization by autoclave. Stock solutions of yeast nitrogen base (YNB) were sterilized with 0.2 μm syringe filters (Chromafils, Macherey-Nagel, Düren, Germany) and inserted into the bottles. The serum bottles were incorporated with CRD and EtOAc extract retentate from the in vitro GIT simulation at a final concentration of 2% (*w*/*v*) and inoculated with fecal slurries of 2% (*v*/*v*) at 37 °C for 48 h without shaking nor pH control. Samples were taken at 0, 12, 24 and 48 h of fermentation. All the experiments were carried out inside an anaerobic cabinet with 5% of H_2, 10% of CO_2 and 85% of N_2 and performed in compliance with the institutional guidelines.

3.7. Gut Microbiota Evaluation

3.7.1. DNA Extraction

Genomic DNA was extracted and purified from stool samples as previously described [33] using NZY Tissue gDNA Isolation Kit (Nzytech, Lisbon, Portugal) with some modifications. Samples were centrifuged at 11,000 *g* during 10 min to separate the supernatant from the pellet. Around 170–200 mg of pellet was taken from the control and test samples for all times. After, the pellets were homogenized in TE buffer (10 mM Tris/HCl; 1 mM EDTA, pH 8.0) and centrifuged again at 4000 *g* for 15 min. The supernatant was discarded, and the pellet was resuspended in 350 μL of buffer NT1. After an incubation step at 95 °C for 10 min, the samples were centrifuged at 11,000 *g* for 1 min. Then, 25 μL of proteinase K was added to 200 μL of supernatant and incubated at 70 °C for 10 min. The remaining steps followed the manufacturer's instructions. The DNA purity and quantification were assessed with a NanoDrop spectrophotometer (ThermoScientific, Wilmington, DE, USA).

3.7.2. Real-Time PCR for Microbial Analysis of Stool

Real-time PCR was performed as described before in [33] in sealed 96-well microplates using a LightCycler FastStart DNA Master SYBR Green kit and a LightCycler instrument (Roche Applied Science, Indianapolis, ID, USA). PCR reaction mixtures (total of 10 μL) contained 5 μL of 2 × Faststart SYBRGreen (Roche Diagnostics Ltd., Burgess Hill, UK), 0.2 μL of each primer (final concentration of 0.2 μM), 3.6 μL of water and 1 μL of DNA (equilibrated to 20 mg). Primer sequences (Sigma-Aldrich, St. Louis, MO, USA) used to target the 16S rRNA gene of the bacteria and the conditions for PCR amplification reactions are reported in Table 4.

Table 4. Primer sequences and real-time PCR conditions used for gut microbiota analysis.

Target Group	Primer Sequence (5′–3′)	Genomic DNA Standard	PCR Product Size (bp)	AT (°C)
Universal	AAA CTC AAA GGA ATT GAC GG ACT TCA CGA GCT GAC	Bacteroides vulgatus ATCC 8482 (DSMZ 1447)	180	45
Firmicutes	ATG TGG TTT AAT TCG AAG CA AGC TGA CGA CAA CCA TGC AC	Lactobacillus gasseri ATCC 33323 (DSMZ 20243)	126	45
Enterococcus spp.	CCC TTA TTG TTA GTT GCC ATC ATT ACT CGT TGT ACT TCC CT TGT	Enterococcus gilvus ATCC BAA-350 (DSMZ 15689)	144	45
Lactobacillus spp.	GAG GCA GCA GTA GGG AAT CTT C GGC CAG TTA CTA CCT CTA TCC TTC TTC	Lactobacillus gasseri ATCC 33323 (DSMZ 20243)	126	55
Bacteroidetes	CAT GTG GTT TAA TTC GAT GAT AGC TGA CGA CAA CCA TGC AG	Bacteroides vulgatus ATCC 8482 (DSMZ 1447)	126	45
Bacteroides spp.	ATA GCC TTT CGA AAG RAA GAT CCA GTA TCA ACT GCA ATT TTA	Bacteroides vulgatus ATCC 8482 (DSMZ 1447)	495	45
Bifidobacterium spp.	CGC GTC TGG TGT GAA AG CCC CAC ATC CAG CAT CCA	Bifidobacterium longum subsp. infantis ATCC 15697 (DSMZ 20088)	244	50

AT—annealing temperature; bp—base pairs; PCR—polymerase chain reaction.

To verify the specificity of the amplicon, a melting curve analysis was performed via monitoring SYBR Green fluorescence in the temperature ramp from 60 to 97 °C. Data were processed and analyzed using the LightCycler software (Roche Applied Science, Penzberg, Germany). Standard curves were constructed using serial tenfold dilutions of bacterial genomic DNA, according to the following webpage http://cels.uri.edu/gsc/cbdna.html (accessed at 31 March 2021). Bacterial genomic DNA used as a standard (Table 4) was obtained from DSMZ (Braunschweig, Germany). Genome size and the copy number of the 16S rRNA gene for each bacterial strain used as a standard was obtained from the NCBI Genome database (http://www.ncbi.nlm.nih.gov, accessed at 31 March 2021). Data are presented as the mean values of duplicate PCR analyses. The F:B ratio was obtained by dividing the number of copies of Firmicutes divisions by the number of copies of Bacteroidetes divisions. Moreover, the relative differences to negative control percentage (only feces fermentation) were calculated using the following equation:

$$Relative\ difference\ to\ control\ \% = \frac{SMC - CMC}{CMC} \times 100$$

where SMC is the mean copy number of the sample at a certain time (12, 24 or 48 h) and CMC is the mean copy number of the control sample at the same time as SMC. Positive % values mean the occurrence of an increase in the number of copies relative to the control sample at that certain time. The higher the value, the higher increase.

3.7.3. Determination of Organic Acids

Supernatants from the batch cultures were filtered through 0.2 μm cellulose acetate membranes. The chromatographic analysis was performed using a Beckman & Coulter 168 series HPLC system with refractive index-RI detector (Knauer, Berlin, Germany). The separation was performed using Aminex HPX-87H column (BioRad, Hercules, CA, USA) operated at 50 °C; mobile phase, 0.003 mol/L H_2SO_4; flow, 0.6 mL/min. Aliquots of the filtered samples were assayed for organic acids (lactic, acetic, succinic, propionic and butyric) using an Agilent 1200 series HPLC system with an RI detector (Agilent, Germany) and a UV detector.

3.8. Statistical Analysis

Data are expressed as mean ± SD of three similar and independent experiments and analyzed using a one-way ANOVA followed by Tukey's post hoc test. The statistical tests were applied using GraphPad Prism, version 7.00 (GraphPad Software, San Diego, CA, USA) and the significance level was $p < 0.05$.

4. Conclusions

Overall, this work provides a great contribution for the understanding of the stability of the phlorotannins of *F. vesiculosus* along the digestive tract, as well as their bioaccessibility and stimulatory effects toward gut microbiota and SCFA production. Similar to plant polyphenols, phlorotannins seem to be susceptible to gut environmental conditions leading to a decrease in their concentration and antioxidant activity along the digestive tract. Moreover, from the portion of phlorotannins that can reach the intestinal lumen intact, only a small fraction of less than 15% will become bioaccessible and available for absorption, which indicates that the majority of these compounds will accumulate in the large intestine where they will be exposed to the metabolic activity of the gut microbiota. Meanwhile, the fermentation of the digested CRD and EtOAc revealed a slight positive effect on the growth of certain commensal bacteria from the human gut, with *Enterococcus* spp. showing the most relevant growth. Moreover, both samples demonstrated an interesting capacity to enhance the production of propionate, while EtOAc caused a notable increase in butyrate levels, both representing important short-chain fatty acids known for their health-promoting status.

In summary, the data gathered herein provide valuable information regarding the behavior of *F. vesiculosus* phlorotannins along their passage through the gastrointestinal tract, and even though the results obtained do not allow to claim *F. vesiculosus* phlorotannin extracts as prebiotics they present clear evidence that these compounds can still positively contribute to the maintenance of a healthy gastrointestinal condition. From here, it would be important to address whether fermentation with human colonic bacteria could affect the antioxidant and other bioactive properties of *F. vesiculosus* CRD and EtOAc. Moreover, it would be particularly relevant to disclose the possible formation of phlorotannin metabolites resultant from the biotransformation and bacterial metabolization in the colon.

Author Contributions: M.D.C. contributed to the conceptualization, investigation, data curation, and writing of the original draft; C.M. and T.B.-L. contributed to the investigation, data curation and writing—reviewing and editing; D.C. contributed to the validation and writing—reviewing and editing; N.M. and A.M.S.S. contributed to the supervision and writing—reviewing and editing; M.M.P. contributed to the conceptualization, supervision, resources and writing—reviewing and editing; S.M.C. contributed to the conceptualization, supervision, writing—reviewing and editing, resources and project administration. All authors have read and agreed to the published version of the manuscript.

Funding: This research was funded by the European Union (FEDER funds through COMPETE POCI-01-0145-FEDER-031015) and national funds (FCT, Fundação para a Ciência e Tecnologia) through project PTDC/BAA-AGR/31015/2017, "Algaphlor—brown algae phlorotannins: from bioavailability to the development of new functional foods".

Institutional Review Board Statement: Ethical review and approval were waived for this study, as it was conducted according to the internal rules legally established, based on the research ethics recommendations and with the informed consent of all subjects involved in the study.

Informed Consent Statement: Informed consent was obtained from all subjects involved in the study.

Data Availability Statement: Data are available from the corresponding author.

Acknowledgments: Thanks to the University of Aveiro (UA) and the Science and Technology Foundation/Ministry of Education and Science (FCT/MEC) for funding the Associated Laboratory for Green Chemistry (LAQV) of the Network of Chemistry and Technology (REQUIMTE) (UIDB/50006/2020), through national funds and, where applicable, co-financed by FEDER, within Portugal 2020. We would like to thank the scientific collaboration under the FCT project UID/Multi/50016/2019. Marcelo D. Catarino's PhD grant (PD/BD/114577/2016) was funded by the FCT.

Conflicts of Interest: The authors declare no conflict of interest. The funders had no role in the design of the study; in the collection, analyses, or interpretation of data; in the writing of the manuscript; or in the decision to publish the results.

References

1. Markowiak, P.; Ślizewska, K. Effects of probiotics, prebiotics, and synbiotics on human health. *Nutrients* **2017**, *9*, 1021. [CrossRef]
2. Wen, L.; Duffy, A. Factors Influencing the Gut Microbiota, Inflammation, and Type 2 Diabetes. *J. Nutr.* **2017**, *147*, 1468S–1475S. [CrossRef]
3. Nishida, A.; Inoue, R.; Inatomi, O.; Bamba, S.; Naito, Y.; Andoh, A. Gut microbiota in the pathogenesis of inflammatory bowel disease. *Clin. J. Gastroenterol.* **2018**, *11*, 1–10. [CrossRef]
4. Demirci, M.; Tokman, H.B.; Uysal, H.K.; Demiryas, S.; Karakullukcu, A.; Saribas, S.; Cokugras, H.; Kocazeybek, B.S. Reduced Akkermansia muciniphila and Faecalibacterium prausnitzii levels in the gut microbiota of children with allergic asthma. *Allergol. Immunopathol.* **2019**, *47*, 365–371. [CrossRef] [PubMed]
5. Hevia, A.; Milani, C.; López, P.; Cuervo, A.; Arboleya, S.; Duranti, S.; Turroni, F.; González, S.; Suárez, A.; Gueimonde, M.; et al. Intestinal dysbiosis associated with systemic lupus erythematosus. *MBio* **2014**, *5*, e01548-14. [CrossRef] [PubMed]
6. Jin, M.; Qian, Z.; Yin, J.; Xu, W.; Zhou, X. The role of intestinal microbiota in cardiovascular disease. *J. Cell. Mol. Med.* **2019**, *23*, 2343–2350. [CrossRef]
7. Li, S.; Hua, D.; Wang, Q.; Yang, L.; Wang, X.; Luo, A.; Yang, C. The Role of Bacteria and Its Derived Metabolites in Chronic Pain and Depression: Recent Findings and Research Progress. *Int. J. Neuropsychopharmacol.* **2020**, *23*, 26–41. [CrossRef]
8. Clapp, M.; Aurora, N.; Herrera, L.; Bhatia, M.; Wilen, E.; Wakefield, S. Gut microbiota's effect on mental health: the gut-brain axis. *Clin. Pract.* **2017**, *7*, 987. [CrossRef]
9. Hirschberg, S.; Gisevius, B.; Duscha, A.; Haghikia, A. Implications of diet and the gut microbiome in neuroinflammatory and neurodegenerative diseases. *Int. J. Mol. Sci.* **2019**, *20*, 3109. [CrossRef] [PubMed]
10. Gibson, G.R.; Roberfroid, M.B. Dietary modulation of the human colonic microbiota: Introducing the concept of prebiotics. *J. Nutr.* **1995**, *125*, 1401–1412. [CrossRef] [PubMed]
11. Gibson, G.R.; Hutkins, R.; Sanders, M.E.; Prescott, S.L.; Reimer, R.A.; Salminen, S.J.; Scott, K.; Stanton, C.; Swanson, K.S.; Cani, P.D.; et al. Expert consensus document: The International Scientific Association for Probiotics and Prebiotics (ISAPP) consensus statement on the definition and scope of prebiotics. *Nat. Rev. Gastroenterol. Hepatol.* **2017**, *14*, 491–502. [CrossRef]
12. Mohanty, D.; Misra, S.; Mohapatra, S.; Sahu, P.S. Prebiotics and synbiotics: Recent concepts in nutrition. *Food Biosci.* **2018**, *26*, 152–160. [CrossRef]
13. Cardona, F.; Andrés-Lacueva, C.; Tulipani, S.; Tinahones, F.J.; Queipo-Ortuño, M.I. Benefits of polyphenols on gut microbiota and implications in human health. *J. Nutr. Biochem.* **2013**, *24*, 1415–1422. [CrossRef]
14. Costantini, L.; Molinari, R.; Farinon, B.; Merendino, N. Impact of omega-3 fatty acids on the gut microbiota. *Int. J. Mol. Sci.* **2017**, *18*, 2645. [CrossRef] [PubMed]
15. Alves-Santos, A.M.; Sugizaki, C.S.A.; Lima, G.C.; Naves, M.M.V. Prebiotic effect of dietary polyphenols: A systematic review. *J. Funct. Foods* **2020**, *74*, 104169. [CrossRef]
16. González-Sarrías, A.; Romo-Vaquero, M.; García-Villalba, R.; Cortés-Martín, A.; Selma, M.V.; Espín, J.C. The Endotoxemia Marker Lipopolysaccharide-Binding Protein is Reduced in Overweight-Obese Subjects Consuming Pomegranate Extract by Modulating the Gut Microbiota: A Randomized Clinical Trial. *Mol. Nutr. Food Res.* **2018**, *62*, 1800160. [CrossRef] [PubMed]
17. Vendrame, S.; Guglielmetti, S.; Riso, P.; Arioli, S.; Klimis-Zacas, D.; Porrini, M. Six-week consumption of a wild blueberry powder drink increases Bifidobacteria in the human gut. *J. Agric. Food Chem.* **2011**, *59*, 12815–12820. [CrossRef]
18. Catarino, D.M.; Silva, M.A.; Cardoso, M.S. Fucaceae: A Source of Bioactive Phlorotannins. *Int. J. Mol. Sci.* **2017**, *18*, 1327. [CrossRef] [PubMed]
19. Charoensiddhi, S.; Conlon, M.A.; Vuaran, M.S.; Franco, C.M.M.; Zhang, W. Polysaccharide and phlorotannin-enriched extracts of the brown seaweed Ecklonia radiata influence human gut microbiota and fermentation in vitro. *J. Appl. Phycol.* **2017**, *29*, 2407–2416. [CrossRef]
20. Yuan, Y.; Zheng, Y.; Zhou, J.; Geng, Y.; Zou, P.; Li, Y.; Zhang, C. Polyphenol-Rich Extracts from Brown Macroalgae Lessonia trabeculata Attenuate Hyperglycemia and Modulate Gut Microbiota in High-Fat Diet and Streptozotocin-Induced Diabetic Rats. *J. Agric. Food Chem.* **2019**, *67*, 12472–12480. [CrossRef]
21. McRae, J.M.; Kennedy, J.A. Wine and grape tannin interactions with salivary proteins and their impact on astringency: A review of current research. *Molecules* **2011**, *16*, 2348–2364. [CrossRef]
22. Quan, W.; Tao, Y.; Lu, M.; Yuan, B.; Chen, J.; Zeng, M.; Qin, F.; Guo, F.; He, Z. Stability of the phenolic compounds and antioxidant capacity of five fruit (apple, orange, grape, pomelo and kiwi) juices during in vitro-simulated gastrointestinal digestion. *Int. J. Food Sci. Technol.* **2018**, *53*, 1131–1139. [CrossRef]
23. Rodríguez-Roque, M.J.; Rojas-Graü, M.A.; Elez-Martínez, P.; Martín-Belloso, O. Changes in vitamin C, phenolic, and carotenoid profiles throughout in vitro gastrointestinal digestion of a blended fruit juice. *J. Agric. Food Chem.* **2013**, *61*, 1859–1867. [CrossRef]
24. Grgić, J.; Šelo, G.; Planinić, M.; Tišma, M.; Bucić-Kojić, A. Role of the encapsulation in bioavailability of phenolic compounds. *Antioxidants* **2020**, *9*, 923. [CrossRef]
25. Dima, C.; Assadpour, E.; Dima, S.; Jafari, S.M. Bioavailability and bioaccessibility of food bioactive compounds; overview and assessment by in vitro methods. *Compr. Rev. Food Sci. Food Saf.* **2020**, *19*, 2862–2884. [CrossRef]
26. Martelli, F.; Favari, C.; Mena, P.; Guazzetti, S.; Ricci, A.; Del Rio, D.; Lazzi, C.; Neviani, E.; Bernini, V. Antimicrobial and fermentation potential of himanthalia elongata in food applications. *Microorganisms* **2020**, *8*, 248. [CrossRef]

27. Lee, S.J.; Lee, D.G.; Park, S.H.; Kim, M.; Kong, C.S.; Kim, Y.Y.; Lee, S.H. Comparison of biological activities in Sargassum siliquanstrum fermented by isolated lactic acid bacteria. *Biotechnol. Bioprocess Eng.* **2015**, *20*, 341–348. [CrossRef]
28. Gupta, S.; Abu-Ghannam, N.; Rajauria, G. Effect of heating and probiotic fermentation on the phytochemical content and antioxidant potential of edible Irish brown seaweeds. *Bot. Mar.* **2012**, *55*, 527–537. [CrossRef]
29. Gupta, S.; Abu-Ghannam, N.; Scannell, A.G.M. Growth and kinetics of Lactobacillus plantarum in the fermentation of edible Irish brown seaweeds. *Food Bioprod. Process.* **2011**, *89*, 346–355. [CrossRef]
30. Corona, G.; Ji, Y.; Anegboonlap, P.; Hotchkiss, S.; Gill, C.; Yaqoob, P.; Spencer, J.P.E.; Rowland, I. Gastrointestinal modifications and bioavailability of brown seaweed phlorotannins and effects on inflammatory markers. *Br. J. Nutr.* **2016**, *15*, 1–14. [CrossRef]
31. Guarner, F.; Malagelada, J.R. Gut flora in health and disease. *Lancet* **2003**, *361*, 512–519. [CrossRef]
32. Madureira, A.R.; Campos, D.; Gullon, B.; Marques, C.; Rodríguez-Alcalá, L.M.; Calhau, C.; Alonso, J.L.; Sarmento, B.; Gomes, A.M.; Pintado, M. Fermentation of bioactive solid lipid nanoparticles by human gut microflora. *Food Funct.* **2016**, *7*, 516–529. [CrossRef] [PubMed]
33. Campos, D.A.; Coscueta, E.R.; Vilas-Boas, A.A.; Silva, S.; Teixeira, J.A.; Pastrana, L.M.; Pintado, M.M. Impact of functional flours from pineapple by-products on human intestinal microbiota. *J. Funct. Foods* **2020**, *67*, 103830. [CrossRef]
34. Qin, J.; Li, R.; Raes, J.; Arumugam, M.; Burgdorf, K.S.; Manichanh, C.; Nielsen, T.; Pons, N.; Levenez, F.; Yamada, T.; et al. A human gut microbial gene catalogue established by metagenomic sequencing. *Nature* **2010**, *464*, 59–65. [CrossRef]
35. Gerritsen, J.; Smidt, H.; Rijkers, G.T.; De Vos, W.M. Intestinal microbiota in human health and disease: The impact of probiotics. *Genes Nutr.* **2011**, *6*, 209–240. [CrossRef] [PubMed]
36. Dubin, K.; Pamer, E.G. Enterococci and Their Interactions with the Intestinal Microbiome. *Bugs Drugs* **2017**, *5*, 1–19. [CrossRef]
37. Allen, S.J.; Martinez, E.G.; Gregorio, G.V.; Dans, L.F. Probiotics for treating acute infectious diarrhoea. *Cochrane Database Syst. Rev.* **2010**, *11*, CD003048. [CrossRef]
38. Wang, C.; Zhao, J.; Zhang, H.; Lee, Y.K.; Zhai, Q.; Chen, W. Roles of intestinal bacteroides in human health and diseases. *Crit. Rev. Food Sci. Nutr.* **2020**, 1–19. [CrossRef]
39. Cockburn, D.W.; Koropatkin, N.M. Polysaccharide Degradation by the Intestinal Microbiota and Its Influence on Human Health and Disease. *J. Mol. Biol.* **2016**, *428*, 3230–3252. [CrossRef]
40. Koliada, A.; Syzenko, G.; Moseiko, V.; Budovska, L.; Puchkov, K.; Perederiy, V.; Gavalko, Y.; Dorofeyev, A.; Romanenko, M.; Tkach, S.; et al. Association between body mass index and Firmicutes/Bacteroidetes ratio in an adult Ukrainian population. *BMC Microbiol.* **2017**, *17*, 4–9. [CrossRef]
41. Larsen, N.; Vogensen, F.K.; Van Den Berg, F.W.J.; Nielsen, D.S.; Andreasen, A.S.; Pedersen, B.K.; Al-Soud, W.A.; Sørensen, S.J.; Hansen, L.H.; Jakobsen, M. Gut microbiota in human adults with type 2 diabetes differs from non-diabetic adults. *PLoS ONE* **2010**, *5*, e9085. [CrossRef]
42. Miquel, S.; Martín, R.; Rossi, O.; Bermúdez-Humarán, L.G.; Chatel, J.M.; Sokol, H.; Thomas, M.; Wells, J.M.; Langella, P. Faecalibacterium prausnitzii and human intestinal health. *Curr. Opin. Microbiol.* **2013**, *16*, 255–261. [CrossRef] [PubMed]
43. Dueñas, M.; Muñoz-González, I.; Cueva, C.; Jiménez-Girón, A.; Sánchez-Patán, F.; Santos-Buelga, C.; Moreno-Arribas, M.V.; Bartolomé, B. A survey of modulation of gut microbiota by dietary polyphenols. *BioMed Res. Int.* **2015**, *2015*, 1–15. [CrossRef] [PubMed]
44. Venegas, D.P.; De La Fuente, M.K.; Landskron, G.; González, M.J.; Quera, R.; Dijkstra, G.; Harmsen, H.J.M.; Faber, K.N.; Hermoso, M.A. Short chain fatty acids (SCFAs)mediated gut epithelial and immune regulation and its relevance for inflammatory bowel diseases. *Front. Immunol.* **2019**, *10*, 1–16. [CrossRef]
45. Chambers, E.S.; Preston, T.; Frost, G.; Morrison, D.J. Role of Gut Microbiota-Generated Short-Chain Fatty Acids in Metabolic and Cardiovascular Health. *Curr. Nutr. Rep.* **2018**, *7*, 198–206. [CrossRef] [PubMed]
46. Fernández-Veledo, S.; Vendrell, J. Gut microbiota-derived succinate: Friend or foe in human metabolic diseases? *Rev. Endocr. Metab. Disord.* **2019**, *20*, 439–447. [CrossRef] [PubMed]
47. Hosseini, E.; Grootaert, C.; Verstraete, W.; Van de Wiele, T. Propionate as a health-promoting microbial metabolite in the human gut. *Nutr. Rev.* **2011**, *69*, 245–258. [CrossRef] [PubMed]
48. Koh, A.; De Vadder, F.; Kovatcheva-Datchary, P.; Bäckhed, F. From dietary fiber to host physiology: Short-chain fatty acids as key bacterial metabolites. *Cell* **2016**, *165*, 1332–1345. [CrossRef]
49. Belenguer, A.; Duncan, S.H.; Holtrop, G.; Anderson, S.E.; Lobley, G.E.; Flint, H.J. Impact of pH on lactate formation and utilization by human fecal microbial communities. *Appl. Environ. Microbiol.* **2007**, *73*, 6526–6533. [CrossRef]
50. Catarino, M.; Silva, A.; Mateus, N.; Cardoso, S. Optimization of Phlorotannins Extraction from Fucus vesiculosus and Evaluation of Their Potential to Prevent Metabolic Disorders. *Mar. Drugs* **2019**, *17*, 162. [CrossRef]
51. Amarante, S.J.; Catarino, M.D.; Marçal, C.; Silva, A.M.S.; Ferreira, R.; Cardoso, S.M. Microwave-Assisted Extraction of Phlorotannins from Fucus vesiculosus. *Mar. Drugs* **2020**, *18*, 559. [CrossRef]
52. Catarino, M.D.; Silva, A.; Cruz, M.T.; Mateus, N.; Silva, A.M.S.; Cardoso, S.M. Phlorotannins from Fucus vesiculosus: Modulation of inflammatory response by blocking NF-κB signaling pathway. *Int. J. Mol. Sci.* **2020**, *21*, 6897. [CrossRef] [PubMed]
53. Pereira, O.; Catarino, M.; Afonso, A.; Silva, A.; Cardoso, S. *Salvia elegans*, *Salvia greggii* and *Salvia officinalis* Decoctions: Antioxidant Activities and Inhibition of Carbohydrate and Lipid Metabolic Enzymes. *Molecules* **2018**, *23*, 3169. [CrossRef] [PubMed]

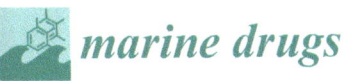

Article

Effect of Phlorofucofuroeckol A and Dieckol Extracted from *Ecklonia cava* on Noise-induced Hearing Loss in a Mouse Model

Hyunjun Woo [1], Min-Kyung Kim [1], Sohyeon Park [1,2], Seung-Hee Han [1], Hyeon-Cheol Shin [3], Byeong-gon Kim [1,4], Seung-Ha Oh [1,4], Myung-Whan Suh [1], Jun-Ho Lee [1,4] and Moo-Kyun Park [1,4,5,*]

1. Department of Otorhinolaryngology-Head and Neck Surgery, Seoul National University College of Medicine, Seoul National University Hospital, Seoul 03080, Korea; junwoo1207@naver.com (H.W.); jkmk928@gmail.com (M.-K.K.); vivihelia@gmail.com (S.P.); hee92h@nate.com (S.-H.H.); byeonggone@naver.com (B.-g.K.); shaoh@snu.ac.kr (S.-H.O.); drmung@naver.com (M.-W.S.); junlee@snu.ac.kr (J.-H.L.)
2. Interdisciplinary Program in Neuroscience, College of Natural Sciences, Seoul National University, Seoul 08826, Korea
3. CEWIT Center for Systems Biology, State University of New York, Incheon 21985, Korea; gerudah@gmail.com
4. Sensory Organ Research Institute, Medical Research Center, Seoul National University, Seoul 03080, Korea
5. Wide River Institute of Immunology, College of Medicine, Seoul National University, Hongcheon 25159, Korea
* Correspondence: aseptic@snu.ac.kr; Tel.: +82-2-2072-2446

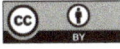

Abstract: One of the well-known causes of hearing loss is noise. Approximately 31.1% of Americans between the ages of 20 and 69 years (61.1 million people) have high-frequency hearing loss associated with noise exposure. In addition, recurrent noise exposure can accelerate age-related hearing loss. Phlorofucofuroeckol A (PFF-A) and dieckol, polyphenols extracted from the brown alga *Ecklonia cava*, are potent antioxidant agents. In this study, we investigated the effect of PFF-A and dieckol on the consequences of noise exposure in mice. In 1,1-diphenyl-2-picrylhydrazyl assay, dieckol and PFF-A both showed significant radical-scavenging activity. The mice were exposed to 115 dB SPL of noise one single time for 2 h. Auditory brainstem response(ABR) threshold shifts 4 h after 4 kHz noise exposure in mice that received dieckol were significantly lower than those in the saline with noise group. The high-PFF-A group showed a lower threshold shift at click and 16 kHz 1 day after noise exposure than the control group. The high-PFF-A group also showed higher hair cell survival than in the control at 3 days after exposure in the apical turn. These results suggest that noise-induced hair cell damage in cochlear and the ABR threshold shift can be alleviated by dieckol and PFF-A in the mouse. Derivatives of these compounds may be applied to individuals who are inevitably exposed to noise, contributing to the prevention of noise-induced hearing loss with a low probability of adverse effects.

Keywords: noise; hearing loss; dieckol; PFF-A; antioxidant

1. Introduction

Hearing loss impairs individuals' communication, comprehension, and quality of life. One of the well-known causes of hearing loss is noise [1]. Noise-induced hearing loss (NIHL) is one of the most common occupational diseases worldwide [2]. Based on the national health and nutrition examination surveys, approximately 12.8% of Americans between the ages of 20 and 69 years have noise-induced hearing threshold shift. [3]. Furthermore, NIHL in teenagers has gathered increasing attention [4]. Considering the substantial medical costs, NIHL is an important social, clinical, and economical issue [5]. Two types of NIHL are known: permanent threshold shift (PTS) and temporary threshold shift (TTS). Because of the reversibility of hearing after TTS, previous studies have considered it less important than PTS. However, a recent study has suggested that TTS can induce synaptopathy, thus accelerating age-related hearing loss [6]. As a result of these considerations, the prevention of TTS has been gaining increased attention [7].

Conventionally, mechanical trauma was thought to be the main cause of NIHL. The total amount of noise is determined by the sound pressure of noise and the duration of exposure over time. Therefore, a low level of noise over a long period of time may have the same damage as a higher level of noise over a short period of time. Recommended precautions for NIHL include avoiding or minimizing exposure to prolonged or loud noise [8]. However, these preventive measures are not applicable to populations that cannot avoid or reduce noise exposure, such as construction workers and soldiers. Recent studies revealed that NIHL is caused by reactive oxygen species (ROS) evoked by excessive noise stimulation. Various studies on the use of antioxidants to prevent NIHL are in progress [8,9]. Although preventive treatments must be applied before the development of NIHL, prescribing preventive medication without any certainty about whether NIHL will develop is risky considering the probable adverse effects of drugs. However, food components can be used with lower risk.

Brown algae are commonly used as dietary supplements and herbal remedies in Asian countries. Among the brown algal species, *Ecklonia cava* produces unique polyphenols named eckols. Although *E. cava* produces various potentially medicinal compounds, such as common sterols (fucosterol, cholesterol, and ergosterols) and phlorotannins (eckol, dieckol, and phlorofucofuroeckol A (PFF-A); Figure 1), eckol and its derivatives are reportedly responsible for the major medicinal properties of this brown alga [10,11]. Recently, various in vitro and in vivo studies indicated that eckols possess a wide spectrum of bioactivities including matrix metalloproteinase inhibitory, protease inhibitory, cytoprotective, anti-inflammatory, and antioxidant effects [12–14]. A previous study has shown a considerable protective effect of a purified polyphenolic extract from *E. cava* against TTS. This extract consists of eckols including dieckol and PFF-A [15]. In this study, we investigated the protective effect of dieckol and PFF-A against TTS in a mouse model of NIHL.

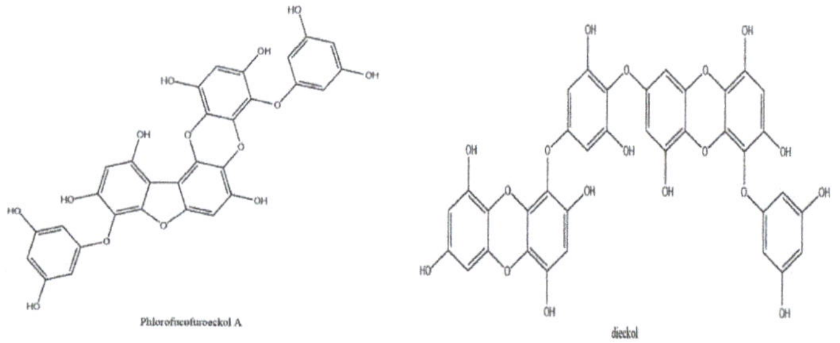

Figure 1. The chemical structures of phlorofucofuroeckol A and dieckol.

2. Results

2.1. Radical Scavenging Activity of Dieckol and PFF-A

The radical-scavenging activity of PFF-A and dieckol increased in a dose-dependent manner (Figure 2). These results suggest that dieckol and PFF-A lowered ROS levels.

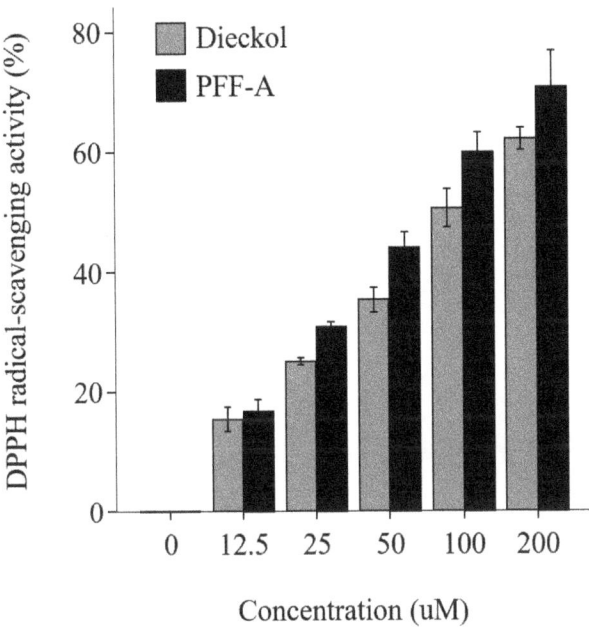

Figure 2. Antioxidant effect of dieckol and phlorofucofuroeckol A (PFF-A), measured as 1,1-diphenyl-2-picrylhydrazyl (DPPH) radical-scavenging activity. Bars represent the mean ± SD.

2.2. ABR Threshold Shifts after Noise Exposure

Saline control showed that ABR thresholds at click and 4 and 16 KHz increased sharply after noise exposure and then gradually decreased at 1 and 3 days. However, the hearing did not return to normal 1 or 3 days after noise exposure. The threshold shift was larger in 16 kHz than click and 4 kHz.

PFF-A (10 mg/kg) showed a lower threshold shift than saline at click 1 day after noise exposure. However, it was not statistically significant. The ABR threshold shifts 1 day after noise exposure were significantly smaller in the high-dose PFF-A (100 mg/kg) with noise group than in the saline with noise group at click stimuli ($p = 0.035$, $t = 2.329$ df = 14). The ABR threshold shifts 1 day after noise exposure were significantly smaller in the high-dose PFF-A (100 mg/kg) with noise group than in the saline with noise group at 16 kHz stimuli ($p = 0.018$, $t = 2.687$ df = 14). Dieckol (10 mg/kg) and high-dieckol (100 mg/kg) groups had lower threshold shifts than the Saline + Noise group at click and 16 kHz, but it was not statistically significant. The ABR threshold shifts in the dieckol with the noise group were significantly smaller than those in the saline with noise group immediately after noise exposure at 4 kHz ($p = 0.042$, $t = 2.250$ df = 13) (Figure 3). ABR amplitudes and latencies after dieckol or PFF-A treatment were not significantly different from those after saline treatment in all waves at 90 dB stimulation (data not shown).

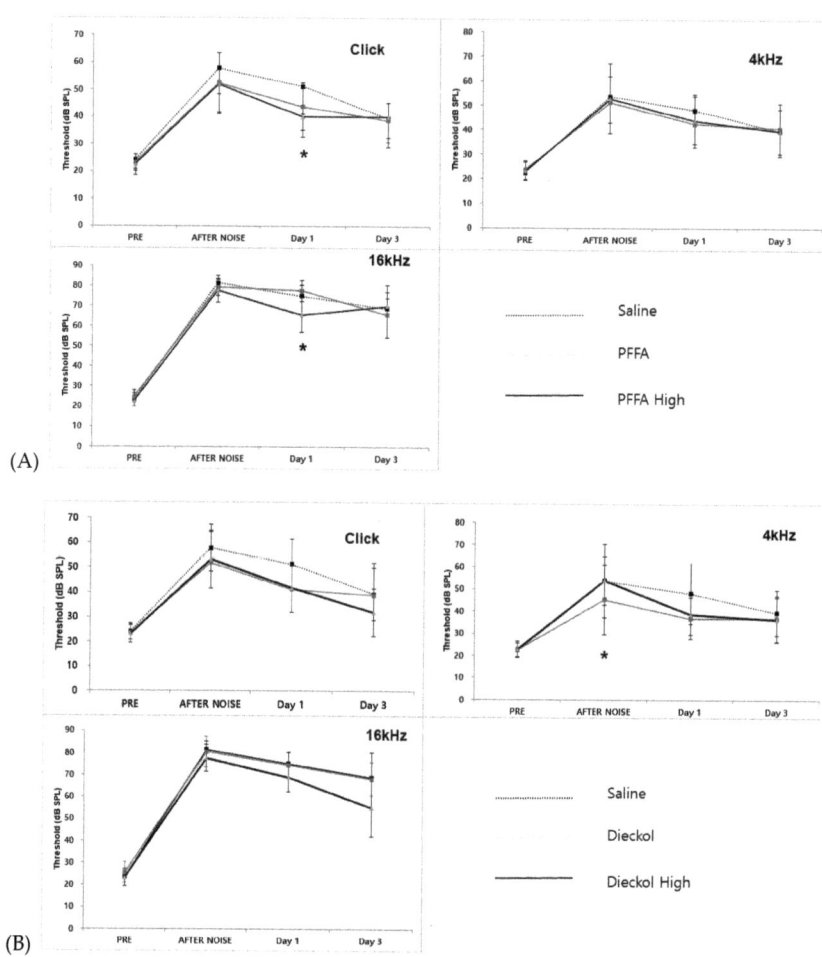

Figure 3. Hearing changes after noise exposure in phlorofucofuroeckol A (PFF-A) and dieckol treatment. Hearing was measured at 4 h and 1 and 3 days after noise exposure at click and 4 and 16 kHz. (**A**) PFFA and High PFF-A treatment; the high-PFF-A group had a significantly lower threshold shift than the Saline + Noise group at click stimuli ($p = 0.015$) and 16 kHz ($p = 0.018$) 1 day after noise exposure. (**B**) Dieckol and High-Dieckol treatment. The Dieckol group showed less threshold shift than the Saline + Noise group at immediately after noise exposure at 4 kHz ($p = 0.042$) (* $p < 0.05$).

2.3. Hair Cell Phalloidin Staining and Counts

Survival at 1 and 3 days after noise exposure was measured. Significant outer hair cell (HC) survival was observed only in the apical turn sections on day 1 of the High-PFF-A group ($p = 0.019$, $t = -2.793$ df = 10). In the basal turn, the High-PFFA group showed better survival than the PFF-A group at 3 days after noise exposure ($p = 0.032$ $t = -2.276$ df = 24) (Figure 4). All three rows of outer HCs from control mice showed no missing hair cells.

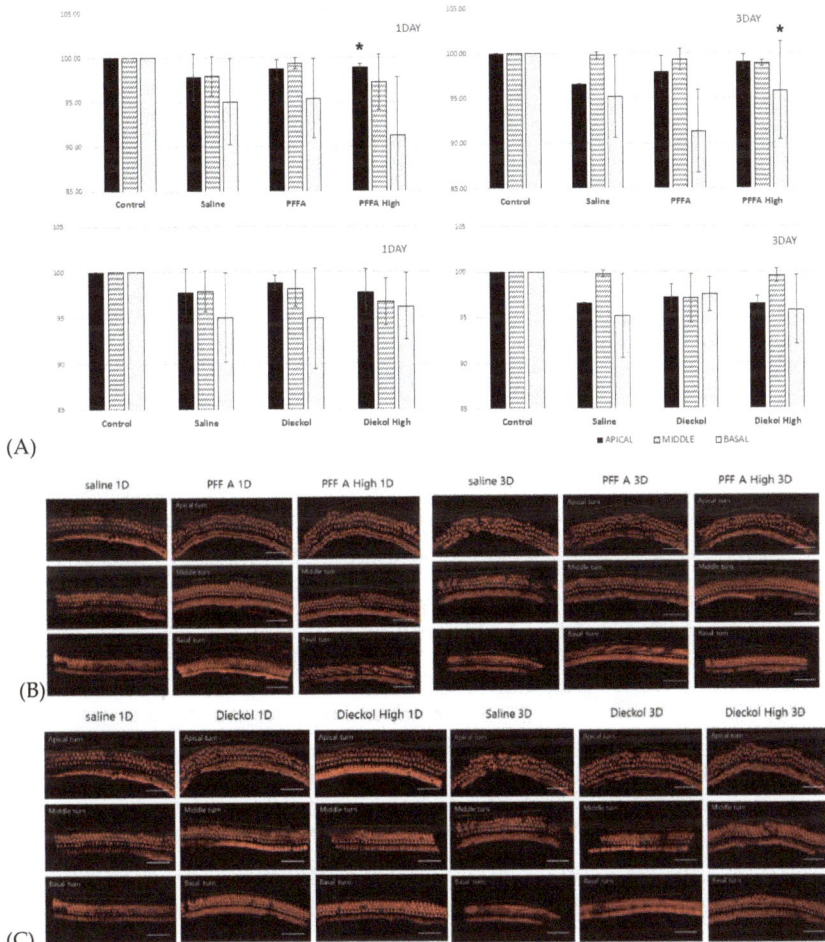

Figure 4. Hair cell (HC) survival and phalloidin staining of outer hair cells. (**A**) Survival rates of outer HCs in each turn section. The surviving HCs per 200 μm along the length of the cochlea in the basal, middle, and apical turn sections were counted. (* $p < 0.05$) (**B**) Fluorescence staining of outer HCs after phlorofucofuroeckol A (PFF A) treatment. (**C**) Fluorescence staining of outer HCs after dieckol treatment. Scale bars are 50 μm. Asterisks indicate the positions of lost HCs. The blue line along the HC line indicates the length of 200 μm.

3. Discussion

This study suggests that PFF-A and dieckol may alleviate the noise-induced temporary threshold shift and HC damage in a mouse model.

The hearing threshold shift was greatest between 1 and 3 days, but OHC loss was observed on days 1 and 3. Therefore, the animal model in this experiment is likely to be a combined threshold shift model rather than a pure TTS model. Broadband (0.2–70 kHz) white noise, which had its peak at 10 kHz, was used to induced hearing loss. Therefore, hearing threshold shifts at 4 and 16 kHz were measured in this study. Click stimulation for hearing threshold shift was used because click stimulation includes the wide frequency on the cochlea. Therefore, the waveform by click stimulation shows the bigger and clearer than other tone burst stimulation. High-frequency stimulation, including 32 kHz, could be more correlated with hair cell loss in basal turn. In a previous study, we used purified polyphenolic extract from *Ecklonia cava* (100 mg/kg) and observed protective effect on noise-induced hearing loss [15]. Purified polyphenolic extract from *Ecklonia cava* includes the 16.85% of dieckol and 3.5% of PFF-A. Therefore, the same (100 mg/kg) and lower dosage (10 mg/kg) of dieckol and PFF-A for this experiment were used.

PFF-A could be a more potent candidate for preventive medication than dieckol because PPF-A shows a stronger radical scavenging activity than dieckol at the same concentration. Dieckol showed a lower threshold shift and hair cell survivable than PFF-A. In addition, high dieckol (100 mg/kg) did not show a greater threshold shift than dieckol (10 mg/kg) at 4 kHz after noise. Paudel et al. reported that PPF-A (phloroglucinol pentamer) could be a more potent antioxidant than dieckol (phloroglucinol hexamer) [16]. The functional effect of PFF-A at tested G-protein coupled receptors is higher than that of dieckol. Dieckol has a higher number of hydroxyl groups, but the structure or orientation of PFF-A could reach the core active site cavity of receptors.

Noise generates ROS in the inner ear, which produce several compounds by peroxidation of polyunsaturated fatty acids [17]. 8-Isoprostaglandin F2a (8-iso-PGF2a), one of these compounds, is a powerful vasoconstrictor that reduces cochlear blood flow and induces cochlear ischemia [18,19]. Subsequently, cochlear ischemia causes excessive release and accumulation of glutamate from the inner hair cells, leading to glutamate excitotoxicity [20,21]. Cochlear ischemia also reduces energy supply to the stria vascularis, leading to decreased endocochlear potential and to HC swelling [22,23]. These processes ultimately lead to dysfunction of HCs and cochlear afferent neurons, resulting in TTS.

Antioxidants protect against NIHL [24,25]. Diverse antioxidants, including N-acetyl-L-cysteine (NAC), acetyl-L-carnitine (ALCAR), 4-hydroxy alpha-phenyl-tert-butylnitrone (4-OHPBN), salicylate, 2,4-disulfonyl a-phenyl tertiary butyl nitrone (HPN-07), HK-2, and others, show protective effect against noise-induced damage in the cochlea [26–30].

PFF-A, a bioactive component of polyphenols extracted from *E. cava*, has been reported to have antioxidant, anti-inflammatory, anti-allergic, and anti-cancer effects [31–35]. PFF-A has an antioxidant effect via scavenging of ROS and eliminating or reducing the ROS production as such. PFF-A also shows an anti-inflammatory effect via inhibition of nitric oxide and prostaglandin E2 (PGE2) synthesis via downregulation of the levels of iNOS and COX-2 proteins [34].

Dieckol, one of the major bioactive components among polyphenols extracted from *E. cava*, has well-documented antioxidant, cytoprotective, and anti-inflammatory effects [36–38]. Dieckol is considered to inhibit ROS activity by removing ROS [31,36,39] and suppressing ROS formation through upregulation of antioxidant enzymes including superoxide dismutase (SOD) and glutathione peroxidase [37], and downregulation of pro-inflammatory enzymes, such as nitric oxide synthase and cyclooxygenase-2 (COX-2) [39].

Considering the pathophysiology of TTS, an effective preventative treatment must be applied before noise exposure. However, potential side effects of drugs make it difficult to administer medication without any certainty on whether the disease will develop. The advantage of using PFF-A and dieckol over the use of medications is that these natural extracts from *E. cava* are as safe as food ingredients. Furthermore, a representative *E. cava* polyphenol extract that contains PFF-A and dieckol was approved by the United States Food and Drug Administration as a new dietary ingredient in 2008 (FDA-1995-S-0039-0176). Therefore, PFF-A and dieckol may be administered for the prevention of TTS to those who are inevitably exposed to noise, with less possibility of adverse effects than in the case of medications.

In this study, mice were administered dieckol and PFF-A via intraperitoneal injection. However, for humans, dieckol and PFF-A would be administered via oral intake. According to our unpublished bioinformatic analysis that was performed during the study, dieckol and PFF-A have low gastrointestinal absorbability and poor water solubility. Although they are potent antioxidant agents and safe materials, additional measures are required before the attempts of oral administration to achieve effective gastrointestinal absorption and significant bioavailability. A report on nanoencapsulation of various polyphenols, including ellagitannins, curcumin, oleuropein, and hydroxytyrosol, has revealed increased gastrointestinal absorption of these polyphenols [40]. In the bioinformatic analysis using SwissADME, both dieckol and PFF-A have high values of WLOGP, which represent lipid solubility, suggesting their high lipid solubility and possible blood–brain barrier (BBB) permeability. However, both compounds also have high values of topological polar surface area. Thus, both dieckol and PFF-A likely show minimal BBB permeability, implying that the effects of both compounds on the inner ear after they enter the systemic circulation may be negligible. To overcome this second obstacle, extra measures to increase BBB permeability are necessary. A study with fluorescein isothiocyanate (FITC)-labeled dieckol and a rhodamine B-labeled dieckol reported effective BBB penetration of these dieckol forms in rats [41]. Further studies are required to establish an effective delivery method of orally applied dieckol and PFF-A into the inner ear.

In vivo study of radical-scavenging activity of PFF-A and dieckol would provide evidence for their antioxidant effects. Further in vivo studies performed in humans would be helpful to demonstrate the protective effect of PFF-A and dieckol against TTS or PTS.

4. Materials and Methods

4.1. Preparation of PFF-A and Dieckol

Purified dieckol and PFF-A were prepared and kindly supplied by BotaMedi, Inc. (Jeju, Korea). Briefly, the whole plant of *E. cava* was collected off the coast of Jeju Island, Korea. Dried *E. cava* powder was extracted with 70% aqueous ethanol and then partitioned between water and ethyl acetate. The ethyl acetate fraction was subjected to octadecylsilyl (ODS) column chromatography followed by gel filtration in a Sephadex LH-20 column equilibrated with methanol. Final purification of individual compounds was accomplished by HPLC (Waters Spherisorb S10 ODS2 column (20 × 250 mm); eluent, 30% methanol; flow rate, 3.5 mL/min) to isolate dieckol (98.5 wt%) and PFF-A (98.0 wt%).

4.2. 1,1-Diphenyl-2-picrylhydrazyl Assay

Dieckol and PFF-A were diluted in distilled water to obtain the experimental concentrations (0, 1, 12.5, 25, 50, 100, and 200 µM). 1,1-Diphenyl-2-picrylhydrazyl (DPPH) powder (Sigma) was dissolved in 95% methanol to create a 1 M stock. PFF-A, dieckol, and 50% methanol were aliquoted into individual wells of a 96-well plate. The DPPH solution was then added to each well. PFF-A and dieckol were allowed to react with DPPH solution in the dark for 30 min at room temperature. Absorbance was measured at 540 nm using a microplate reader. Two wells were used for each concentration, and the experiment was repeated twice.

4.3. Noise Exposure

Six-week-old male C57BL/6 mice weighing 18–20 g were purchased from Koatech Inc. (Pyeongtaek, Korea). The mice were fed a standard commercial diet and housed in a facility with an ambient temperature of 20–22 °C and a relative humidity of 50 ± 5% under 12/12 h day/light cycle conditions. All of the animal experiments described here were approved by the Institutional Animal Care and Use Committee of Seoul National University Hospital (Seoul, Korea; 18-0025-C1A0), which is endorsed by the Association for the Assessment and Accreditation of Laboratory Animal Care International.

A total of 46 mice were randomly assigned to the following groups: Saline (n = 6), Saline + Noise (n = 8), PFF-A (10 mg/kg) + Noise (n = 8), High PFF-A (100 mg/kg) + Noise (n = 8), Dieckol (10 mg/kg) + Noise (n = 8), and High- dieckol (100 mg/kg) + Noise (n = 8) (Figure 5). Mice were administered dieckol and PFF-A via intraperitoneal injection. The mice were treated on 3 consecutive days starting 1 day before the noise exposure. The mice were exposed to 115 dB SPL of noise one single time for 2 h.

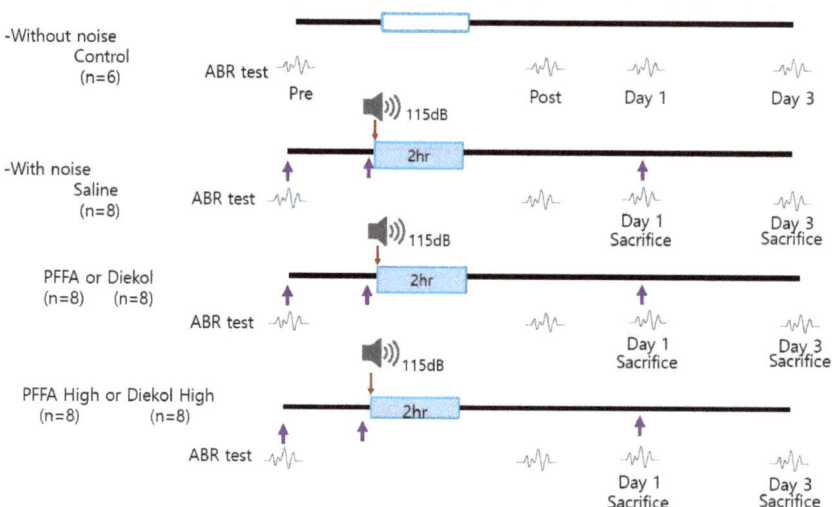

Figure 5. Noise exposure protocol. Empty box indicates control condition without noise exposure. ABR: auditory brainstem response; PPF-A: phlorofucofuroeckol A. Purple arrow: intraperitoneal injection.

Mice were anesthetized via an intramuscular injection before noise exposure using a mixture of 40 mg/kg Zoletil (Zoletil 50; Virbac, Bogotá, Colombia) and 10 mg/kg xylazine (Rumpun; Bayer-Korea, Seoul, Korea). Each mouse was placed in a separate wire cage to avoid uneven noise exposure. Experiment was performed in a specially designed acrylic box in a sound-attenuating laboratory booth with an electromagnetic shield. The mice were exposed to broadband white noise at 115 dB SPL using a 2446-J compression driver (JBL Professional, Los Angeles, CA, USA) with an MA-620 power amplifier (Inkel, Incheon, Korea).

4.4. Auditory Brainstem Response Recordings

Audiometry was conducted 4 h after the termination of noise exposure to perform as stable measurements as possible (Figure 2). Then, mice were divided into 2 equal subgroups (n = 4 each). Hearing was evaluated in one subgroup at 1 day after the noise exposure (Day 1 group) and in the other subgroup at 3 days after the noise exposure (Day 3 group).

The mice were anesthetized and placed in sound-attenuating booths. The sound stimuli applied were tone-bursts of clicks (4 and 16 kHz, duration, 1562 µm; CoS shaping, 21 Hz). High-frequency software (ver. 3.30; Intelligent Hearing Systems, Miami, FL, USA) and high-frequency transducers (HFT9911-20-0035; Intelligent Hearing Systems) were used to measure the auditory brainstem response (ABR). Before obtaining the electroencephalography signal, the impedance between the electrodes was evaluated to determine whether this was less than 2 kΩ. Responses to the signal were amplified approximately 100,000-fold and band-pass filtered (100–1500 Hz). The intensity of the stimuli covered from 20 to 90 dB SPL in 5 dB increments; 512 sweeps in total were averaged at each intensity level. Additional ABRs were measured at 4 h, day 1, and day 3 after noise exposure. The ABR threshold was defined as the lowest stimulus intensity level that produced an evident waveform for wave II or IV. Latency of waves II–IV and amplitude of waves II and IV at 90 dB stimuli were also analyzed and compared between experimental groups.

4.5. Outer Hair Cell Staining

All mice were sacrificed under anesthesia on the day of their hearing evaluation. The cochlea was detached from the temporal bone and fixed in 4% paraformaldehyde solution for 24 h at 4 °C. The thin layer of laminar bone surrounding the cochlea was carefully decorticated using a 2 mm diameter diamond burr drill (Strong 90; Saeshin Precision,

Daegu, Korea) and the thinned laminar bone was then removed using a conventional 1 mm syringe needle. Next, the stria vascularis and Reissner's membrane were removed. Phalloidin was used to stain F-actin, and the photostable orange fluorescent Alexa Fluor 546 dye was used to visualize the cuticular plate and stereocilia within the hair cells (HCs). After surface preparation, the isolated spiral structure of the organ of Corti was incubated in a solution containing 0.3% Triton X-100 and Alexa Fluor 546 phalloidin (1:100 dilution; Invitrogen, Carlsbad, CA, USA) for 60 min at room temperature in a light-proof box [29]. The sample was separated into three segments using Vannas capsulotomy scissors (E-3386; Karl Storz SE & Co. KG, Tuttlingen, Germany). The first complete turn from the top of the organ of Corti was named apical section, the second complete turn was named middle section, and the final half-turn was named basal section. Then, the sections were mounted on a slide using ProLong Gold Antifade mountant (P36930; Invitrogen). Hair cells were measured in five different areas of each section with the images obtained using a STED CW confocal laser scanning system (Leica, Wetzlar, Germany).

4.6. Statistical Analyses

All data were expressed as the mean ± standard error of the mean and analyzed using SPSS software (ver. 25; IBM, Armonk, NY, USA). An F-test was performed to determine whether the levels of variation within the groups were equal. After the F-test, the data were analyzed using Student's t-tests to identify significant differences between groups. A p-value of < 0.05 was considered statistically significant.

5. Conclusions

Our investigation of the effect of PFF-A and dieckol against TTS in mice revealed that these compounds isolated from *E. cava* prevented TTS through their antioxidant activity. Since these compounds are dietary ingredients approved by USFDA, they may be used with less possibility of adverse effects than in the case of medications.

Author Contributions: Conceptualization, M.-K.P.; methodology, M.-K.P.; validation, S.P., S.-H.H., B.-g.K., and M.-K.P.; formal analysis, H.W., S.P., S.-H.H. and M.-K.P.; investigation, S.P., S.-H.H. and B.-g.K.; resources, H.-C.S.; writing—original draft preparation, H.W., M.-K.K.; writing—review and editing, M.-K.P.; visualization, H.W., S.P., S.-H.H. and B.-g.K.; supervision, S.-H.O., M.-W.S., and J.-H.L.; project administration, M.-K.P.; funding acquisition, M.-K.P. All authors have read and agreed to the published version of the manuscript.

Funding: This research was a part of the project titled "Drug development for prevention of noise induced hearing loss using *Ecklonia cava*", funded by the Ministry of Oceans and Fisheries, Korea. (20200364).

Institutional Review Board Statement: The study was approved by the Institutional Animal Care and Use Committee of Seoul National University Hospital (Seoul, Korea; 18-0025-C1A0), which is endorsed by the Association for the Assessment and Accreditation of Laboratory Animal Care International.

Informed Consent Statement: Not applicable.

Data Availability Statement: The datasets generated during and/or analyzed during the current study are available from the corresponding author on reasonable request.

Conflicts of Interest: The authors declare no conflict of interest.

References

1. Concha-Barrientos, M.; Steenland, K.; Pruss-Ustun, A.; Campbell-Lendrum, D.H.; Corvalán, C.F.; Woodward, A.; WHO. Occupational Noise: Assessing the Burden of Disease from Work-related Hearing Impairment at National and Local Levels/Marisol Concha-Barrientos, Diarmid Campbell-Lendrum, Kyle Steenland. 2004. Available online: https://apps.who.int/iris/handle/10665/43001 (accessed on 20 June 2021).
2. Henderson, D.; Bielefeld, E.C.; Harris, K.C.; Hu, B.H. The role of oxidative stress in noise-induced hearing loss. *Ear Hear.* **2006**, *27*, 1–19. [CrossRef] [PubMed]

3. Mahboubi, H.; Zardouz, S.; Oliaei, S.; Pan, D.; Bazargan, M.; Djalilian, H.R. Noise-induced hearing threshold shift among US adults and implications for noise-induced hearing loss: National Health and Nutrition Examination Surveys. *Eur. Arch. Otorhinolaryngol.* **2013**, *270*, 461–467. [CrossRef] [PubMed]
4. Rhee, J.; Lee, D.; Lim, H.J.; Park, M.K.; Suh, M.W.; Lee, J.H.; Hong, Y.C.; Oh, S.H. Hearing loss in Korean adolescents: The prevalence thereof and its association with leisure noise exposure. *PLoS ONE* **2019**, *14*, e0209254. [CrossRef] [PubMed]
5. Nelson, D.I.; Nelson, R.Y.; Concha-Barrientos, M.; Fingerhut, M. The global burden of occupational noise-induced hearing loss. *Am. J. Ind. Med.* **2005**, *48*, 446–458. [CrossRef]
6. Kujawa, S.G.; Liberman, M.C. Acceleration of age-related hearing loss by early noise exposure: Evidence of a misspent youth. *J. Neurosci.* **2006**, *26*, 2115–2123. [CrossRef]
7. Liberman, M.C. Noise-Induced Hearing Loss: Permanent Versus Temporary Threshold Shifts and the Effects of Hair Cell Versus Neuronal Degeneration. *Adv. Exp. Med. Biol.* **2016**, *875*, 1–7. [CrossRef] [PubMed]
8. Le, T.N.; Straatman, L.V.; Lea, J.; Westerberg, B. Current insights in noise-induced hearing loss: A literature review of the underlying mechanism, pathophysiology, asymmetry, and management options. *J. Otolaryngol. Head Neck Surg.* **2017**, *46*, 41. [CrossRef]
9. Doosti, A.; Lotfi, Y.; Moossavi, A.; Bakhshi, E.; Talasaz, A.H.; Hoorzad, A. Comparison of the effects of N-acetyl-cysteine and ginseng in prevention of noise induced hearing loss in male textile workers. *Noise Health* **2014**, *16*, 223–227. [CrossRef] [PubMed]
10. Li, Y.; Qian, Z.J.; Ryu, B.; Lee, S.H.; Kim, M.M.; Kim, S.K. Chemical components and its antioxidant properties in vitro: An edible marine brown alga, Ecklonia cava. *Bioorg. Med. Chem.* **2009**, *17*, 1963–1973. [CrossRef]
11. Li, Y.; Lee, S.H.; Le, Q.T.; Kim, M.M.; Kim, S.K. Anti-allergic effects of phlorotannins on histamine release via binding inhibition between IgE and Fc epsilonRI. *J. Agric. Food Chem.* **2008**, *56*, 12073–12080. [CrossRef]
12. Heo, S.J.; Kim, J.P.; Jung, W.K.; Lee, N.H.; Kang, H.S.; Jun, E.M.; Park, S.H.; Kang, S.M.; Lee, Y.J.; Park, P.J.; et al. Identification of chemical structure and free radical scavenging activity of diphlorethohydroxycarmalol isolated from a brown alga, Ishige okamurae. *J. Microbiol. Biotechnol.* **2008**, *18*, 676–681. [PubMed]
13. Iwai, K. Antidiabetic and antioxidant effects of polyphenols in brown alga Ecklonia stolonifera in genetically diabetic KK-A(y) mice. *Plant Foods Hum. Nutr.* **2008**, *63*, 163–169. [CrossRef] [PubMed]
14. Kang, K.; Park, Y.; Hwang, H.J.; Kim, S.H.; Lee, J.G.; Shin, H.C. Antioxidative properties of brown algae polyphenolics and their perspectives as chemopreventive agents against vascular risk factors. *Arch. Pharm. Res.* **2003**, *26*, 286–293. [CrossRef] [PubMed]
15. Chang, M.Y.; Han, S.Y.; Shin, H.C.; Byun, J.Y.; Rah, Y.C.; Park, M.K. Protective effect of a purified polyphenolic extract from Ecklonia cava against noise-induced hearing loss: Prevention of temporary threshold shift. *Int. J. Pediatric Otorhinolaryngol.* **2016**, *87*, 178–184. [CrossRef]
16. Paudel, P.; Seong, S.H.; Park, S.E.; Ryu, J.H.; Jung, H.A.; Choi, J.S. In Vitro and In Silico Characterization of G-Protein Coupled Receptor (GPCR) Targets of Phlorofucofuroeckol-A and Dieckol. *Marine Drugs* **2021**, *19*, 326. [CrossRef]
17. Morrow, J.D.; Awad, J.A.; Kato, T.; Takahashi, K.; Badr, K.F.; Roberts, L.J., 2nd; Burk, R.F. Formation of novel non-cyclooxygenase-derived prostanoids (F2-isoprostanes) in carbon tetrachloride hepatotoxicity. An animal model of lipid peroxidation. *J. Clin. Investg.* **1992**, *90*, 2502–2507. [CrossRef] [PubMed]
18. Miller, J.M.; Brown, J.N.; Schacht, J. 8-iso-prostaglandin F(2alpha), a product of noise exposure, reduces inner ear blood flow. *Audiol. Neurootol.* **2003**, *8*, 207–221. [CrossRef]
19. Ohinata, Y.; Miller, J.M.; Altschuler, R.A.; Schacht, J. Intense noise induces formation of vasoactive lipid peroxidation products in the cochlea. *Brain Res.* **2000**, *878*, 163–173. [CrossRef]
20. Hakuba, N.; Gyo, K.; Yanagihara, N.; Mitani, A.; Kataoka, K. Efflux of glutamate into the perilymph of the cochlea following transient ischemia in the gerbil. *Neurosci. Lett.* **1997**, *230*, 69–71. [CrossRef]
21. Hakuba, N.; Koga, K.; Shudou, M.; Watanabe, F.; Mitani, A.; Gyo, K. Hearing loss and glutamate efflux in the perilymph following transient hindbrain ischemia in gerbils. *J. Comp. Neurol.* **2000**, *418*, 217–226. [CrossRef]
22. Perlman, H.B.; Kimura, R.; Fernandez, C. Experiments on temporary obstruction of the internal auditory artery. *Laryngoscope* **1959**, *69*, 591–613. [CrossRef]
23. Tabuchi, K.; Tsuji, S.; Fujihira, K.; Oikawa, K.; Hara, A.; Kusakari, J. Outer hair cells functionally and structurally deteriorate during reperfusion. *Hear. Res.* **2002**, *173*, 153–163. [CrossRef]
24. Fetoni, A.R.; De Bartolo, P.; Eramo, S.L.; Rolesi, R.; Paciello, F.; Bergamini, C.; Fato, R.; Paludetti, G.; Petrosini, L.; Troiani, D. Noise-induced hearing loss (NIHL) as a target of oxidative stress-mediated damage: Cochlear and cortical responses after an increase in antioxidant defense. *J. Neurosci.* **2013**, *33*, 4011–4023. [CrossRef]
25. Alvarado, J.C.; Fuentes-Santamaría, V.; Juiz, J.M. Antioxidants and Vasodilators for the Treatment of Noise-Induced Hearing Loss: Are They Really Effective? *Front. Cell Neurosci.* **2020**, *14*, 226. [CrossRef] [PubMed]
26. Choi, C.H.; Du, X.; Floyd, R.A.; Kopke, R.D. Therapeutic effects of orally administrated antioxidant drugs on acute noise-induced hearing loss. *Free Radic. Res.* **2014**, *48*, 264–272. [CrossRef] [PubMed]
27. Chen, G.D.; Daszynski, D.M.; Ding, D.; Jiang, H.; Woolman, T.; Blessing, K.; Kador, P.F.; Salvi, R. Novel oral multifunctional antioxidant prevents noise-induced hearing loss and hair cell loss. *Hear. Res.* **2020**, *388*, 107880. [CrossRef]
28. Kopke, R.D.; Weisskopf, P.A.; Boone, J.L.; Jackson, R.L.; Wester, D.C.; Hoffer, M.E.; Lambert, D.C.; Charon, C.C.; Ding, D.L.; McBride, D. Reduction of noise-induced hearing loss using L-NAC and salicylate in the chinchilla. *Hear. Res.* **2000**, *149*, 138–146. [CrossRef]

9. Ewert, D.L.; Lu, J.; Li, W.; Du, X.; Floyd, R.; Kopke, R. Antioxidant treatment reduces blast-induced cochlear damage and hearing loss. *Hear. Res.* **2012**, *285*, 29–39. [CrossRef] [PubMed]
10. Kopke, R.; Bielefeld, E.; Liu, J.; Zheng, J.; Jackson, R.; Henderson, D.; Coleman, J.K. Prevention of impulse noise-induced hearing loss with antioxidants. *Acta. Otolaryngol.* **2005**, *125*, 235–243. [CrossRef]
11. Chang, M.Y.; Byon, S.H.; Shin, H.C.; Han, S.E.; Kim, J.Y.; Byun, J.Y.; Lee, J.D.; Park, M.K. Protective effects of the seaweed phlorotannin polyphenolic compound dieckol on gentamicin-induced damage in auditory hair cells. *Int. J. Pediatric Otorhinolaryngol.* **2016**, *83*, 31–36. [CrossRef] [PubMed]
12. Kang, H.S.; Chung, H.Y.; Jung, J.H.; Son, B.W.; Choi, J.S. A new phlorotannin from the brown alga Ecklonia stolonifera. *Chem. Pharm. Bull.* **2003**, *51*, 1012–1014. [CrossRef] [PubMed]
13. Kang, H.S.; Chung, H.Y.; Kim, J.Y.; Son, B.W.; Jung, H.A.; Choi, J.S. Inhibitory phlorotannins from the edible brown alga Ecklonia stolonifera on total reactive oxygen species (ROS) generation. *Arch. Pharm. Res.* **2004**, *27*, 194–198. [CrossRef]
14. Kim, A.R.; Shin, T.S.; Lee, M.S.; Park, J.Y.; Park, K.E.; Yoon, N.Y.; Kim, J.S.; Choi, J.S.; Jang, B.C.; Byun, D.S.; et al. Isolation and identification of phlorotannins from Ecklonia stolonifera with antioxidant and anti-inflammatory properties. *J. Agric. Food Chem.* **2009**, *57*, 3483–3489. [CrossRef]
15. Eo, H.J.; Kwon, T.H.; Park, G.H.; Song, H.M.; Lee, S.J.; Park, N.H.; Jeong, J.B. In Vitro Anticancer Activity of Phlorofucofuroeckol A via Upregulation of Activating Transcription Factor 3 against Human Colorectal Cancer Cells. *Mar. Drugs* **2016**, *14*, 69. [CrossRef]
16. Lee, S.H.; Kim, J.Y.; Yoo, S.Y.; Kwon, S.M. Cytoprotective effect of dieckol on human endothelial progenitor cells (hEPCs) from oxidative stress-induced apoptosis. *Free Radic. Res.* **2013**, *47*, 526–534. [CrossRef]
17. Kang, M.C.; Kang, S.M.; Ahn, G.; Kim, K.N.; Kang, N.; Samarakoon, K.W.; Oh, M.C.; Lee, J.S.; Jeon, Y.J. Protective effect of a marine polyphenol, dieckol against carbon tetrachloride-induced acute liver damage in mouse. *Environ. Toxicol. Pharmacol.* **2013**, *35*, 517–523. [CrossRef]
18. Kang, M.C.; Kim, K.N.; Kang, S.M.; Yang, X.; Kim, E.A.; Song, C.B.; Nah, J.W.; Jang, M.K.; Lee, J.S.; Jung, W.K.; et al. Protective effect of dieckol isolated from Ecklonia cava against ethanol caused damage in vitro and in zebrafish model. *Environ. Toxicol. Pharmacol.* **2013**, *36*, 1217–1226. [CrossRef] [PubMed]
19. Lee, S.H.; Han, J.S.; Heo, S.J.; Hwang, J.Y.; Jeon, Y.J. Protective effects of dieckol isolated from Ecklonia cava against high glucose-induced oxidative stress in human umbilical vein endothelial cells. *Toxicol. Vitr.* **2010**, *24*, 375–381. [CrossRef]
20. Yang, B.; Dong, Y.; Wang, F.; Zhang, Y. Nanoformulations to Enhance the Bioavailability and Physiological Functions of Polyphenols. *Molecules* **2020**, *25*, 4613. [CrossRef]
21. Kwak, J.H.; Yang, Z.; Yoon, B.; He, Y.; Uhm, S.; Shin, H.C.; Lee, B.H.; Yoo, Y.C.; Lee, K.B.; Han, S.Y.; et al. Blood-brain barrier-permeable fluorone-labeled dieckols acting as neuronal ER stress signaling inhibitors. *Biomaterials* **2015**, *61*, 52–60. [CrossRef] [PubMed]

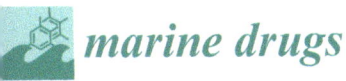

Review

Brown Algae Carbohydrates: Structures, Pharmaceutical Properties, and Research Challenges

Yanping Li [1], Yuting Zheng [1], Ye Zhang [1], Yuanyuan Yang [1], Peiyao Wang [1], Balázs Imre [2], Ann C. Y. Wong [2], Yves S. Y. Hsieh [2,3,*] and Damao Wang [1,*]

1. College of Food Science, Southwest University, Chongqing 400715, China; lyp0702@email.swu.edu.cn (Y.L.); zyt20040817@email.swu.edu.cn (Y.Z.); swuzhangye@email.swu.edu.cn (Y.Z.); yyy798620096@email.swu.edu.cn (Y.Y.); wpy20075@email.swu.edu.cn (P.W.)
2. School of Pharmacy, College of Pharmacy, Taipei Medical University, Taipei 110301, Taiwan; lalazsimre@tmu.edu.tw (B.I.); annwong.sverige@gmail.com (A.C.Y.W.)
3. Division of Glycoscience, Department of Chemistry, School of Engineering Sciences in Chemistry, Biotechnology and Health, Royal Institute of Technology (KTH), AlbaNova University Centre, 11421 Stockholm, Sweden
* Correspondence: yvhsieh@kth.se (Y.S.Y.H.); wangdamao@swu.edu.cn (D.W.)

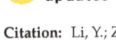

Citation: Li, Y.; Zheng, Y.; Zhang, Y.; Yang, Y.; Wang, P.; Imre, B.; Wong, A.C.Y.; Hsieh, Y.S.Y.; Wang, D. Brown Algae Carbohydrates: Structures, Pharmaceutical Properties, and Research Challenges. *Mar. Drugs* **2021**, *19*, 620. https://doi.org/10.3390/md19110620

Academic Editor: Roland Ulber

Received: 8 October 2021
Accepted: 29 October 2021
Published: 31 October 2021

Publisher's Note: MDPI stays neutral with regard to jurisdictional claims in published maps and institutional affiliations.

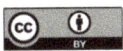

Copyright: © 2021 by the authors. Licensee MDPI, Basel, Switzerland. This article is an open access article distributed under the terms and conditions of the Creative Commons Attribution (CC BY) license (https:// creativecommons.org/licenses/by/ 4.0/).

Abstract: Brown algae (*Phaeophyceae*) have been consumed by humans for hundreds of years. Current studies have shown that brown algae are rich sources of bioactive compounds with excellent nutritional value, and are considered functional foods with health benefits. Polysaccharides are the main constituents of brown algae; their diverse structures allow many unique physical and chemical properties that help to moderate a wide range of biological activities, including immunomodulation, antibacterial, antioxidant, prebiotic, antihypertensive, antidiabetic, antitumor, and anticoagulant activities. In this review, we focus on the major polysaccharide components in brown algae: the alginate, laminarin, and fucoidan. We explore how their structure leads to their health benefits, and their application prospects in functional foods and pharmaceuticals. Finally, we summarize the latest developments in applied research on brown algae polysaccharides.

Keywords: brown algae; alginate; laminarin; fucoidan; bioactivity

1. Introduction

Algae is an important food source consumed by humans since ancient times. Marine macroalgae, in particular, are important food sources in the coastal regions of East Asia such as China, Korea, Japan, and Indonesia [1]. The global commercial seaweed market was calculated at USD 5.9 billion in 2019 and is anticipated to a compound annual growth rate of 9.1% [2]. Health benefits of seaweed food and snack products are gaining spotlight as vegan sources of protein, lipid and carbohydrates, and demand is expected to boost both for consumption and for further applications. For example, microalgae polysaccharide extracts are used as thickening and gelling agents in the cosmetic and food industries, and the demand is growing particularly in North America and Europe [3]. Among their many uses, the portion directly consumed (excluding thickeners and hydrogels used in food and beverage processing) alone have reached 24 million tons per year, accounting for about 40% of the annual seaweed production [4]. Indeed, the concept of seaweed as healthy food is deeply rooted in many people's minds. While new applications of polysaccharides derived from marine algae are constantly being discovered, the raising awareness of this ecofriendly, organic, and environmentally sustainable food source further promotes its consumption. Macroalgae are also used in biorefineries; the carbohydrates are converted to high-value byproducts with metabolic engineering approach [5]. The prospects of algae as green, healthy food, and a bioresource is being actively explored.

Macroalgae are classified into green, red, and brown algae [6]. Brown algae is comprised of 20 classes; the class *Phaeophyceae* alone accounts for over 1800 species and 66%

of the total algae consumption [7]. The most common species are the kelps *Laminaria* (kombu), *Undaria* (wakame), and *Macrocystis* [8]. The polysaccharides alginate, laminarin, and fucoidan (Figure 1) account for more than 50% of the total dry weight of brown algae, and can reach up to 70% in some species. Cellulose is the only crystalline component which has been reported in the walls from brown algae so far and it only occurs at 1–8% of algal dry weight [9].Mannitol exists in 2% of laminarin in M-chains, and can also be found on its own, out of the M-chains, in a range of 5–25% of dry weight [10]. It is a sugar alcohol derived from the six carbon sugar D-mannose [11] and appears to be the primary product of photosynthesis [12]. Mixed-linkage-(1,3)-(1,4)-β-D-glucan (MLG) is common in brown algal cell walls. MLG may perform a distinct role in strengthening the cell wall of brown algae [13].The polysaccharides' proportions and structures vary among species, with some showing markable difference depending on cultivation conditions and harvest seasons [14]. Such heterogeneity may reflect in their diverse biological activities, including anti-inflammatory, antiviral, antioxidant, antitumor, anticoagulant, and hypolipidemic activities, as reported in the literature. This review examines the current knowledge of the biological activity of brown algae polysaccharides and their derivatives as functional foods and bioactive substances. Furthermore, we aim to provide practical strategies and references for developing brown algae-based functional foods and dietary supplements.

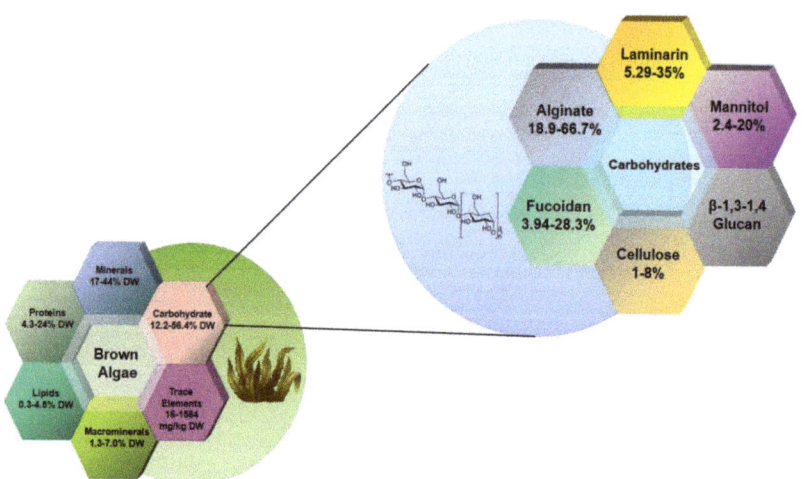

Figure 1. Schematic diagram of the dry matter and carbohydrate composition of brown algae; data summarized from references [9,15–17].

2. Alginate and Alginate Lyase

Alginate is the predominant polysaccharide component found in the cell walls and intercellular matrix of brown macroalgae. It is a linear polysaccharide composed of two conformational isomer residues: β-D-mannuronic acid (M) and α-L-guluronic acid (G) connected through 1,4-glycosidic linkages [18]. Therefore, the polymer may consist of three types of blocks: homopolymeric sections of consecutive Ms, consecutive Gs, or heteropolymeric sections of randomly arranged M and G units (Figure 2). The ratio of M to G is generally 1:1. Nevertheless, the relative proportions of M and G, as well as their arrangement in the polymer chain, vary according to numerous factors such as the algae species, growth conditions, season, and part of the algae [19]. The M/G ratio of alginate from *Ascophyllum nodosum*, for instance, is about 2:1 [20]. Alginates rich in G residues have higher water solubility than those rich in M residues [21] which also exhibit stronger stiffness and gelling properties due to the presence of metal ions such as Ca^{2+} [22].

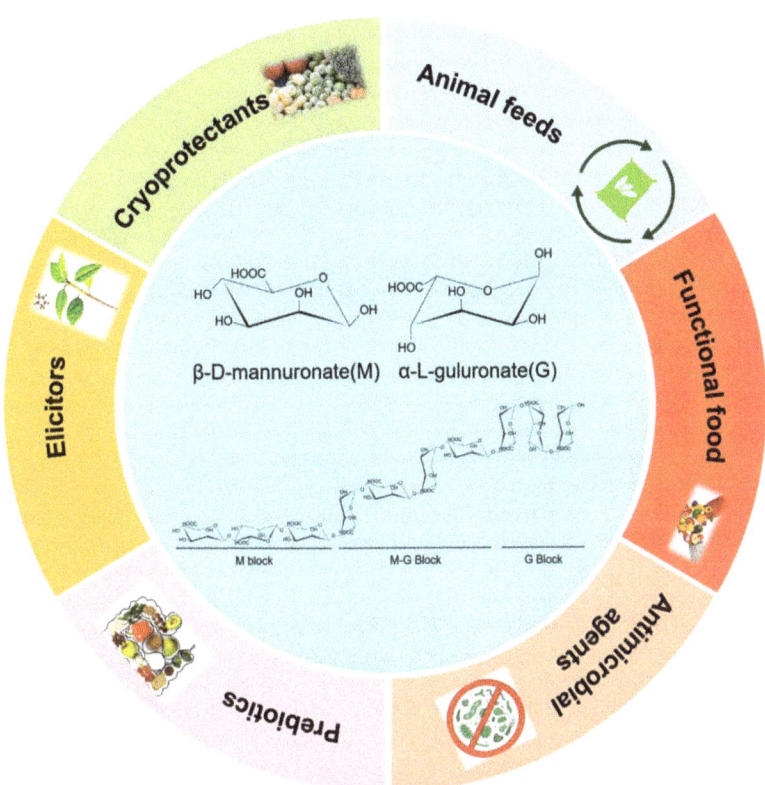

Figure 2. The structure of alginate and the potential applications of alginate oligosaccharides.

Alginate oligosaccharides (AOS) are oligomers with a degree of polymerization of 2 to 25, commonly obtained by chemical degradation (such as acid hydrolysis, alkali hydrolysis), physical degradation (such as microwave degradation), enzymatic degradation (alginate lyase), or chemical synthesis. Compared with physicochemical methods, enzymatic degradation of alginate is eco-friendly, energy-saving, selective, and the products are biologically more active [23]. Alginate lyase degrade alginate through β-elimination and produce unsaturated oligosaccharides with double bonds at the non-reducing end [24]. Endolytic alginate lyase have been widely used to produce AOSs with various DPs. For instance, Li et al. found a high activity endo-type alginate lyase from *Pseudomonas* sp. HZJ216 and efficiently produced AOSs with DP of 2–7 [25]. Kim et al. reported an endo-type alginate lyase Alg7D from a marine bacterium *Saccharophagus degradans* 2-40^T, which produces AOSs DP3–5 [26]. Endo-type alginate lyase Algb from *Vibrio* sp. W13 mainly released oligosaccharides DP of 2–5 [27]. Zhu et al. prepared series of AOSs with DP of 2-5 by using a new alginate lyase Cel32 from *Cellulophaga* sp. NJ-1 [28]. Alginate lyase have the advantage of controlling the predominant DP of AOS products between two and nine without significant amounts of monomers or larger oligomers (DP > 10).

AOSs have been reported to modulate a variety of biological activities and are beneficial to health. Studies have shown that AOSs with different degrees of polymerization have differential biological activity. Therefore, they can be used as antimicrobial, antioxidant, prebiotic, antihypertensive, antidiabetic, antitumor, and anticoagulant agents; their many applications are further discussed below. [29–35].

2.1. Antioxidant Activity

AOSs can scavenge free radicals. The AOS produced by the alginate lyase from *Microbulbifer* (DP: 2–5) was capable to scavenge free radicals (DPPH (2,2-Diphenyl-1-picrylhydrazyl), ABTS+ (2,2′-Azinobis-(3-ethylbenzthiazoline-6-sulphonate), and hydroxyl) and was non-toxic even at high concentrations [36]. Mia et al. found that the AOS prepared by enzymatic method has good antioxidant properties and can completely inhibit the formation of thiobarbituric acid-reactive substances (TBARS) during the iron-induced oxidation of emulsified linoleic acid. In comparison, traditional antioxidant ascorbic acid has only 89% inhibition. For the free radicals ABTS•, •OH, and O•$_{2-}$, polymeric alginate scavenged up to 23, 46, and <1%, while monomeric alginate (represented by glucuronic acid) scavenged up to <1, 25, and 99%, respectively [37]. Due to the conjugated alkenoic acid structure formed during enzymatic depolymerization, AOSs have a higher scavenging ability than similar carbohydrates [37]. The possible mechanism for free radicals scavenging may be a combination of hydrogen abstraction (presumably of hydrogen-bonded hydrogens) and free radical addition to the conjugated olefin acid, resulting in an adduct that is stable through resonance [38].

Compared to chitosan and fucoidan-derived oligosaccharides, AOSs showed higher free radical scavenging capacity [39]. Studies have shown AOSs to play a role in preventing lipid oxidation in skincare emulsions and to scavenge hydroxyl radicals and superoxide anion radicals [40]. In the neuronal PC12 cell model, it was found that AOS pretreatment can block caspase-dependent production of endoplasmic reticulum and mitochondria induced by H_2O_2 stress [41]. In mice injured by doxorubicin, AOS pretreatment increases the survival rate through reducing the oxidative stress and inhibiting the expression of gp91phox and 4-hydroxynonenal in the heart [42]. Furthermore, AOSs are also introduced as a new additive in livestock and poultry feed formulation which can effectively improve cellular antioxidative capacity [43]. The free radical scavenging activity of AOSs is tentatively dose-dependent, and that their molecular weight and M/G ratio modulate antioxidative activities. Studies have shown antioxidative activity is negatively correlated with the molecular weight of the oligosaccharide [44,45].

2.2. Antimicrobial Activity

Hu et al. found that oligo-G and oligo-M (DP: 1–5) obtained by enzymatic hydrolysis had in vitro antibacterial activity against 19 bacterial strains. The antibacterial spectrum of the M oligomer fractions was wider than that of the G oligomers. Within the former, mannuronic acid oligomers with a molecular weight of 4.2 kDa had the highest antibacterial activity and a strong inhibitory effect on *Escherichia coli*, *Salmonella paratyphi*, *Staphylococcus aureus*, and *Bacillus subtilis* [46].

The drug candidate OligoG CF-5/20 is developed by the Norway-based biotech company AlgiPharma. It is a G-enriched alginate oligosaccharide composed of G (85%) and M (15%) blocks. The OligoG CF-5/20 is effective in disrupting and destroying biofilms in a dose-dependent manner. The number of colony-forming units (CFU) in the lungs of infected mice was reduced by 2.5 log; furthermore, 5% OligoG CF-5/20 significantly reduced the minimum biofilm eradication concentration (MBEC) of colistin from 512 to 4 µg/mL after 8 h [47]. OligoG CF-5/20 treatment also reduced *Candida albicans* mycelial infiltration in an in vitro epithelial cell model. OligoG CF-5/20 reduced the expression of *C. albicans* virulence proteins (phospholipase B (PLB2), SAP4 and SAP6) [35], but the mechanism is unclear. Powell et al. also reported AOS exposure to cause changes in biofilm structure, lowering Young's modulus compared to untreated biofilm. In the untreated control, surface irregularity was higher and resistance to hydrodynamic shear was lower [48]. The results suggested that the observed effect might be caused by OligoG induced changes in the structural characteristics of the extracellular polymers in the bacterial biofilm [48]. Similar effects were found with mucociliary clearance, where lower molecular weight negatively charged G oligomers was found to disrupt the intermolecular interactions of mucus, weakened the viscoelastic properties of mucus, and led to rheological deformation [49].

OligoG CF-5/20 has been proposed as inhalation therapy for the treatment of chronic bacterial respiratory diseases [50]. The oligosaccharides can bind to respiratory mucin, altering its surface charge and the porosity of the three-dimensional mucin network in cystic fibrosis sputum. It has been found that AOSs can act synergistically with the antibiotic azithromycin on wild-type antibiotic-resistant *Pseudomonas aeruginosa*. Azithromycin combined with 2 mg/mL enzymatically produced AOS inhibited the growth of *Pseudomonas aeruginosa*, virulence factors, and biofilm formation controlled by quorum sensing [51]. Pritchard et al. found OligoG CF-5/20 (2%) treatment to induce the destruction of *Pseudomonas aeruginosa* biofilm and colistin to maintain its antibacterial activity. OligoG CF-5/20 did not change the orientation of the alginate carboxyl groups, while mass spectrometry analysis showed the oligomers to reduce pseudomonal quorum-sensing signaling [52]. The gelation of alginate in the presence of divalent cations, such as Ca^{2+}, in homopolyguluronic acid, is known to induce changes in coordination of the carboxylate groups [53], which resulting in formation of robust biofilms [54]. However, CD spectra indicated that the orientation of the carboxy groups monitored at ~210 nm were not changed upon mixing OligoG CF-5/20 with high-Mw alginate. This shows that OligoG CF-5/20 combines with Ca^{2+}, avoiding the formation of a strong biofilm, so that the colistin can better play an antibacterial effect [52]. Tøndervik et al. found that OligoG (>0.5%) also showed a significant inhibitory effect on mycelial growth in embryonic tube analysis. OligoG (≥2%) alone or in combination with fluconazole significantly hindered fungal biofilm formation. Through the combined treatment, the surface roughness of the cells also increased significantly ($p < 0.001$) [55].

2.3. Immunomodulatory and Antitumor Activity

AOSs can enhance immune activity and regulate the function of the immune system in a variety of ways, including regulating the secretion of cytokines and immune-complement molecules. The AOSs produced by depolymerization with alginate lyase increased TNF-α-inducing activity compared to untreated alginate, including the expressions of cytokine-induced TNF-α, granulocyte colony-stimulating factor (CSF), single nuclear cell chemotactic protein-1 (regulated after activating normal T cell expression and secretion), granulocyte macrophages (GM)-CSF, and eosinophil chemokine [56]. AOSs can readily activate macrophages and stimulate TLR4/Akt/NF-κB, TLR4/Akt/mTOR, and MAPK signaling pathways to exert their immune activity [31]. According to the Bio-Plex analysis in RAW264.7 cells, M-rich AOSs tend to have higher immune activity than G-rich oligomers [57]. Uno et al. found that AOSs introduced orally can inhibit the production of IgE and prevent allergic reactions in mice [58]. When administered intraperitoneally, AOSs stimulated the production of 20 cytokines such as granulocyte CSF, monocyte chemoattractant protein-1, IL-6, keratinocyte chemotactic factor, IL-12, and RANTES [59]. AOSs can also induce the production of nitric oxide (NO) by increasing the expression of NO synthase in cells. NO is a multifunctional molecule that can act as a vasodilator, neurotransmitter, inflammatory mediator, and specific immunomodulator [60]. The immunomodulatory activity of AOSs is affected by many factors, e.g., degree of polymerization, purity, M/G ratio, and MG sequence. The unsaturated end-structure achieved by the enzymatic degradation of alginate plays a key role in determining the immunomodulatory activity, as saturated AOSs prepared by acid hydrolysis showed much lower activity. Xu et al. showed that the unsaturated end-structure, molecular size, and M/G ratio of enzymatically produced AOSs affect the activation of macrophages through the NF-κB and MAPK signaling pathways [61–63].

Recent studies have also shown AOSs to have antitumor effects. They exert, for instance, an inhibitory effect on the proliferation of human leukemia U-937 cells and produced cytotoxins in human monocytes [56]. AOSs themselves, however, have no direct cytotoxicity to tsFT210 cells. Sulfated AOS derivative with a molecular weight of 3798 Da (sulfation degree of 1.3) has been reported to suppress the growth of solid sarcoma 180 tumor [64]; adding 100 mg/kg AOS, the inhibition rate of solid sarcoma 180 tumor reached 70.4%. It is likely that the AOS and other sulfated derivatives may trigger antitumor effects through organ-mediated immune defense response, especially the immune defense response of the spleen. The AOS of DP 2–10 showed a significant inhibitory effect on the growth of prostate cancer cells. Studies on molecular mechanisms have shown AOSs to attenuate derivatization (α-2,6-sialylation) and reduce ST6Gal-1 promoter activity through the Hippo/YAP/c-Jun signaling pathway [65]. At present, the molecular mechanisms of the contribution of various chemical structural modifications to the antitumor activity of AOSs have not been clarified. Further studies are also needed on the structure-function relationships of antitumor AOSs in targeted cancer therapy.

3. Laminarin

Laminarin is another major storage carbohydrate of brown macroalgae. It is commonly found in the fronds of *Laminaria* and *Saccharina* macroalgae, although it is also found in *Ascophyllum*, *Fucus* and *Undaria* [7]. Laminarin is a β-glucan, mainly composed of β-1,3-D-glucopyranose residues; the majority of glucose is 6-O-branched, while a part of it has β-1,6-intrachain links [66]. Laminarin linked to D-mannitol at the reducing end of the chain is called an M chain, while laminarin without mannitol at the reducing end is a G chain [67] (Figure 3). The ratio of β-1,3- and β-1,6-glycosidic bonds in the polysaccharide depends on the type of algae. For example, laminarin from *Eisenia bicyclis* has a ratio of 2:1 of (1–3) and (1–6) linkage [68]. Laminariales are known to produce high amounts of laminarins, with contents reaching up to 35% of total dry weight, particularly in *L. saccharina* and *L. digitata* [14]. Other reported values of laminarin contents include those of *A. esculenta*, *U. pinnatifida*, *A. nodosum* and *F. serratus* (11.1, 3, 4.5, and up to 19% of total dry weight, respectively) [69–71]. The molecular weight of laminarin is about 5 kDa, with a degree of polymerization between 20 and 25 [72,73]. Laminarinases are the enzymes that degrade β-1,3 and β-1,6 glycosidic bonds of laminarin and produce oligosaccharides and glucose, which were classified into endolytic (EC3.2.1.39) and exolytic (EC3.2.1.58) enzymes [74]. The endo-β-1,3-glucanases hydrolyze β-1,3 bonds between adjacent glucose subunits to release oligosaccharides while exo-β-1,3-glucosidase can hydrolyze laminarin by sequentially cleaving glucose residues from the non-reducing end and releasing glucose [75]. For debranching of laminarin, β-1,6-glucanases randomly hydrolyze β-1,6 glycosidic bonds and release gentio-oligosaccharides or glucose [76]. Endo laminarinases were widely applied to produce oligosaccharides. Recently, Kumar et al. reported a thermostable laminarinase belongs to GH81 from *C. thermocellum* which can hydrolyze laminarin into a series of oligosaccharides (DP2 to DP7) [77]. Badur et al. reported four laminarinases from *Vibrio breoganii* 1C10, of which *Vb*GH16C can hydrolyze laminarin to oligosaccharides of DP8 and DP9, and *Vb*GH17A can hydrolyze laminarin into a series of laminarin oligosaccharides (DP4 to DP9) [78]. Wang et al. characterized a bifunctional enzyme from GH5 subfamily 47 (GH5_47) in *Saccharophagus degradans* 2-40^T and identified as a novel β-1,3-endoglucanase (EC 3.2.1.39) and bacterial β-1,6-glucanase (EC 3.2.1.75). This bifunctional laminarinase can degrade both the backbone and branch chain of laminarin, and is also active on hydrolyzing pustulan which is a linear β-1,6-glucan. This enzyme also showed transglycosylase activity toward β-1,3-oligosaccharides when laminarioligosaccharides were used as the substrates [79]. The above findings provide more possibilities for the green preparation of biologically active oligosaccharides.

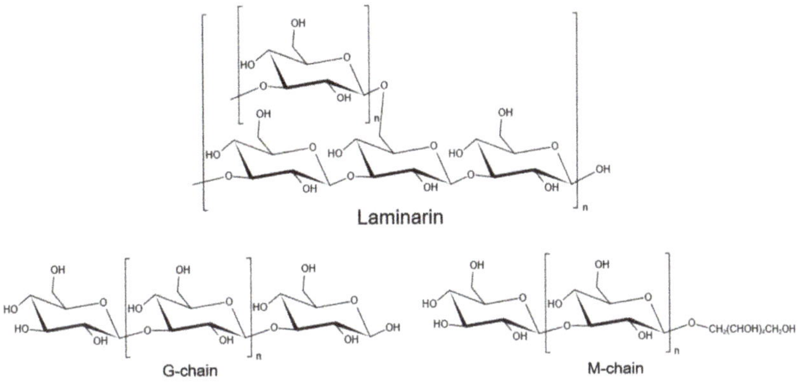

Figure 3. Structures of laminarin.

Laminarins and laminarin oligosaccharides are recognized for their various biological activities; they have shown to stimulate innate immunity [80], stimulate antitumor responses [81,82], increase resistance to infections [83], promote wound repair [84], and enhance the immune response of macrophages [85]. Laminarins can be used to activate macrophages, leading to immune stimulation, antitumor, and wound-healing activities [86]. Furthermore, they can be partially or fully fermented by endogenous gut microbiota [87]. Consequently, they have good prospects for application in the field of functional foods and biomedicine.

3.1. Antioxidant and Antimicrobial Activities

Studies have shown of the crude extracts of laminarin from *L. hyperborea* and *A. nodosum* to remove DPPH free radicals effectively, with clearance rates of 87.6 and 93.2%, respectively. Compared to extracts obtained with water solvents, acid-extracted laminarin was showed to have higher antioxidant activity [88].

Laminarin-rich seaweed extracts are found to have inhibitory effects against both Gram-positive (such as *Staphylococcus aureus* and *Listeria monocytogenes*) and Gram-negative (*E. coli* and *Salmonella typhimurium*) bacterial strains. Notably, the inhibitory rate of *A. nodosum* extract against *Salmonella typhimurium* can reach 100%. Laminarin-rich extracts obtained using ultrasound and acid solvents had minimum inhibitory concentrations (MIC) of 13.1 mg/mL for *E. coli* and *S. typhimurium* and 6.6 and 3.3 mg/mL for *S. aureus* and *L. monocytogenes*, respectively [88]. Therefore, the polysaccharide can be applied in the preparation of antibacterial products such as edible packaging materials and even wound dressings.

3.2. Antitumor and Anticoagulant Activity

Several studies have demonstrated the significant antitumor and anticancer activities of laminarin and laminarin oligosaccharides [89]. The underlying mechanisms include apoptosis and the inhibition of cancer cell colony formation [90]. Different concentrations of laminarin have been used to treat human colon cancer LoVo cells and the intracellular reactive oxygen species (ROS), pH, intracellular calcium ion concentration, mitochondrial permeability transition pore, mitochondrial membrane potential, and Cyt-C, Caspase-9 and Caspase-3 expression levels were analyzed. The studies have found kelp polysaccharides to induce the apoptosis of human colon cancer LoVo cells through the mitochondrial pathway [91,92]. The polysaccharide did not show direct cytotoxicity, but exhibited significant antitumor activity on SK-MEL-28 human melanoma cells and it could effectively inhibit the colony formation of HT-29 cells [93,94].

Laminarin oligosaccharides can inhibit the proliferation of human tissue lymphoma cell line (U937 cells) by stimulating monocytes to produce cytokines [95]. Specific enzyme products with high content of 1,6-linked glucopyranose residues (laminarin oligosaccharides with DP 9–23) have shown significant anticancer activity and can inhibit the colony formation of melanoma and colon cancer cells [96,97]. Sulfated laminarins (LAMS) with a sulfate content of 45.92% proved to inhibit the growth of LoVo cells more significantly than laminarin, suggesting the better antitumor activity of LAMS. Accordingly, enzymatic hydrolysis and molecular modification provide new ideas for the production of laminarin derivatives with high antitumor activity [98].

The anticoagulant activity of *Laminaria* sp. extract was first reported in 1941 [99]. Although laminarin is a non-sulfated polysaccharide in seaweed, its sulfated products showed anticoagulant activity [100]. Many studies have been published on the extraction and modification of laminarin sulfate from algae in the genus *Laminaria*. If each glucose residue has an average of two sulfate groups, the anticoagulant activity of the preparation reaches 25–30% of that of standard heparin [101], while the activity of sulfonic acid derivatives appears to be higher than that of sulfate esters [102]. A derivative of laminarin with 1.83 sulfate groups per glucose unit showed 33% of the potency of heparin in rabbits, although it was extremely toxic to guinea pigs [103]. This suggests that laminarin sulphate might be effective in the prevention and treatment of cerebrovascular diseases.

3.3. Anti-Inflammatory and Immunostimulatory Activity

Studies have shown that β-glucans cause reduced recruitment of inflammatory cells and decreased secretion of inflammatory mediators in liver tissues through direct effects on immune cells or indirect effects as dietary fibers [104]. Laminarin significantly increases the release of inflammatory mediators, such as hydrogen peroxide, calcium, nitric oxide, monocyte chemoattractant protein-1, vascular endothelial growth factor, leukemia-inhibitory factor, and granulocyte colony-stimulating factor, and enhances the expression of signal transducer and transcriptional activators [86]. Recent studies have found laminarin to induce positive effect of decreasing mitochondrial activities without cytotoxicity caused by oxidative stress by regulating the interaction between glycans and receptors on the skin cell surface [105].

3.4. Prebiotic Activity

The prebiotic properties of algae polysaccharides enable them to play an important role in regulating human intestinal health [106]. For laminarin, it has been confirmed in vitro that it cannot be hydrolyzed by hydrochloric acid under physiological conditions, nor by homogenates of the human digestive system [14,107]. Since laminarin is resistant to hydrolytic enzymes in the human upper digestive tract, it can reach the intestinal flora [108]. Animal experiments have shown that adding laminarin to the diet of mice can significantly reduce the Firmicutes to Bacteroidetes ratio in the intestines, indicating that it can enhance the high-energy metabolism of the intestinal microbiota to reduce the side-effects of high-fat diets [109]. In addition, laminarin oligosaccharides are beneficial for the growth of *Bifidobacterium animalis* and *Lactobacillus casei*, also increasing the production of short-chain fatty acids, such as lactic acid and acetic acid [110].

4. Fucoidan

Fucoidan is a sulfated polysaccharide that consists mainly of fucose repeating units besides several other monosaccharide residues. It is commonly found in brown seaweed [111,112], and has also been reported in echinoderms and some lower plants [113]. Fucoidan typically acts as a structural polysaccharide in the cell walls of brown macroalgae, with its relative amount ranging between 4 and 8% of the total dry weight [114]. Since fucoidan was first isolated in 1913, the structure of fucoidans from different brown seaweeds has been studied. Seaweed fucoidan is a heterogeneous material, with varying composition of carbohydrate units and non-carbohydrate substituents [115]. Fucoidan is mainly composed of fucose and sulfate groups (Figure 4). For example, the fucoidan from bladder wrack (*Fucus vesiculosus*) has a simple composition and contains only fucose and sulfate groups (44.1% fucose, 26.3% sulfate) [116]. In addition, it might also contain other monosaccharides (mannose, galactose, glucose, xylose, etc.), uronic acid, and even acetyl groups and proteins. For example, the fucoidan from *Fucus vesiculosus* contains 84% fucose, 6% xylose, 7.3% galactose, and 2% mannose [117]. The fucoidan found in *Fucus distichus* is composed of 51.6% fucose, 2.7% xylose, 1.5% galactose, 0.7% mannose, and 0.2% glucose [118]. Comprehensive analysis concluded that the fucose content of fucoidans is in the range of 4.45–84%, besides 1.44–49% galactose, 0.2–45% glucose, and 0.3% to 16% xylose and mannose. As a heterogeneous polymer, fucoidan exhibits considerable structural diversity that makes it difficult to draw general conclusions. Moreover, its structure cannot be described solely based on monosaccharide composition.

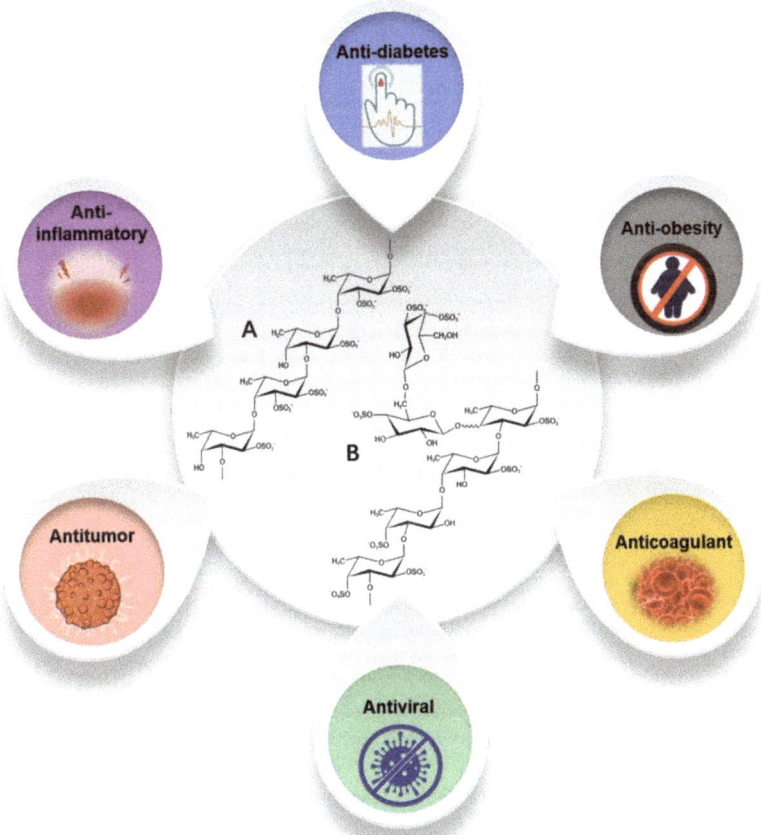

Figure 4. Structure and biological effects of fucoidan (A: *Ascophyllum nodosum* and *Fucus vesiculosus*; B: *Saccharina japonica*, adapted from literature [119–121]).

The structural variety of fucoidans is to a large extent related to the different types of brown algae they are found in. Generally, α (1→3) and/or (1→4) glycosidic bonds constitute the main chain of the macromolecules, dominating in most backbone structures. The presence of sulfate groups at the C-2, C-4 and or C-3 position is another important feature [94,122–127]. Due to the structural heterogeneity of fucoidans, the degradation of fucoidan requires a large set of enzymes of different activities and specificities [128]. Fucoidanase are mainly from marine bacteria, invertebrates and sometimes fungi. Similar to the above mentioned polysaccharide-degrading enzymes, endo-type fucoidanase produce fuco-oligosaccharides while exo-type fucosidase leads to the formation of mono- or oligosaccharides with a small degree of polymerization [129]. Natalie et al. purified a new fucoidanase and hydrolyzed fucoidan without desulfation to form oligosaccharides ranging from 10 to 2 fucose units plus fucose [130]. Dong et al. discovered a new α-L-fucosidase from marine bacterium *Wenyingzhuangia fucanilytica*, and found that Alf1_Wf was capable of hydrolyzing α-1,4-fucosidic linkage and synthetic substrate. Besides, Alf1_Wf could act on partially degraded fucoidan [131]. Compared to other brown polysaccharides, there are few studies on the enzymatic degradation of fucoidan and the function of fuco-oligosaccharides, whereas the functional investigation of biological activities, such as anti-obesity, antivirus, antitumor, antidiabetic, and antioxidative effects has been widely proven. It is generally believed that fucoidan can become an important substance in the functional food and nutrition and health industries [132,133].

4.1. Antitumor Activity

Fucoidan has significant antitumor activity against liver cancer, stomach cancer, cervical cancer, lung cancer, and breast cancer [113,134–138]. The underlying mechanism includes the inhibition of tumor cell proliferation, stimulating tumor cell apoptosis, blocking tumor cell metastasis, and enhancing various immune responses [136,139–141]. Low molecular weight fucoidan (LMWF), for instance, triggers G1-block and apoptosis in human colon cancer cells (HCT116 cells) through ap53-independent mechanisms [142]. Through the assessment of microtubule-associated proteins and the accumulation of Beclin-1, fucoidan is also found to induce autophagy in human gastric cancer cells (AGS cells) [143]. The polysaccharide induces the apoptosis of HTLV-1-infected T-cell lines mediated by cytostatics that downregulate apoptosis protein-2. The use of fucoidan in vivo thus severely inhibits the tumor growth of subcutaneously transplanted HTHT-1-infected T-cell lines in immunodeficient mice [138]. In addition, fucoidan activates the caspase-independent apoptotic pathway in MCF-7 cancer cells by activating ROS-mediated MAP kinase and regulating the mitochondrial pathway mediated by Bcl-2 family proteins [144]. Similarly, fucoidan has shown antitumor activity against PC-3 (prostate cancer), HeLa (cervical cancer), A549 (alveolar cancer), and HepG2 (hepatocellular carcinoma) cells [145].

4.2. Antiviral and Anti-Inflammatory Activity

Fucoidans isolated from different seaweed species have potential antiviral activity. For instance, they can inhibit the replication of enveloped viruses, including the human immunodeficiency virus (HIV) and the herpes simplex virus (HSV) [146]. According to Queiroz et al. [147], fucoidans from *Dictyota mertensii*, *Lobophora variegata*, *Spatoglossum schroederi*, and *Fucus vesiculosus* inhibit the HIV reverse transcriptase (RT) enzyme, while other studies have shown that they also reduce the amount of the HIV-1 p24 antigen [148]. Compared with other antiviral drugs currently used in clinical medicine, the inhibitory effect of fucoidan is accompanied by lower cytotoxicity. According to one potential mechanism, fucoidan prevents viruses from entering the cells by changing the characteristics of the cell surface. The polysaccharide may also directly interact with viral enzymes or viral proteins on the surface of the pathogen.

Many studies have reported the blocking effect of fucoidan on HSV infection. Fledman et al. isolated different fucoidan components from *Leathesia difformis* and verified the selective antiviral activity of different components against HSV-1 and HSV-2 [149]. Fucoidan extracted from *Undaria pinnatifida* has shown antiviral activity against 32 HSV clinical strains, including 12 ACV-resistant (4 HSV-1 and 8 HSV-2) and 20 ACV-susceptible ones. Judging by the survival rate and lesion score, oral fucoidan can protect mice from HSV-1 infection by stimulating cytotoxic T lymphocytes, natural killer activity, and neutralizing antibodies [150].

The above findings clearly indicate the potential antiviral activity of seaweed fucoidans, which can also strengthen the immune response of the host and achieve multi-channel and multi-level regulation of the immune system [151,152]. The polysaccharide is able to prevent virus transmission by directly inhibiting virus replication and stimulating innate and adaptive immune defense functions. The immunomodulatory activity of fucoidan is another hot research topic. Numerous studies have already confirmed fucoidan to exhibit an anti-inflammatory effect through immune regulation (Table 1). This involves the polysaccharide binding to different receptors, e.g., the Toll-like receptors (TLRs) of monocytes, such as dendritic cells (DCs) and macrophages, and thereby initiating the release of pro-inflammatory factors: cytokines and chemokines. They also suppress the expression of NO synthase (iNOS) and cyclooxygenase (COX)-2 at the protein level, and dose-dependently inhibit the production of nitric oxide (NO) and prostaglandin E2 (PGE2).

Table 1. Monosaccharide composition, molecular weight, concentration, sulfation degree and anti-inflammatory mechanism of different fucoidans.

Brown Seaweed	Monosaccharide Composition	Molecular Weight	Concentration	Sulphate Content (%)	Mechanisms	References
Cladosiphon novae-caledoniae	Fucose 73 mol%, Xylose 12 mol% Mannose 7 mol%	-	19.35 ng/μL; 80.64 ng/μL	14.5%	Inhibited COX-1 and COX-2	[153]
Sargassum horneri	Polyphenols 3.9%	Mw > 30 kDa	25–100 μg/mL	12%	Decreased production of TNF-α, IL-6, NO and PGE2	[154]
Laminaria japonica	Fucose 79.49% Xylose 1.08% Mannose 1.84% Galactose 16.76% Rhamnose 0.82%	104.3 kDa	25 μg/mL	30.72%	Decreased production of TNF-α, IL-1β, IL-6, NO, iNOS, and COX-2 expression; downregulation of MAPK and NF-κB signaling pathways	[155]
Turbinaria decurrens	Fucose 59.3% Xylose 11.4% Galactose 12.6% Mannose 9.6%	-	50 mg/kg	23.51%	Reduced the expression of genes of COX-2, IL-1β, the NF-κB signaling pathway	[156]
Turbinaria ornata	Fucose 86.4 mol% Rhamnose 0.4 mol% Galactose 1.7 mol% Glucose 0.8 mol%	-	25–100 μg/mL	38.3%	Suppressed the expression of COX-2 and pro-inflammatory cytokines in LPS-induced RAW 264.7 macrophages	[157]
Undaria pinnatifida	Fucose 50.9% Xylose 4.2% Galactose 44.6% Mannose 0.3%	-	50 mg/kg;150 mg/kg		Reduced the COX-2 expression dose dependently	[112]
Ecklonia cava	Fucose 77.9 mol% Rhamnose 2.3 mol% Galactose 10.1 mol% Glucose 2.2 mol% Xylose 7.5 mol%	-	50–100 μg/mL	39.1%	Reduced NO production and levels of TNF-α, IL-1β, and IL-6	[158]
Fucus vesiculosus	Molar rate 1:0.03:0.02:0.04:0.2:1.2 for Fucose, Galactose, Mannose, Xylose, Uronic acid, and sulfate	-	30–60 mg/kg	27%	Inhibition of COX, hyaluronidase, and MAPK p38 enzymes.	[159]
Cladosiphon okamuranus	Fucose 30.9% Xylose 0.7% Glucose 2.2% Uronic acid 23.4%	-	4.0 mg/kg	15.1%	Inhibition of neutrophil extravasation into peritoneal cavity	[115]
Fucus vesiculosus	Fucoidan	-	0–100 mg/mL		Inhibited the release of nitric oxide, IL-1b, TNF-a, prostaglandin E2 and monocyte chemoattractant protein-1 by inhibiting NF-κB, Akt and MAPK kinases activation	[160]
Sargassum hemiphyllum	Fucose 210.99 mmol/g	-	100 mg/mL	38.99.4%	Inhibition of IL-1b, TNF-a, and reduction of IL-10, IFN-c in production LPS treated cells	[161]
Macrocystis pyrifera	Fucose 25.77% Galactose 3.93% Glucose 1.14% Mannose 1.12% Xylose 0.84% Uronic acid 5.54%	-	5-100 μg/mL	27.32%	Delayed the apoptosis and promote pro-inflammatory cytokine production in human neutrophils	[151]
Ascophyllum nodosum	Fucose 39.8% Galactose 3.37% Glucose 0.88% Mannose 0.72% Xylose 3.68% Uronic acid 1.72%	-	50–100 μg/mL	24.07%	Delayed the apoptosis and promote pro-inflammatory cytokine production in human neutrophils	[151]

Fucoidan can enhance the various beneficial effects of lactic acid bacteria on immune function by improving Th1/Th2 immune balance [162], and can also treat gastric mucosal damage caused by oral aspirin through its ability to regulate immune response and reduce ulcers' inflammation [163]. During in vivo experiments, Li et al. evaluated the potential inhibitory activity of fucoidan on the myocardial ischemia-reperfusion (I/R) model in rats. The results showed a significant effect by modulating the inflammatory response through the inactivation of high mobility group box 1 (HMGB1) and nuclear factor kappa B (NF-κB) [164].

It has been reported that the destruction of connective tissue during inflammatory diseases such as chronic wounds, chronic inflammation, or rheumatoid arthritis is a result of a continuous supply of inflammatory cells and increased production of inflammatory cytokines and matrix proteases [165]. Selectins expressed on endothelial cells, leukocytes, and platelets contribute to the interaction of leukocytes and platelets on the side of vascular injury, thereby enhancing the inflammatory response during the arterial response to injury [166]. Fucoidan can effectively inhibit the interaction between selectins and their ligands leading to reduced inflammation at an early stage. Therefore, fucoidan use seems beneficial for treating certain inflammations accompanied by uncontrolled extracellular matrix degradation. The above studies have laid the preclinical foundation for the development of fucoidans as a new generation of polysaccharide immunomodulators.

4.3. Antidiabetic Activity

Studies have shown that fucoidan can also exhibit antidiabetic effects by reducing postprandial hyperglycemia and pancreatic β-cell damage, increasing insulin secretion, and regulating glucose metabolism to reduce blood sugar [167,168]. Fucoidan has a significant inhibitory effect on the three starch-hydrolyzing enzymes; it is a non-competitive inhibitor of α-amylase and amyloglucosidase, while being a competitive inhibitor of α-glucosidase [169]. Its inhibitory mechanism lies in the formation of hydrogen bonds [170]: the hydroxyl groups of fucoidan, especially the ones at the C-terminus that may be connected to fucose, can easily form hydrogen bonds with the amino acids of the two enzymes. The negatively charged oxygens of the sulfated groups of the polysaccharide (and the ones connected to C-2 and/or C-3 in particular) further facilitate the formation of hydrogen bonds or salt bridges with the proteins, resulting in strong interactions, thereby inhibiting the enzyme. Furthermore, inhibition of dipeptidyl peptidase-IV (DPP-IV) is one of the possible mechanisms involved in the antihyperglycemic activity of fucoidan. Dipeptidyl peptidase-IV (DPP-IV) is an enzyme that is involved in the inhibition of the rapid degradation of incretin hormones, which prevents postprandial hyperglycemia. Inhibiting DPP-IV prolongs the action of incretins, which reduces glucose production and increases insulin production [171]. Fucoidan can be used as a dipeptidyl peptidase-IV (DPP-IV) inhibitor to block DPP-IV action thereby prolonging the half-life and biological activity of incretin hormones [172], which play a crucial role in glucose homeostasis by promoting α and β cell function [173]. It also downregulates the gastric emptying and gastric acid secretion to reduce the postprandial glucose level [174,175]. Olga N. Pozharitskaya et al. have found a concentration-dependent inhibition of the enzyme DPP-IV by fucoidan at the concentration range of 0.02–200 µg/mL, The IC50 was 11.1 µg/mL and the maximum inhibition degree was 60–75% [176].

In addition, fucoidan may have a positive effect on antidiabetics by reducing β cell damage in the pancreas and increasing insulin secretion. According to a complex mechanism, the polysaccharide enhances the activity of sirtuin 1, thereby inducing deacetylation and upregulation of FOXA2 and p-FOXO-1 to promote the expression of PDX-1 and its regulation of insulin synthesis, thereby reducing β cell apoptosis and dysfunction in mice [177]. Furthermore, fucoidan is able to prevent the occurrence of diabetic nephropathy (DN) associated with spontaneous diabetes by inhibiting the NF-κB signaling pathway and lowering blood sugar in a non-toxic way [178]. It has also been found that a combination of fucoidan and traditional Chinese medicine has a beneficial effect on hyperglycemia and DN in rats [179].

4.4. Other Biological Activities

Heparin is a highly sulfated polysaccharide found in mammalian tissues and has been used as an anticoagulant for more than 50 years [180]. However, the clinical use of heparin is known to cause various side effects, such as excessive bleeding, thrombocytopenia, mild transaminase elevation, and hyperkalemia [181]. Therefore, it is necessary to find alternative drugs with safe and effective anticoagulant properties. It is worth noting that fucoidan has shown effectiveness for blood clotting, and many studies suggest it as an alternative to heparin [182,183]. Through studying the anticoagulant activity of fucoidans isolated from nine species of brown seaweed, the ones from *Ecklonia kurome* and *Hijikia fusiforme* were found to have the strongest effect in terms of thromboplastin time (TT) and activated partial thromboplastin time (aPTT) [184]. The mechanism of fucoidan action differs from that of heparin since it can be used in the cases where the application of heparin itself, for some reason or other, is ineffective. The anticoagulant action of fucoidans (as well as that of heparin) can be quickly blocked by the intravenous introduction of biocompatible cationic polymers such as protamine sulfate and VIM-DEMC (a synthetic copolymer of 1-vinylimidazole with diethyl maleate) [185]. Fucoidans may inhibit thrombin activity by directly acting on the enzyme or through the activation of thrombin inhibitors, including antithrombin III and heparin cofactor II [186]. The position of the sulfate group on the sugar residues was found to be an important factor, with the concentration of C-2 sulfated and C-2,3 disulfated residues considerably affecting anticoagulant activity [123].

Fucoidan also has a positive effect in treating and preventing obesity. It has been shown to suppress the formation of 3T3-L1 adipocytes, thus inhibiting fat accumulation, by downregulating fatty acid binding proteins, acetyl-CoA carboxylase, and peroxisome proliferation-activated receptor γ. [187]. Furthermore, *Fucus vesiculosus*-derived fucoidan was found to hinder fat accumulation in 3T3-L1 adipocytes by stimulating lipolysis through increased hormone-sensitive lipase expression and reduced glucose uptake [188].

At present, there is limited information available regarding the antiallergic effect of fucoidan. Recent studies have shown that the orally administered polysaccharide suppresses allergic symptoms by promoting the expression of galectin-9 mRNA and serum galectin-9 levels, thereby preventing immunoglobulin E (IgE) binding to mast cells [189].

5. Conclusions

This review summarized the physicochemical and structural properties of polysaccharides and oligosaccharides derived from brown algae. Their structure and composition determine their biological activity and thereby their nutritional and therapeutic potentials. Although more is now known regarding their biological activities in vitro and significant advance has been made in their extraction from natural sources and modifications, further structural-activity investigation is necessary. Sustainable technologies must be established for the purification of the polysaccharides and the production of oligosaccharides, minimizing energy and chemical consumption while allowing upscaling of consistent quality and freedom from side-effect causing impurities. Lastly, research on catalytic enzymes, including alginate lyase, laminarinase, fucoidanase, and fucosidase, with high stability and desired substrate specificity is needed to enable the production of high-purity oligosaccharides with uniform structure and degrees of polymerization. Progress in enzyme and metabolic engineering will further promote the utilization of brown algae polysaccharides in the food and pharmaceutical industries.

Author Contributions: D.W. and Y.S.Y.H. conceived and designed the project. Y.L., Y.Z. (Yuting Zheng), A.C.Y.W. and B.I. wrote the article. Y.Z. (Ye Zhang), Y.Y. and P.W. collected the literature. All authors have read and agreed to the published version of the manuscript.

Funding: This work was supported by "the Fundamental Research Funds for the Central Universities, Southwest University" (No. SWU019034), Chongqing Science and Technology Bureau (cstc2020jcyj-msxmX0463), "Innovation and entrepreneurship project for returned overseas talents in Chongqing" (CX2019016), Postgraduate mentor team-building program of Southwest University (XYDS201905), Knut and Alice Wallenberg Foundation, and the Swedish Foundation for International Cooperation in Research and Higher Education (KO2018-7936).

Conflicts of Interest: The authors declare no conflict of interest.

References

1. Wells, M.L.; Potin, P.; Craigie, J.S.; Raven, J.A.; Merchant, S.S.; Helliwell, K.E.; Smith, A.G.; Camire, M.E.; Brawley, S.H. Algae as nutritional and functional food sources: Revisiting our understanding. *J. Appl. Phycol.* **2017**, *29*, 949–982. [CrossRef]
2. Commercial Seaweeds Market Size, Share & Trends Analysis Report by Product (Brown Seaweeds, Red Seaweeds, Green Seaweeds), by Form (Liquid, Powdered, Flakes), by Application, by Region, and Segment Forecasts, 2020–2027. Available online: https://www.grandviewresearch.com/industry-analysis/commercial-seaweed-market (accessed on 25 April 2021).
3. Lourenço-Lopes, C.; Fraga-Corral, M.; Jimenez-Lopez, C.; Pereira, A.G.; Garcia-Oliveira, P.; Carpena, M.; Prieto, M.A.; Simal-Gandara, J. Metabolites from Macroalgae and Its Applications in the Cosmetic Industry: A Circular Economy Approach. *Resources* **2020**, *9*, 101. [CrossRef]
4. Radulovich, R.; Neori, A.; Valderrama, D.; Reddy, C.R.K.; Cronin, H.; Forster, J. Chapter 3—Farming of seaweeds. In *Seaweed Sustainability*; Tiwari, B.K., Troy, D.J., Eds.; Academic Press: San Diego, CA, USA, 2015; pp. 27–59.
5. Lü, J.; Sheahan, C.; Fu, P. Metabolic engineering of algae for fourth generation biofuels production. *Energ. Environ. Sci.* **2011**, *4*, 2451–2466. [CrossRef]
6. Sudhakar, K.; Mamat, R.; Samykano, M.; Azmi, W.H.; Ishak, W.F.W.; Yusaf, T. An overview of marine macroalgae as bioresource. *Renew. Sustain. Energy Rev.* **2018**, *91*, 165–179. [CrossRef]
7. Holdt, S.L.; Kraan, S. Bioactive compounds in seaweed: Functional food applications and legislation. *J. Appl. Phycol.* **2011**, *23*, 543–597. [CrossRef]
8. Rioux, L.-E.; Turgeon, S.L. Chapter 7—Seaweed carbohydrates. In *Seaweed Sustainability*; Tiwari, B.K., Troy, D.J., Eds.; Academic Press: San Diego, CA, USA, 2015; pp. 141–192.
9. Salmeán, A.; Duffieux, D.; Harholt, J.; Qin, F.; Michel, G.; Czjzek, M.; Willats, W.; Hervé, C. Insoluble (1→3), (1→4)-β-D-glucan is a component of cell walls in brown algae (Phaeophyceae) and is masked by alginates in tissues. *Sci. Rep.* **2017**, *7*, 2880. [CrossRef]
10. Lewis, D.H.; Smith, D.C. Sugar alcohols (polyols) in fungi and green plants. I. Distribution, physiology and metabolism. *New Phytol.* **1967**, *66*, 143–184. [CrossRef]
11. Tada, B.; Bv, A.; Am, B. A review of the biochemistry of heavy metal biosorption by brown algae. *Water Res.* **2003**, *37*, 4311–4330.
12. Black, W.A.P. The seasonal variation in the cellulose content of the common Scottish Laminariaceae and Fucaceae. *J. Mar. Biol. Assoc. UK* **2010**, *29*, 379–387. [CrossRef]
13. Kloareg, B.; Quattrano, R.S. Structure of the cell walls of marine algae and ecophysiological functions of the matrix polysaccharides. *Oceanogr. Mar. Biol.* **1988**, *26*, 259–315.
14. Kadam, S.U.; Tiwari, B.K.; O'Donnell, C.P. Extraction, structure and biofunctional activities of laminarin from brown algae. *Int. J. Food Sci. Technol.* **2015**, *50*, 24–31. [CrossRef]
15. Dobrinčić, A.; Balbino, S.; Zorić, Z.; Pedisić, S.; Bursać Kovačević, D.; Elez Garofulić, I.; Dragović-Uzelac, V. Advanced Technologies for the Extraction of Marine Brown Algal Polysaccharides. *Mar. Drugs* **2020**, *18*, 168. [CrossRef]
16. Olsson, J.; Toth, G.B.; Albers, E. Biochemical composition of red, green and brown seaweeds on the Swedish west coast. *J. Appl. Phycol.* **2020**, *32*, 3305–3317. [CrossRef]
17. Cronshaw, J.; Myers, A.; Preston, R.D. A chemical and physical investigation of the cell walls of some marine algae. *Biochim. Biophys. Acta* **1958**, *27*, 89–103. [CrossRef]
18. Brownlee, I.A.; Allen, A.; Pearson, J.P.; Dettmar, P.W.; Havler, M.E.; Atherton, M.R.; Onsøyen, E. Alginate as a source of dietary fiber. *Crit. Rev. Food Sci. Nutr.* **2005**, *45*, 497–510. [CrossRef] [PubMed]
19. Usman, A.; Khalid, S.; Usman, A.; Hussain, Z.; Wang, Y. Chapter 5—Algal Polysaccharides, Novel Application, and Outlook. In *Algae Based Polymers, Blends, and Composites*; Zia, K.M., Zuber, M., Ali, M., Eds.; Elsevier: Amsterdam, The Netherlands, 2017; pp. 115–153.
20. Moen, E.; Larsen, B.; Østgaard, K.; Jensen, A. Alginate Stability during High Salt Preservation of *Ascophyllum nodosum*. In Proceedings of the Sixteenth International Seaweed Symposium, Cebu City, Philippines, 12–17 April 1998; Kain, J.M., Brown, M.T., Lahaye, M., Eds.; Springer: Dordrecht, The Netherlands, 1999; pp. 535–539.
21. Jiménez-Escrig, A.; Sánchez-Muniz, F.J. Dietary fibre from edible seaweeds: Chemical structure, physicochemical properties and effects on cholesterol metabolism. *Nutr. Res.* **2000**, *20*, 585–598. [CrossRef]
22. Radwan, A.; Davies, G.; Fataftah, A.; Ghabbour, E.A.; Jansen, S.A.; Willey, R.J. Isolation of humic acid from the brown algae *Ascophyllum nodosum, Fucus vesiculosus, Laminaria saccharina* and the marine angiosperm *Zostera marina*. *J. Appl. Phycol.* **1996**, *8*, 553–562. [CrossRef]
23. Cheng, D.; Jiang, C.; Xu, J.; Liu, Z.; Mao, X. Characteristics and applications of alginate lyases: A review. *Int. J. Biol. Macromol.* **2020**, *164*, 1304–1320. [CrossRef] [PubMed]

4. Gacesa, P. Alginate-modifying Enzymes—A proposed unified mechanism of action for the lyases and epimerases. *FEBS Lett.* **1987**, *212*, 199–202. [CrossRef]
5. Li, L.; Jiang, X.; Guan, H.; Wang, P. Preparation, purification and characterization of alginate oligosaccharides degraded by alginate lyase from *Pseudomonas* sp. HZJ 216. *Carbohydr. Res.* **2011**, *346*, 794–800. [CrossRef] [PubMed]
6. Kim, H.T.; Ko, H.-J.; Kim, N.; Kim, D.; Lee, D.; Choi, I.-G.; Woo, H.C.; Kim, M.D.; Kim, K.H. Characterization of a recombinant endo-type alginate lyase (Alg7D) from *Saccharophagus degradans*. *Biotechnol. Lett.* **2012**, *34*, 1087–1092. [CrossRef]
7. Zhu, B.; Tan, H.; Qin, Y.; Xu, Q.; Du, Y.; Yin, H. Characterization of a new endo-type alginate lyase from *Vibrio* sp. W13. *Int. J. Biol. Macromol.* **2015**, *75*, 330–337. [CrossRef]
8. Zhu, B.; Chen, M.; Yin, H.; Du, Y.; Ning, L. Enzymatic Hydrolysis of Alginate to Produce Oligosaccharides by a New Purified Endo-Type Alginate Lyase. *Mar. Drugs* **2016**, *14*, 108. [CrossRef] [PubMed]
9. Wang, X.; Wang, L.; Che, J.; Li, X.; Li, J.; Wang, J.; Xu, Y. In vitro non-specific immunostimulatory effect of alginate oligosaccharides with different molecular weights and compositions on sea cucumber (*Apostichopus japonicus*) coelomocytes. *Aquaculture* **2014**, *434*, 434–441. [CrossRef]
10. Chen, J.; Hu, Y.; Zhang, L.; Wang, Y.; Wang, S.; Zhang, Y.; Guo, H.; Ji, D.; Wang, Y. Alginate Oligosaccharide DP5 Exhibits Antitumor Effects in Osteosarcoma Patients following Surgery. *Front. Pharmacol.* **2017**, *8*, 623. [CrossRef] [PubMed]
11. Fang, W.; Bi, D.; Zheng, R.; Cai, N.; Xu, H.; Zhou, R.; Lu, J.; Wan, M.; Xu, X. Identification and activation of TLR4-mediated signalling pathways by alginate-derived guluronate oligosaccharide in RAW264.7 macrophages. *Sci. Rep.* **2017**, *7*, 1663. [CrossRef] [PubMed]
12. Hao, J.; Hao, C.; Zhang, L.; Liu, X.; Zhou, X.; Dun, Y.; Li, H.; Li, G.; Zhao, X.; An, Y.; et al. OM2, a Novel Oligomannuronate-Chromium(III) Complex, Promotes Mitochondrial Biogenesis and Lipid Metabolism in 3T3-L1 Adipocytes via the AMPK-PGC1α Pathway. *PLoS ONE* **2015**, *10*, e0131930. [CrossRef]
13. Hu, Y.; Feng, Z.; Feng, W.; Hu, T.; Guan, H.; Mao, Y. AOS ameliorates monocrotaline-induced pulmonary hypertension by restraining the activation of P-selectin/p38MAPK/NF-κB pathway in rats. *Biomed. Pharmacother.* **2019**, *109*, 1319–1326. [CrossRef]
14. Li, S.; Wang, L.; Han, F.; Gong, Q.; Yu, W. Cloning and characterization of the first polysaccharide lyase family 6 oligoalginate lyase from marine *Shewanella* sp. Kz7. *J. Biochem.* **2016**, *159*, 77–86. [CrossRef]
15. Pritchard, M.F.; Jack, A.A.; Powell, L.C.; Sadh, H.; Rye, P.D.; Hill, K.E.; Thomas, D.W. Alginate oligosaccharides modify hyphal infiltration of *Candida albicans* in an in vitro model of invasive human candidosis. *J. Appl. Microbiol.* **2017**, *123*, 625–636. [CrossRef]
16. Zhu, Y.; Wu, L.; Chen, Y.; Ni, H.; Xiao, A.; Cai, H. Characterization of an extracellular biofunctional alginate lyase from marine *Microbulbifer* sp. ALW1 and antioxidant activity of enzymatic hydrolysates. *Microbiol. Res.* **2016**, *182*, 49–58. [CrossRef]
17. Falkeborg, M.; Cheong, L.-Z.; Gianfico, C.; Sztukiel, K.M.; Kristensen, K.; Glasius, M.; Xu, X.; Guo, Z. Alginate oligosaccharides: Enzymatic preparation and antioxidant property evaluation. *Food Chem.* **2014**, *164*, 185–194. [CrossRef]
18. Liu, M.; Liu, L.; Zhang, H.-f.; Yi, B.; Everaert, N. Alginate oligosaccharides preparation, biological activities and their application in livestock and poultry. *J. Integr. Agric.* **2021**, *20*, 24–34. [CrossRef]
19. Wang, P.; Jiang, X.; Jiang, Y.; Hu, X.; Mou, H.; Li, M.; Guan, H. In vitro antioxidative activities of three marine oligosaccharides. *Nat. Prod. Res.* **2007**, *21*, 646–654. [CrossRef]
20. Zhao, X.; Li, B.; Xue, C.; Sun, L. Effect of molecular weight on the antioxidant property of low molecular weight alginate from *Laminaria japonica*. *J. Appl. Phycol.* **2012**, *24*, 295–300. [CrossRef]
21. Tusi, S.K.; Khalaj, L.; Ashabi, G.; Kiaei, M.; Khodagholi, F. Alginate oligosaccharide protects against endoplasmic reticulum- and mitochondrial-mediated apoptotic cell death and oxidative stress. *Biomaterials* **2011**, *32*, 5438–5458. [CrossRef] [PubMed]
22. Guo, J.-J.; Ma, L.-L.; Shi, H.-T.; Zhu, J.-B.; Wu, J.; Ding, Z.-W.; An, Y.; Zou, Y.-Z.; Ge, J.-B. Alginate Oligosaccharide Prevents Acute Doxorubicin Cardiotoxicity by Suppressing Oxidative Stress and Endoplasmic Reticulum-Mediated Apoptosis. *Mar. Drugs* **2016**, *14*, 231. [CrossRef]
23. Jacobsen, C.; Sørensen, A.M.; Holdt, S.L.; Akoh, C.C.; Hermund, D.B. Source, Extraction, Characterization, and Applications of Novel Antioxidants from Seaweed. *Annu. Rev. Food Sci. Technol.* **2019**, *10*, 541–568. [CrossRef]
24. Şen, M. Effects of molecular weight and ratio of guluronic acid to mannuronic acid on the antioxidant properties of sodium alginate fractions prepared by radiation-induced degradation. *Appl. Radiat. Isot.* **2011**, *69*, 126–129. [CrossRef]
25. Ueno, M.; Hiroki, T.; Takeshita, S.; Jiang, Z.; Kim, D.; Yamaguchi, K.; Oda, T. Comparative study on antioxidative and macrophage-stimulating activities of polyguluronic acid (PG) and polymannuronic acid (PM) prepared from alginate. *Carbohydr. Res.* **2012**, *352*, 88–93. [CrossRef] [PubMed]
26. Hu, X.; Jiang, X.; Gong, J.; Hwang, H.; Liu, Y.; Guan, H. Antibacterial activity of lyase-depolymerized products of alginate. *J. Appl. Phycol.* **2005**, *17*, 57–60. [CrossRef]
27. Hengzhuang, W.; Song, Z.; Ciofu, O.; Onsøyen, E.; Rye, P.D.; Høiby, N. OligoG CF-5/20 Disruption of Mucoid *Pseudomonas aeruginosa* Biofilm in a Murine Lung Infection Model. *Antimicrob. Agents Chemother.* **2016**, *60*, 2620–2626. [CrossRef] [PubMed]
28. Powell, L.C.; Sowedan, A.; Khan, S.; Wright, C.J.; Hawkins, K.; Onsøyen, E.; Myrvold, R.; Hill, K.E.; Thomas, D.W. The effect of alginate oligosaccharides on the mechanical properties of Gram-negative biofilms. *Biofouling* **2013**, *29*, 413–421. [CrossRef] [PubMed]
29. Nordgård, C.T.; Draget, K.I. Oligosaccharides as modulators of rheology in complex mucous systems. *Biomacromolecules* **2011**, *12*, 3084–3090. [CrossRef]

50. Pritchard, M.F.; Powell, L.C.; Menzies, G.E.; Lewis, P.D.; Hawkins, K.; Wright, C.; Doull, I.; Walsh, T.R.; Onsøyen, E.; Dessen, A.; et al. A New Class of Safe Oligosaccharide Polymer Therapy to Modify the Mucus Barrier of Chronic Respiratory Disease. *Mol. Pharm.* **2016**, *13*, 863–872. [CrossRef]
51. He, X.; Hwang, H.M.; Aker, W.G.; Wang, P.; Lin, Y.; Jiang, X.; He, X. Synergistic combination of marine oligosaccharides and azithromycin against *Pseudomonas aeruginosa*. *Microbiol. Res.* **2014**, *169*, 759–767. [CrossRef]
52. Pritchard, M.F.; Powell, L.C.; Jack, A.A.; Powell, K.; Beck, K.; Florance, H.; Forton, J.; Rye, P.D.; Dessen, A.; Hill, K.E.; et al. A Low-Molecular-Weight Alginate Oligosaccharide Disrupts Pseudomonal Microcolony Formation and Enhances Antibiotic Effectiveness. *Antimicrob. Agents Chemother.* **2017**, *61*, e00762-17. [CrossRef]
53. Grant, G.T.; Morris, E.R.; Rees, D.A.; Smith, P.J.C.; Thom, D. Biological interactions between polysaccharides and divalent cations: The egg-box model. *FEBS Lett.* **1973**, *32*, 195–198. [CrossRef]
54. Flemming, H.C.; Wingender, J. The biofilm matrix. *Nat. Rev. Microbiol.* **2010**, *8*, 623–633. [CrossRef]
55. Tøndervik, A.; Sletta, H.; Klinkenberg, G.; Emanuel, C.; Powell, L.C.; Pritchard, M.F.; Khan, S.; Craine, K.M.; Onsøyen, E.; Rye, P.D.; et al. Alginate Oligosaccharides Inhibit Fungal Cell Growth and Potentiate the Activity of Antifungals against *Candida* and *Aspergillus* spp. *PLoS ONE* **2014**, *9*, e112518. [CrossRef]
56. Iwamoto, Y.; Xu, X.; Tamura, T.; Oda, T.; Muramatsu, T. Enzymatically depolymerized alginate oligomers that cause cytotoxic cytokine production in human mononuclear cells. *Biosci. Biotechnol. Biochem.* **2003**, *67*, 258–263. [CrossRef]
57. Yamamoto, Y.; Kurachi, M.; Yamaguchi, K.; Oda, T. Induction of multiple cytokine secretion from RAW264.7 cells by alginate oligosaccharides. *Biosci. Biotechnol. Biochem.* **2007**, *71*, 238–241. [CrossRef] [PubMed]
58. Uno, T.; Hattori, M.; Yoshida, T. Oral Administration of Alginic Acid Oligosaccharide Suppresses IgE Production and Inhibits the Induction of Oral Tolerance. *Biosci. Biotechnol. Biochem.* **2006**, *70*, 3054–3057. [CrossRef]
59. Yamamoto, Y.; Kurachi, M.; Yamaguchi, K.; Oda, T. Stimulation of multiple cytokine production in mice by alginate oligosaccharides following intraperitoneal administration. *Carbohydr. Res.* **2007**, *342*, 1133–1137. [CrossRef] [PubMed]
60. Ueno, M.; Cho, K.; Nakazono, S.; Isaka, S.; Abu, R.; Takeshita, S.; Yamaguchi, K.; Kim, D.; Oda, T. Alginate oligomer induces nitric oxide (NO) production in RAW264.7 cells: Elucidation of the underlying intracellular signaling mechanism. *Biosci. Biotechnol. Biochem.* **2015**, *79*, 1787–1793. [CrossRef]
61. Xu, X.; Bi, D.-C.; Li, C.; Fang, W.-S.; Zhou, R.; Li, S.-M.; Chi, L.-L.; Wan, M.; Shen, L.-M. Morphological and Proteomic Analyses Reveal that Unsaturated Guluronate Oligosaccharide Modulates Multiple Functional Pathways in Murine Macrophage RAW264.7 Cells. *Mar. Drugs* **2015**, *13*, 1798–1818. [CrossRef]
62. Xu, X.; Bi, D.; Wu, X.; Wang, Q.; Wei, G.; Chi, L.; Jiang, Z.; Oda, T.; Wan, M. Unsaturated guluronate oligosaccharide enhances the antibacterial activities of macrophages. *FASEB J. Off. Publ. Fed. Am. Soc. Exp. Biol.* **2014**, *28*, 2645–2654. [CrossRef]
63. Xu, X.; Wu, X.; Wang, Q.; Cai, N.; Zhang, H.; Jiang, Z.; Wan, M.; Oda, T. Immunomodulatory Effects of Alginate Oligosaccharides on Murine Macrophage RAW264.7 Cells and Their Structure-Activity Relationships. *J. Agric. Food Chem.* **2014**, *62*, 3168–3176. [CrossRef]
64. Hu, X.; Jiang, X.; Hwang, H.; Liu, S.; Guan, H. Antitumour activities of alginate-derived oligosaccharides and their sulphated substitution derivatives. *Eur. J. Phycol.* **2004**, *39*, 67–71. [CrossRef]
65. Han, Y.; Zhang, L.; Yu, X.; Wang, S.; Xu, C.; Yin, H.; Wang, S. Alginate oligosaccharide attenuates α2,6-sialylation modification to inhibit prostate cancer cell growth via the Hippo/YAP pathway. *Cell Death Dis.* **2019**, *10*, 374. [CrossRef] [PubMed]
66. Peat, S.; Whelan, W.J.; Lawley, H.G. 141. The structure of laminarin. Part I. The main polymeric linkage. *J. Chem. Soc.* **1958**, 724–728. [CrossRef]
67. Stark, J.R. A new method fot the analysis of laminarins and for preparative-scale fractionation of their components. *Carbohydr. Res.* **1976**, *47*, 176–178. [CrossRef]
68. Shin, H.J.; Oh, S.J.; Kim, S.I.; Won Kim, H.; Son, J.-H. Conformational characteristics of β-glucan in laminarin probed by terahertz spectroscopy. *Appl. Phys. Lett.* **2009**, *94*, 111911. [CrossRef]
69. Je, J.-Y.; Park, P.-J.; Kim, E.-K.; Park, J.-S.; Yoon, H.-D.; Kim, K.-R.; Ahn, C.-B. Antioxidant activity of enzymatic extracts from the brown seaweed *Undaria pinnatifida* by electron spin resonance spectroscopy. *LWT—Food Sci. Technol.* **2009**, *42*, 874–878. [CrossRef]
70. Schiener, P.; Black, K.D.; Stanley, M.S.; Green, D.H. The seasonal variation in the chemical composition of the kelp species *Laminaria digitata, Laminaria hyperborea, Saccharina latissima* and *Alaria esculenta*. *J. Appl. Phycol.* **2015**, *27*, 363–373. [CrossRef]
71. Stiger-Pouvreau, V.; Bourgougnon, N.; Deslandes, E. Chapter 8—Carbohydrates from Seaweeds. In *Seaweed in Health and Disease Prevention*; Fleurence, J., Levine, I., Eds.; Academic Press: San Diego, CA, USA, 2016; pp. 223–274.
72. Nelson, T.E.; Lewis, B.A. Separation and characterization of the soluble and insoluble components of insoluble laminaran. *Carbohydr. Res.* **1974**, *33*, 63–74. [CrossRef]
73. Alderkamp, A.C.; van Rijssel, M.; Bolhuis, H. Characterization of marine bacteria and the activity of their enzyme systems involved in degradation of the algal storage glucan laminarin. *FEMS Microbiol. Ecol.* **2007**, *59*, 108–117. [CrossRef] [PubMed]
74. Davies, G.; Henrissat, B. Structures and Mechanisms of Glycosyl Hydrolases. *Structure* **1995**, *3*, 853–859. [CrossRef] [PubMed]
75. Bara, M.T.F.; Lima, A.L.; Ulhoa, C.J. Purification and characterization of an exo-beta-1,3-glucanase produced by *Trichoderma asperellum*. *Fems Microbiol. Lett.* **2003**, *219*, 81–85. [CrossRef]
76. Wang, D.; Kim, D.H.; Yun, E.J.; Park, Y.-C.; Seo, J.-H.; Kim, K.H. The first bacterial beta-1,6-endoglucanase from *Saccharophagus degradans* 2-40^T for the hydrolysis of pustulan and laminarin. *Appl. Microbiol. Biotechnol.* **2017**, *101*, 197–204. [CrossRef] [PubMed]

77. Kumar, K.; Correia, M.A.S.; Pires, V.M.R.; Dhillon, A.; Sharma, K.; Rajulapati, V.; Fontes, C.M.G.A.; Carvalho, A.L.; Goyal, A. Novel insights into the degradation of beta-1,3-glucans by the cellulosome of *Clostridium thermocellum* revealed by structure and function studies of a family 81 glycoside hydrolase. *Int. J. Biol. Macromol.* **2018**, *117*, 890–901. [CrossRef]
78. Badur, A.H.; Ammar, E.M.; Yalamanchili, G.; Hehemann, J.-H.; Rao, C.V. Characterization of the GH16 and GH17 laminarinases from *Vibrio breoganii* 1C10. *Appl. Microbiol. Biotechnol.* **2020**, *104*, 161–171. [CrossRef] [PubMed]
79. Wang, D.; Kim, D.H.; Seo, N.; Yun, E.J.; An, H.J.; Kim, J.H.; Kim, K.H. A Novel Glycoside Hydrolase Family 5 β-1,3-1,6-Endoglucanase from *Saccharophagus degradans* 2-40^T and Its Transglycosylase Activity. *Appl. Environ. Microbiol.* **2016**, *82*, 4340–4349. [CrossRef]
80. Williams, D.L. Overview of (1→3)-beta-D-glucan immunobiology. *Mediat. Inflamm.* **1997**, *6*, 247–250. [CrossRef]
81. Cheung, N.K.; Modak, S.; Vickers, A.; Knuckles, B. Orally administered beta-glucans enhance anti-tumor effects of monoclonal antibodies. *Cancer Immunol. Immunother.* **2002**, *51*, 557–564. [CrossRef]
82. Hong, F.; Yan, J.; Baran, J.T.; Allendorf, D.J.; Hansen, R.D.; Ostroff, G.R.; Xing, P.X.; Cheung, N.K.; Ross, G.D. Mechanism by which orally administered beta-1,3-glucans enhance the tumoricidal activity of antitumor monoclonal antibodies in murine tumor models. *J. Immunol.* **2004**, *173*, 797–806. [CrossRef] [PubMed]
83. Williams, D.L.; Mueller, A.; Browder, W. Glucan-Based Macrophage Stimulators. *Clin. Immunother.* **1996**, *5*, 392–399. [CrossRef]
84. Wei, D.; Zhang, L.; Williams, D.L.; Browder, I.W. Glucan stimulates human dermal fibroblast collagen biosynthesis through a nuclear factor-1 dependent mechanism. *Wound Repair Regen.* **2002**, *10*, 161–168. [CrossRef]
85. Schepetkin, I.A.; Quinn, M.T. Botanical polysaccharides: Macrophage immunomodulation and therapeutic potential. *Int. Immunopharmacol.* **2006**, *6*, 317–333. [CrossRef] [PubMed]
86. Lee, J.Y.; Kim, Y.-J.; Kim, H.J.; Kim, Y.-S.; Park, W. Immunostimulatory Effect of Laminarin on RAW 264.7 Mouse Macrophages. *Molecules* **2012**, *17*, 5404–5411. [CrossRef] [PubMed]
87. Devillé, C.; Damas, J.; Forget, P.; Dandrifosse, G.; Peulen, O. Laminarin in the dietary fibre concept. *J. Sci. Food Agric.* **2004**, *84*, 1030–1038. [CrossRef]
88. Kadam, S.U.; O'Donnell, C.P.; Rai, D.K.; Hossain, M.B.; Burgess, C.M.; Walsh, D.; Tiwari, B.K. Laminarin from Irish Brown Seaweeds *Ascophyllum nodosum* and *Laminaria hyperborea*: Ultrasound Assisted Extraction, Characterization and Bioactivity. *Mar. Drugs* **2015**, *13*, 4270–4280. [CrossRef] [PubMed]
89. Park, H.K.; Kim, I.H.; Kim, J.; Nam, T.J. Induction of apoptosis by laminarin, regulating the insulin-like growth factor-IR signaling pathways in HT-29 human colon cells. *Int. J. Mol. Med.* **2012**, *30*, 734–738. [CrossRef]
90. Zargarzadeh, M.; Amaral, A.J.R.; Custódio, C.A.; Mano, J.F. Biomedical applications of laminarin. *Carbohyd. Polym.* **2020**, *232*, 115774. [CrossRef]
91. Ji, Y.B.; Ji, C.F.; Zhang, H. Laminarin induces apoptosis of human colon cancer LOVO cells through a mitochondrial pathway. *Molecules* **2012**, *17*, 9947–9960. [CrossRef]
92. Ji, C.F.; Ji, Y.B. Laminarin-induced apoptosis in human colon cancer LoVo cells. *Oncol. Lett.* **2014**, *7*, 1728–1732. [CrossRef]
93. Ermakova, S.; Men'shova, R.; Vishchuk, O.; Kim, S.-M.; Um, B.-H.; Isakov, V.; Zvyagintseva, T. Water-soluble polysaccharides from the brown alga *Eisenia bicyclis*: Structural characteristics and antitumor activity. *Algal Res.* **2013**, *2*, 51–58. [CrossRef]
94. Usoltseva Menshova, R.V.; Anastyuk, S.D.; Shevchenko, N.M.; Zvyagintseva, T.N.; Ermakova, S.P. The comparison of structure and anticancer activity in vitro of polysaccharides from brown algae *Alaria marginata* and *A. angusta*. *Carbohydr. Polym.* **2016**, *153*, 258–265. [CrossRef]
95. Pang, Z.; Otaka, K.; Maoka, T.; Hidaka, K.; Ishijima, S.; Oda, M.; Ohnishi, M. Structure of beta-glucan oligomer from laminarin and its effect on human monocytes to inhibit the proliferation of U937 cells. *Biosci. Biotechnol. Biochem.* **2005**, *69*, 553–558. [CrossRef]
96. Menshova, R.V.; Ermakova, S.P.; Anastyuk, S.D.; Isakov, V.V.; Dubrovskaya, Y.V.; Kusaykin, M.I.; Um, B.H.; Zvyagintseva, T.N. Structure, enzymatic transformation and anticancer activity of branched high molecular weight laminaran from brown alga *Eisenia bicyclis*. *Carbohydr. Polym.* **2014**, *99*, 101–109. [CrossRef]
97. Ji, C.F.; Ji, Y.B.; Meng, D.Y. Sulfated modification and anti-tumor activity of laminarin. *Exp. Ther. Med.* **2013**, *6*, 1259–1264. [CrossRef]
98. Huang, Y.; Jiang, H.; Mao, X.; Ci, F. Laminarin and Laminarin Oligosaccharides Originating from Brown Algae: Preparation, Biological Activities, and Potential Applications. *J. Ocean Univ. China* **2021**, *20*, 641–653. [CrossRef]
99. Shanmugam, M.; Mody, K.H. Heparinoid-active sulphated polysaccharides from marine algae as potential blood anticoagulant agents. *Curr. Sci.* **2000**, *79*, 1672–1683.
100. Hoffman, J.; Larm, O.; Larsson, K.; Andersson, L.O.; Holmer, E.; Söderström, G. Studies on the blood-anticoagulant activity of sulphated polysaccharides with different uronic acid content. *Carbohyd. Polym.* **1982**, *2*, 115–121. [CrossRef]
101. O'Neill, A.N. Sulphated derivatives of laminarin. *Can. J. Chem.* **1955**, *33*, 1097–1101. [CrossRef]
102. Hawkins, W.W.; O'Neill, A.N. The anticoagulant action in blood of sulphated derivatives of laminarin. *Can. J. Biochem. Physiol.* **1955**, *33*, 545–552. [CrossRef]
103. Adams, S.S.; Thorpe, H.M. The anticoagulant activity and toxicity of laminarin sulphate K. *J. Pharm. Pharmacol.* **1957**, *9*, 459–463. [CrossRef]
104. Goodridge, H.S.; Wolf, A.J.; Underhill, D.M. Beta-glucan recognition by the innate immune system. *Immunol. Rev.* **2009**, *230*, 38–50. [CrossRef]

105. Ozanne, H.; Toumi, H.; Roubinet, B.; Landemarre, L.; Lespessailles, E.; Daniellou, R.; Cesaro, A. Laminarin Effects, a β-(1,3)-Glucan, on Skin Cell Inflammation and Oxidation. *Cosmetics* **2020**, *7*, 66. [CrossRef]
106. Ramnani, P.; Chitarrari, R.; Tuohy, K.; Grant, J.; Hotchkiss, S.; Philp, K.; Campbell, R.; Gill, C.; Rowland, I. In vitro fermentation and prebiotic potential of novel low molecular weight polysaccharides derived from agar and alginate seaweeds. *Anaerobe* **2012**, *18*, 1–6. [CrossRef]
107. Walsh, A.M.; Sweeney, T.; O'Shea, C.J.; Doyle, D.N.; 'Doherty, J.V.O. Effect of supplementing varying inclusion levels of laminarin and fucoidan on growth performance, digestibility of diet components, selected faecal microbial populations and volatile fatty acid concentrations in weaned pigs. *Anim. Feed Sci. Technol.* **2013**, *183*, 151–159. [CrossRef]
108. Devillé, C.; Gharbi, M.; Dandrifosse, G.; Peulen, O. Study on the effects of laminarin, a polysaccharide from seaweed, on gut characteristics. *J. Sci. Food Agric.* **2007**, *87*, 1717–1725. [CrossRef]
109. Nguyen, S.G.; Kim, J.; Guevarra, R.B.; Lee, J.H.; Kim, E.; Kim, S.I.; Unno, T. Laminarin favorably modulates gut microbiota in mice fed a high-fat diet. *Food Funct.* **2016**, *7*, 4193–4201. [CrossRef]
110. Leal, B.E.S.; Prado, M.R.; Grzybowski, A.; Tiboni, M.; Koop, H.S.; Scremin, L.B.; Sakuma, A.C.; Takamatsu, A.A.; Santos, A.F.d.; Cavalcanti, V.F.; et al. Potential prebiotic oligosaccharides from aqueous thermopressurized phosphoric acid hydrolysates of microalgae used in treatment of gaseous steakhouse waste. *Algal Res.* **2017**, *24*, 138–147. [CrossRef]
111. Fitton, J.H.; Stringer, D.N.; Karpiniec, S.S. Therapies from Fucoidan: An Update. *Mar. Drugs* **2015**, *13*, 5920–5946. [CrossRef] [PubMed]
112. Phull, A.-R.; Majid, M.; Haq, I.-u.; Khan, M.R.; Kim, S.J. In vitro and in vivo evaluation of anti-arthritic, antioxidant efficacy of fucoidan from *Undaria pinnatifida* (Harvey) Suringar. *Int. J. Biol. Macromol.* **2017**, *97*, 468–480. [CrossRef]
113. Atashrazm, F.; Lowenthal, R.M.; Woods, G.M.; Holloway, A.F.; Dickinson, J.L. Fucoidan and Cancer: A Multifunctional Molecule with Anti-Tumor Potential. *Mar. Drugs* **2015**, *13*, 2327–2346. [CrossRef] [PubMed]
114. Black, W.A.P. The seasonal variation in the combined L-fucose content of the common British Laminariaceae and fucaceae. *J. Sci. Food Agric.* **1954**, *5*, 445–448. [CrossRef]
115. Cumashi, A.; Ushakova, N.A.; Preobrazhenskaya, M.E.; D'Incecco, A.; Piccoli, A.; Totani, L.; Tinari, N.; Morozevich, G.E.; Berman, A.E.; Bilan, M.I.; et al. A comparative study of the anti-inflammatory, anticoagulant, antiangiogenic, and antiadhesive activities of nine different fucoidans from brown seaweeds. *Glycobiology* **2007**, *17*, 541–552. [CrossRef]
116. Nishino, T.; Nishioka, C.; Ura, H.; Nagumo, T. Isolation and partial characterization of a novel amino sugar-containing fucan sulfate from commercial *Fucus vesiculosus* fucoidan. *Carbohydr. Res.* **1994**, *255*, 213–224. [CrossRef]
117. Lahrsen, E.; Schoenfeld, A.K.; Alban, S. Size-dependent pharmacological activities of differently degraded fucoidan fractions from *Fucus vesiculosus*. *Carbohydr. Polym.* **2018**, *189*, 162–168. [CrossRef]
118. Bilan, M.I.; Grachev, A.A.; Ustuzhanina, N.E.; Shashkov, A.S.; Nifantiev, N.E.; Usov, A.I. A highly regular fraction of a fucoidan from the brown seaweed *Fucus distichus* L. *Carbohydr. Res.* **2004**, *339*, 511–517. [CrossRef]
119. Ale, M.T.; Meyer, A.S. Fucoidans from brown seaweeds: An update on structures, extraction techniques and use of enzymes as tools for structural elucidation. *RSC Adv.* **2013**, *3*, 8131–8141. [CrossRef]
120. Chevolot, L.; Foucault, A.; Chaubet, F.; Kervarec, N.; Sinquin, C.; Fisher, A.M.; Boisson-Vidal, C. Further data on the structure of brown seaweed fucans: Relationships with anticoagulant activity. *Carbohydr. Res.* **1999**, *319*, 154–165. [CrossRef]
121. Fedorov, S.N.; Ermakova, S.P.; Zvyagintseva, T.N.; Stonik, V.A. Anticancer and cancer preventive properties of marine polysaccharides: Some results and prospects. *Mar. Drugs* **2013**, *11*, 4876–4901. [CrossRef]
122. Bilan, M.I.; Grachev, A.A.; Shashkov, A.S.; Kelly, M.; Sanderson, C.J.; Nifantiev, N.E.; Usov, A.I. Further studies on the composition and structure of a fucoidan preparation from the brown alga *Saccharina latissima*. *Carbohydr. Res.* **2010**, *345*, 2038–2047. [CrossRef] [PubMed]
123. Chevolot, L.; Mulloy, B.; Ratiskol, J.; Foucault, A.; Colliec-Jouault, S. A disaccharide repeat unit is the major structure in fucoidans from two species of brown algae. *Carbohydr. Res.* **2001**, *330*, 529–535. [CrossRef]
124. Lim, S.J.; Wan Aida, W.M.; Schiehser, S.; Rosenau, T.; Böhmdorfer, S. Structural elucidation of fucoidan from *Cladosiphon okamuranus* (Okinawa mozuku). *Food Chem.* **2019**, *272*, 222–226. [CrossRef]
125. Menshova, R.V.; Anastyuk, S.D.; Ermakova, S.P.; Shevchenko, N.M.; Isakov, V.I.; Zvyagintseva, T.N. Structure and anticancer activity in vitro of sulfated galactofucan from brown alga *Alaria angusta*. *Carbohydr. Polym.* **2015**, *132*, 118–125. [CrossRef]
126. Shevchenko, N.M.; Anastyuk, S.D.; Menshova, R.V.; Vishchuk, O.S.; Isakov, V.I.; Zadorozhny, P.A.; Sikorskaya, T.V.; Zvyagintseva, T.N. Further studies on structure of fucoidan from brown alga *Saccharina gurjanovae*. *Carbohydr. Polym.* **2015**, *121*, 207–216. [CrossRef]
127. Sun, Q.-L.; Li, Y.; Ni, L.-Q.; Li, Y.-X.; Cui, Y.-S.; Jiang, S.-L.; Xie, E.-Y.; Du, J.; Deng, F.; Dong, C.-X. Structural characterization and antiviral activity of two fucoidans from the brown algae *Sargassum henslowianum*. *Carbohydr. Polym.* **2020**, *229*, 115487. [CrossRef] [PubMed]
128. Zvyagintseva, T.N.; Usoltseva, R.V.; Shevchenko, N.M.; Surits, V.V.; Imbs, T.I.; Malyarenko, O.S.; Besednova, N.N.; Ivanushko, L.A.; Ermakova, S.P. Structural diversity of fucoidans and their radioprotective effect. *Carbohydr. Polym.* **2021**, *273*, 118551. [CrossRef] [PubMed]
129. Kusaykin, M.I.; Silchenko, A.S.; Zakharenko, A.M.; Zvyagintseva, T.N. Fucoidanases. *Glycobiology* **2016**, *26*, 3–12. [CrossRef] [PubMed]

30. Wang, Y.; Li, B.; Zhao, X.; Piao, M. Isolation and characterization of a fucoidan-degrading bacterium from *Laminaria japonica*. *J. Ocean Univ. China* **2014**, *13*, 153–156. [CrossRef]
31. Dong, S.; Chang, Y.; Shen, J.; Xue, C.; Chen, F. Purification, expression and characterization of a novel alpha-L-fucosidase from a marine bacteria *Wenyingzhuangia fucanilytica*. *Protein Expr. Purif.* **2017**, *129*, 9–17. [CrossRef]
32. Wijesinghe, W.A.J.P.; Jeon, Y.-J. Biological activities and potential industrial applications of fucose rich sulfated polysaccharides and fucoidans isolated from brown seaweeds: A review. *Carbohydr. Polym.* **2012**, *88*, 13–20. [CrossRef]
33. Vo, T.-S.; Ngo, D.-H.; Kim, S.-K. Marine algae as a potential pharmaceutical source for anti-allergic therapeutics. *Process Biochem.* **2012**, *47*, 386–394. [CrossRef]
34. Yamasaki-Miyamoto, Y.; Yamasaki, M.; Tachibana, H.; Yamada, K. Fucoidan induces apoptosis through activation of caspase-8 on human breast cancer MCF-7 cells. *J. Agric. Food Chem.* **2009**, *57*, 8677–8682. [CrossRef]
35. Xie, J.H.; Liu, X.; Shen, M.Y.; Nie, S.P.; Zhang, H.; Li, C.; Gong, D.M.; Xie, M.Y. Purification, physicochemical characterisation and anticancer activity of a polysaccharide from *Cyclocarya paliurus* leaves. *Food Chem.* **2013**, *136*, 1453–1460. [CrossRef] [PubMed]
36. Zong, A.; Cao, H.; Wang, F. Anticancer polysaccharides from natural resources: A review of recent research. *Carbohydr. Polym.* **2012**, *90*, 1395–1410. [CrossRef] [PubMed]
37. Aisa, Y.; Miyakawa, Y.; Nakazato, T.; Shibata, H.; Saito, K.; Ikeda, Y.; Kizaki, M. Fucoidan induces apoptosis of human HS-Sultan cells accompanied by activation of caspase-3 and down-regulation of ERK Pathways. *Am. J. Hematol.* **2005**, *78*, 7–14. [CrossRef]
38. Haneji, K.; Matsuda, T.; Tomita, M.; Kawakami, H.; Ohshiro, K.; Uchihara, J.-N.; Masuda, M.; Takasu, N.; Tanaka, Y.; Ohta, T.; et al. Fucoidan Extracted From Cladosiphon Okamuranus Tokida Induces Apoptosis of Human T-Cell Leukemia Virus Type 1-Infected T-Cell Lines and Primary Adult T-Cell Leukemia Cells. *Nutr. Cancer* **2005**, *52*, 189–201. [CrossRef]
39. Hyun, J.-H.; Kim, S.-C.; Kang, J.-I.; Kim, M.-K.; Boo, H.-J.; Kwon, J.-M.; Koh, Y.-S.; Hyun, J.-W.; Park, D.-B.; Yoo, E.-S.; et al. Apoptosis Inducing Activity of Fucoidan in HCT-15 Colon Carcinoma Cells. *Biol. Pharm. Bull.* **2009**, *32*, 1760–1764. [CrossRef] [PubMed]
40. Jin, J.-O.; Song, M.-G.; Kim, Y.-N.; Park, J.-I.; Kwak, J.-Y. The mechanism of fucoidan-induced apoptosis in leukemic cells: Involvement of ERK1/2, JNK, glutathione, and nitric oxide. *Mol. Carcinog.* **2010**, *49*, 771–782. [CrossRef] [PubMed]
41. Yu, Y.; Shen, M.; Song, Q.; Xie, J. Biological activities and pharmaceutical applications of polysaccharide from natural resources: A review. *Carbohydr. Polym.* **2018**, *183*, 91–101. [CrossRef] [PubMed]
42. Park, H.Y.; Park, S.-H.; Jeong, J.-W.; Yoon, D.; Han, M.H.; Lee, D.-S.; Choi, G.; Yim, M.-J.; Lee, J.M.; Kim, D.-H.; et al. Induction of p53-Independent Apoptosis and G1 Cell Cycle Arrest by Fucoidan in HCT116 Human Colorectal Carcinoma Cells. *Mar. Drugs* **2017**, *15*, 154. [CrossRef]
43. Park, H.S.; Kim, G.-Y.; Nam, T.-J.; Deuk Kim, N.; Hyun Choi, Y. Antiproliferative Activity of Fucoidan Was Associated with the Induction of Apoptosis and Autophagy in AGS Human Gastric Cancer Cells. *J. Food Sci.* **2011**, *76*, T77–T83. [CrossRef] [PubMed]
44. Zhang, Z.; Teruya, K.; Eto, H.; Shirahata, S. Fucoidan extract induces apoptosis in MCF-7 cells via a mechanism involving the ROS-dependent JNK activation and mitochondria-mediated pathways. *PLoS ONE* **2011**, *6*, e27441. [CrossRef]
45. Synytsya, A.; Kim, W.-J.; Kim, S.-M.; Pohl, R.; Synytsya, A.; Kvasnička, F.; Čopíková, J.; Il Park, Y. Structure and antitumour activity of fucoidan isolated from sporophyll of Korean brown seaweed *Undaria pinnatifida*. *Carbohydr. Polym.* **2010**, *81*, 41–48. [CrossRef]
46. Jiao, G.; Yu, G.; Zhang, J.; Ewart, H.S. Chemical structures and bioactivities of sulfated polysaccharides from marine algae. *Mar. Drugs* **2011**, *9*, 196–223. [CrossRef]
47. Queiroz, K.C.; Medeiros, V.P.; Queiroz, L.S.; Abreu, L.R.; Rocha, H.A.; Ferreira, C.V.; Jucá, M.B.; Aoyama, H.; Leite, E.L. Inhibition of reverse transcriptase activity of HIV by polysaccharides of brown algae. *Biomed. Pharmacother.* **2008**, *62*, 303–307. [CrossRef]
48. Dinesh, S.; Menon, T.; Hanna, L.E.; Suresh, V.; Sathuvan, M.; Manikannan, M. In vitro anti-HIV-1 activity of fucoidan from *Sargassum swartzii*. *Int. J. Biol. Macromol.* **2016**, *82*, 83–88. [CrossRef]
49. Feldman, S.C.; Reynaldi, S.; Stortz, C.A.; Cerezo, A.S.; Damont, E.B. Antiviral properties of fucoidan fractions from *Leathesia difformis*. *Phytomedicine Int. J. Phytother. Phytopharm.* **1999**, *6*, 335–340. [CrossRef]
50. Hayashi, K.; Nakano, T.; Hashimoto, M.; Kanekiyo, K.; Hayashi, T. Defensive effects of a fucoidan from brown alga *Undaria pinnatifida* against herpes simplex virus infection. *Int. Immunopharmacol.* **2008**, *8*, 109–116. [CrossRef]
51. Zhang, W.; Oda, T.; Yu, Q.; Jin, J.-O. Fucoidan from *Macrocystis pyrifera* Has Powerful Immune-Modulatory Effects Compared to Three Other Fucoidans. *Mar. Drugs* **2015**, *13*, 1084–1104. [CrossRef] [PubMed]
52. Akira, S.; Uematsu, S.; Takeuchi, O. Pathogen recognition and innate immunity. *Cell* **2006**, *124*, 783–801. [CrossRef]
53. Oka, S.; Okabe, M.; Tsubura, S.; Mikami, M.; Imai, A. Properties of fucoidans beneficial to oral healthcare. *Odontology* **2020**, *108*, 34–42. [CrossRef] [PubMed]
54. Sanjeewa, K.; Fernando, I.; Kim, E.; Kim, S.Y.; Jeon, Y.J. Anti-inflammatory activity of a fucose rich sulfated polysaccharide isolated from an enzymatic digest of brown seaweed Sargassum horneri. In Proceedings of the 2016 KFN International Symposium and Annual Meeting, Jeju, Korea, 31 October–2 November 2016; p. 476.
55. Ln, A.; Lei, W.; Xf, A.; Ddd, E.; Yjjb, C.; Jx, A.; Xin, G.A. In vitro and in vivo anti-inflammatory activities of a fucose-rich fucoidan isolated from *Saccharina japonica*. *Int. J. Biol. Macromol.* **2020**, *156*, 717–729.
56. Rm, A.; Dp, A.; Km, A.; Mb, B.; Ma, A.; Sj, A.; Spc, D.; Sgyc, D.; Nmp, E. Studies on isolation, characterization of fucoidan from brown algae *Turbinaria decurrens* and evaluation of it's in vivo and in vitro anti-inflammatory activities. *Int. J. Biol. Macromol.* **2020**, *160*, 1263–1276.

157. Jayawardena, T.U.; Fernando, I.; Lee, W.W.; Sanjeewa, K.; Kim, H.S.; Lee, D.S.; Jeon, Y.J. Isolation and purification of fucoidan fraction in *Turbinaria ornata* from the Maldives; Inflammation inhibitory potential under LPS stimulated conditions in in-vitro and in-vivo models. *Int. J. Biol. Macromol.* **2019**, *131*, 614–623. [CrossRef]
158. Lee, S.H.; Ko, C.I.; Ahn, G.; You, S.G.; Kim, J.S.; Min, S.H.; Kim, J.I.; Jee, Y.; Jeon, Y.J. Molecular characteristics and anti-inflammatory activity of the fucoidan extracted from *Ecklonia cava*. *Carbohydr. Polym.* **2012**, *89*, 599–606. [CrossRef]
159. Lim, J.D.; Lee, S.R.; Kim, T.; Jang, S.-A.; Kang, S.C.; Koo, H.J.; Sohn, E.; Bak, J.P.; Namkoong, S.; Kim, H.K.; et al. Fucoidan from *Fucus vesiculosus* Protects against Alcohol-Induced Liver Damage by Modulating Inflammatory Mediators in Mice and HepG2 Cells. *Mar. Drugs* **2015**, *13*, 1051–1067. [CrossRef]
160. Park, H.Y.; Han, M.H.; Park, C.; Jin, C.Y.; Kim, G.Y.; Choi, I.W.; Kim, N.D.; Nam, T.J.; Kwon, T.K.; Choi, Y.H. Anti-inflammatory effects of fucoidan through inhibition of NF-kB, MAPK and Akt activation in lipopolysaccharide-induced BV2 microglia cells. *Food Chem. Toxicol.* **2011**, *49*, 1745–1752. [CrossRef]
161. Hwang, P.A.; Phan, N.N.; Lu, W.J.; Hieu, B.T.N.; Lin, Y.C. Low-molecular-weight fucoidan and high-stability fucoxanthin from brown seaweed exert prebiotics and anti-inflammatory activities in Caco-2 cells. *Food Nutr. Res.* **2016**, *60*, 32033. [CrossRef] [PubMed]
162. Jin, J.-O.; Zhang, W.; Du, J.-Y.; Wong, K.-W.; Oda, T.; Yu, Q. Fucoidan Can Function as an Adjuvant In Vivo to Enhance Dendritic Cell Maturation and Function and Promote Antigen-Specific T Cell Immune Responses. *PLoS ONE* **2014**, *9*, e99396.
163. Raghavendran, H.R.B.; Srinivasan, P.; Rekha, S. Immunomodulatory activity of fucoidan against aspirin-induced gastric mucosal damage in rats. *Int. Immunopharmacol.* **2011**, *11*, 157–163. [CrossRef]
164. Li, C.; Gao, Y.; Xing, Y.; Zhu, H.; Shen, J.; Tian, J. Fucoidan, a sulfated polysaccharide from brown algae, against myocardial ischemia–reperfusion injury in rats via regulating the inflammation response. *Food Chem. Toxicol.* **2011**, *49*, 2090–2095. [CrossRef]
165. Senni, K.; Gueniche, F.; Foucault-Bertaud, A.; Igondjo-Tchen, S.; Fioretti, F.; Colliec-Jouault, S.; Durand, P.; Guezennec, J.; Godeau, G.; Letourneur, D. Fucoidan a sulfated polysaccharide from brown algae is a potent modulator of connective tissue proteolysis. *Arch. Biochem. Biophys.* **2006**, *445*, 56–64. [CrossRef]
166. Ley, K. The role of selectins in inflammation and disease. *Trends Mol. Med.* **2003**, *9*, 263–268. [CrossRef]
167. Bordone, L.; Motta, M.C.; Picard, F.; Robinson, A.; Jhala, U.S.; Apfeld, J.; McDonagh, T.; Lemieux, M.; McBurney, M.; Szilvasi, A.; et al. Sirt1 regulates insulin secretion by repressing UCP2 in pancreatic beta cells. *PLoS Biol.* **2006**, *4*, e31. [CrossRef]
168. Lorenzati, B.; Zucco, C.; Miglietta, S.; Lamberti, F.; Bruno, G. Oral Hypoglycemic Drugs: Pathophysiological Basis of Their Mechanism of ActionOral Hypoglycemic Drugs: Pathophysiological Basis of Their Mechanism of Action. *Pharmaceuticals* **2010**, *3*, 3005–3020. [CrossRef] [PubMed]
169. Koh, H.S.A.; Lu, J.; Zhou, W. Structural Dependence of Sulfated Polysaccharide for Diabetes Management: Fucoidan From *Undaria pinnatifida* Inhibiting α-Glucosidase More Strongly Than α-Amylase and Amyloglucosidase. *Front. Pharmacol.* **2020**, *11*, 831. [CrossRef] [PubMed]
170. Raghu, C.; Arjun, H.A.; Anantharaman, P. In vitro and in silico inhibition properties of fucoidan against α-amylase and α-D-glucosidase with relevance to type 2 diabetes mellitus. *Carbohydr. Polym.* **2019**, *209*, 350–355. [CrossRef]
171. Havale, S.H.; Pal, M. Medicinal chemistry approaches to the inhibition of dipeptidyl peptidase-4 for the treatment of type 2 diabetes. *Bioorganic Med. Chem.* **2009**, *17*, 1783–1802. [CrossRef] [PubMed]
172. Sanjeewa, A.; Jayawardena, T.U.; Kim, H.S.; Kim, S.Y.; Jeon, Y.J. Fucoidan isolated from Padina commersonii inhibit LPS-induced inflammation in macrophages blocking TLR/NF-κB signal pathway. *Carbohydr. Polym.* **2019**, *224*, 115195. [CrossRef] [PubMed]
173. Wang, J.; Zhang, Q.; Zhang, Z.; Li, Z. Antioxidant activity of sulfated polysaccharide fractions extracted from *Laminaria japonica*. *Int. J. Biol. Macromol.* **2008**, *42*, 127–132. [CrossRef]
174. Wang, Y.; Xing, M.; Cao, Q.; Ji, A.; Liang, H.; Song, S. Biological Activities of Fucoidan and the Factors Mediating Its Therapeutic Effects: A Review of Recent Studies. *Mar. Drugs* **2019**, *17*, 183. [CrossRef]
175. Hui, S.; Lu, J.; Zhou, W. Structure characterization and antioxidant activity of fucoidan isolated from *Undaria pinnatifida* grown in New Zealand. *Carbohydr. Polym.* **2019**, *212*, 178–185.
176. Pozharitskaya, O.N.; Obluchinskaya, E.D.; Shikov, A.N. Mechanisms of Bioactivities of Fucoidan from the Brown Seaweed *Fucus vesiculosus* L. of the Barents Sea. *Mar. Drugs* **2020**, *18*, 275. [CrossRef] [PubMed]
177. Yu, W.-C.; Chen, Y.-L.; Hwang, P.-A.; Chen, T.-H.; Chou, T.-C. Fucoidan ameliorates pancreatic β-cell death and impaired insulin synthesis in streptozotocin-treated β cells and mice via a Sirt-1-dependent manner. *Mol. Nutr. Food Res.* **2017**, *61*, 1700136. [CrossRef]
178. Wang, Y.; Nie, M.; Lu, Y.; Wang, R.; Li, J.; Yang, B.; Xia, M.; Zhang, H.; Li, X. Fucoidan exerts protective effects against diabetic nephropathy related to spontaneous diabetes through the NF-κB signaling pathway in vivo and in vitro. *Int. J. Mol. Med.* **2015**, *35*, 1067–1073. [CrossRef]
179. Peng, Y.; Ren, D.; Song, Y.; Hu, Y.; Wu, L.; Wang, Q.; He, Y.; Zhou, H.; Liu, S.; Cong, H. Effects of a combined fucoidan and traditional Chinese medicine formula on hyperglycaemia and diabetic nephropathy in a type II diabetes mellitus rat model. *Int. J. Biol. Macromol.* **2020**, *147*, 408–419. [CrossRef]
180. Lindahl, U. 'Heparin'—From anticoagulant drug into the new biology. *Glycoconj. J.* **2000**, *17*, 597–605. [CrossRef] [PubMed]
181. Tolwani, A.J.; Wille, K.M. Anticoagulation for continuous renal replacement therapy. *Semin. Dial.* **2009**, *22*, 141–145. [CrossRef] [PubMed]

182. Mourão, P.A. Use of sulfated fucans as anticoagulant and antithrombotic agents: Future perspectives. *Curr. Pharm. Des.* **2004**, *10*, 967–981. [CrossRef]
183. Mourão, P.A.; Pereira, M.S. Searching for alternatives to heparin: Sulfated fucans from marine invertebrates. *Trends Cardiovasc. Med.* **1999**, *9*, 225–232. [CrossRef]
184. Nishino, T.; Nagumo, T. Anticoagulant and antithrombin activities of oversulfated fucans. *Carbohydr. Res.* **1992**, *229*, 355–362. [CrossRef]
185. Usov, A.I.; Bilan, M.I. Fucoidans—Sulfated polysaccharides of brown algae. *Russ. Chem. Rev.* **2009**, *78*, 846–862. [CrossRef]
186. Grauffel, V.; Kloareg, B.; Mabeau, S.; Durand, P.; Jozefonvicz, J. New natural polysaccharides with potent antithrombic activity: Fucans from brown algae. *Biomaterials* **1989**, *10*, 363–368. [CrossRef]
187. Kim, M.-J.; Chang, U.-J.; Lee, J.-S. Inhibitory Effects of Fucoidan in 3T3-L1 Adipocyte Differentiation. *Mar. Biotechnol.* **2009**, *11*, 557–562. [CrossRef]
188. Park, M.K.; Jung, U.; Roh, C. Fucoidan from Marine Brown Algae Inhibits Lipid Accumulation. *Mar. Drugs* **2011**, *9*, 1359–1367. [CrossRef] [PubMed]
189. Tanino, Y.; Hashimoto, T.; Ojima, T.; Mizuno, M. F-fucoidan from *Saccharina japonica* is a novel inducer of galectin-9 and exhibits anti-allergic activity. *J. Clin. Biochem. Nutr.* **2016**, *59*, 25–30. [CrossRef] [PubMed]

MDPI
St. Alban-Anlage 66
4052 Basel
Switzerland
Tel. +41 61 683 77 34
Fax +41 61 302 89 18
www.mdpi.com

Marine Drugs Editorial Office
E-mail: marinedrugs@mdpi.com
www.mdpi.com/journal/marinedrugs

www.ingramcontent.com/pod-product-compliance
Lightning Source LLC
LaVergne TN
LVHW070702100526
838202LV00013B/1014